Volunteer Nurses & Doctors

Volunteer Nurses & Doctors
In the Serbo-Turkish War of 1876

Service in Servia Under the Red Cross
Emma Maria Pearson and Louisa Elisabeth McLaughlin

Adventures in Servia
Alfred Wright

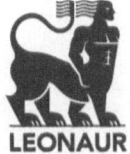

*Volunteer Nurses & Doctors
In the Serbo-Turkish War of 1876
Service in Servia Under the Red Cross*
by Emma Maria Pearson and Louisa Elisabeth McLaughlin
and
Adventures in Servia
by Alfred Wright

FIRST EDITION

First published under the titles
Service in Servia Under the Red Cross
and
Adventures in Servia

Leonaur is an imprint of Oakpast Ltd

Copyright in this form © 2022 Oakpast Ltd

ISBN: 978-1-78282-980-5 (hardcover)
ISBN: 978-1-78282-981-2 (softcover)

http://www.leonaur.com

Publisher's Notes

The views expressed in this book are not necessarily those of the publisher.

Contents

Service in Servia Under the Red Cross 7
Adventures in Servia 191

Service in Servia Under the Red Cross

Contents

Off to the War	11
On the Danube	15
Belgrade	19
Our Life in Belgrade	20
Sketches Taken in Belgrade	25
On the Save	30
The Army of the Drina	35
To Badovinsky	39
Headquarters in Badovinsky	43
The Camp on the Drina	47
A Dinner in Bosnia	52
A Servian Ambulance	58
The Return to Schabatz	62
A Great Mistake	66
A Wrong Letter of Introduction	73
Once More on the Danube	78
Our Country Town	82
Our Doctor and the Ambulance	87

Our Sick and Wounded	92
Life Upcountry in Servia	97
The Préfet of Négotin	104
Wine and Caviare	109
The Pass of Kazan	113
Servia and Roumania	118
The Russians on the Danube	123
A Day with the Russians	128
The Turks in Belgrade	133
On the Road to Paratjin	140
The Ambulance at Paratjin	145
Servia's Last Battle	151
The Retreat	158
From Jagodina to Semendria	164
Belgrade Under the Russians	173
From Belgrade to Venice	183

CHAPTER 1

Off to the War

Starting on a foreign tour, to the Tyrol, the Italian Lakes, or Switzerland, is an every-day occurrence. Each recurring August witnesses an exodus of all who can afford to cross the seas, and find mental rest, and bodily fatigue in climbing snow mountains, crossing high passes, and roughing it in hotels, good or bad, as the case may be; for, after all, it is roughing it in hotel life, compared with the quiet and comfort of an English home.

But our start on that sunny August day, 1876, was something more to us. We were off to Belgrade, for service with the Red Cross Society of Servia, but our geography, as regarded the Slav provinces, was somewhat hazy.

We had not bought a war map, and stuck it all over with pins bearing the flags of the combatants. The telegrams from the seat of war had been contradictory and confusing, and even *Bradshaw's Continental Railway Guide* gave no route to Servia.

We only knew that we must get to Belgrade, and that Vienna was the point to be first attained, but the exact situation of the Servian capital, with reference to the other Slav provinces, and to the other parts of Servia itself, was the puzzle.

But we learned our way to Belgrade, and up country in Servia, in many a weary day and night of travel, and we penetrated far inland, where the very sight of an Englishwoman caused quite an excitement amongst the natives.

This may be easily imagined when we know that the resident English population of Belgrade itself does not amount to a dozen, though at the time we arrived it rose as high as twenty-two, owing to the presence of two or three doctors, and some newspaper correspondents.

We left England on the 8th of August, 1876. Many kind friends came to wish us Godspeed, and we reached the shores of France at midnight, after a most lovely voyage.

From Calais we went on direct to Brussels, and here, by some mysterious arrangement of the Belgian railway authorities, instead of there being a train ready to take on the passengers to Cologne, we had to wait a couple of hours.

But Cologne was reached at last, and here our troubles began. The officials at the station made themselves most obnoxious, and insisted on opening every box, though addressed to ourselves at Belgrade, and marked with the Red Cross, on the ground that they looked as if they contained arms.

Now, to open trunks or boxes containing clothes is a very light matter, but to knock open chests containing bottles, carefully packed in hay, and to turn them all out, is a very serious thing, and we strongly objected to the process.

Fortunately for us, a Hessian officer was standing there, he recognised the decoration of the "*Sanitats Kreuz Militar*" of Hesse Darmstadt, which both of us wore. He most kindly stepped forward, and addressed us by name, saying that he was perfectly sure the boxes only contained medical stores, and that he would take it upon himself to answer for that.

After an animated discussion with the stationmaster, it was arranged that the chests should be sealed down and sent on to Vienna.

We claimed the right of Red Cross baggage to pass at half-price; this the officials denied, and we promised to return next morning, and pay the five *francs* which were demanded for sealing down, as well as the cost of carriage to Vienna.

But the official in charge of the sealing department demanded the five *francs*, then and there, which we paid.

The truth was, we had a friend in reserve. A kind adviser in London told us, if the Cologne stationmaster made himself disagreeable, as he most probably would, to go to M. Niessen, and to him we repaired next morning. To our astonishment, we found no stranger, but an old friend of Sedan days. He at once most generously took all the trouble upon himself; the officials came to utter grief, and had to return the five *francs*, which it seems was an illegal charge, and our baggage was sent on half-price to Vienna.

Up the Rhine and down the Danube are beaten tracks, well known to all who have travelled to Vienna; and certainly if there is no reason for haste, the last part of the journey, from Sassan to Vienna, should be made by the Danube boats, for some of the loveliest and grandest scenery on the Danube is to be found there. Below Vienna the scenery is monotonous for a long way, but below Belgrade again, and down to the far-famed Iron Gates, it Is most magnificent.

We had only time to go from Linz to Vienna by the river; the next Belgrade boat was on Tuesday, and one day in Vienna would be enough for us, and this for business purposes, such as claiming our baggage, and sending it on board for Belgrade.

All we saw of the famous city, except the streets through which we drove, was the cathedral of St. Stephen. We were disappointed in its size, but one service we witnessed there can never be forgotten.

Twilight was coming on, the long grey twilight of a bright August day. The columns of the cathedral grew obscure in the gloom, a soft darkness seemed to fill nave and aisle, but the choir was all one flood of silver light, pure as the snow on the Alpine mountain-tops under the rays of an unclouded sun.

It was the eve of the great festival of the Catholic Church—the Feast of the Assumption. The silver altar was uncovered, and shone brilliantly in the light that flashed upon it. The central point of all the shrine itself was half veiled in curtains of cloth of silver, and wreathed with white flowers, touched here and there with a cool green leaf. All around the choir were similar hangings, caught back by long wreaths of the same pure white blossoms and green leaves.

A line of priests knelt in solemn adoration before the altar, their vestments all of silver cloth with silver embroidery—no tinge of colour anywhere; while the incense went up in pale clouds and softened down the glare of the innumerable lights, into one glorious wave of silver light. As the darkness came on it grew brighter and brighter, till the whole choir shone with an almost unearthly radiance. Dead silence pervaded the church, only broken by the sounds of soft, sweet, plaintive music, that seemed to float trembling up to Heaven.

To come out from so exquisite and solemn a scene, into the noise, and glare of the streets of a great city, was like the shock of plunging into the sea. It was leaving the regions of peace and quiet for the turmoil of the world. But on such an errand as was ours, there was no time to stay dreaming, and our next care was to find Herr Pollitzer, a gentleman who had acted as agent for all the English goods sent to the Vienna Exhibition, and our true-hearted old friend Major de Winton had sent us a letter of introduction to him.

We found him at once a most gentlemanly and most business-like man. He begged us to leave it to him to claim the baggage; he would send it on to Belgrade to meet us, and in the day or two which would probably elapse before it reached that place, we should find out where we were going, and the baggage would go straight to that destination from the wharf at Belgrade. He was of opinion that we ought to start by the steamer next morning, or the war would be over before we got there. The opinion in Austria was all along (and after-events fully justified it) that Servia alone could not resist Turkey, that Herzegovina and Montenegro had enough to do to hold their own, and that unless Bosnia and Bulgaria rose against their Moslem ruler there was no use in prolonging the struggle, and that this rising was not probable, owing to the jealousies which existed between the different provinces.

We took his advice, and thanked him for his great kindness and for the interest which he felt in us and our errand; and next morning, early, embarked on board the small steamer which was to convey us to the Pesth boat; for only the Sunday boat went direct to Belgrade, and we could not wait a week for that. The little steamer was certainly very small, and very full of passengers. We were a long time getting off, but at last swung clear of the shore, and started down the river.

Chapter 2

On the Danube

Our little steamer made its way quietly down the stream, which ran past high stone banks, surmounted by houses. Then came grass banks, and then open country with trees scattered over it: a very dull and prosaic bit of river this was. Very shallow too here and there, with banks of sand and pebble appearing above the water.

Through these, and round them, we found our path; and all went well till our captain was seized with an idea that he would go straight ahead, over a sandbank, and of course we stuck there.

Upon this he tore his hair, cursed his fate, and expressed his intense indignation at the sand-bank, for daring to stick in the way and impede the progress of His Imperial Majesty's Companies steamers and mails; but as this did not float her, he ordered all the passengers to go aft, that he might slip off the bank backwards. This failed, and then everybody was told to go forward, that we might pitch over in front. This too was not successful, and there we might have remained for hours, had it not been for two tug-steamers, which were evidently lying in wait there for such disasters; and which, having waited till all our efforts were exhausted, came steaming up to us—which they might as well have done at first—and towed us off the bank backwards. All this took up a couple of hours, and we reached the large steamer very late indeed.

These Danube boats are very comfortable. The cabin on the deck is all devoted to one large saloon, surrounded by broad sofas covered with red velvet, and with velvet cushions; down below are the sleeping cabins. The quarter-deck is on the roof of the saloon; two easy ladders lead up to it, and there is also a walk round the cabin, which is under cover from the flooring of the deck above, extending to the bulwarks.

The fore-part of the vessel is arranged in a similar manner, and as all the vessel is floored over, as it were at the sides, it is possible to pass from the aft to the fore-deck, without going down to the main-deck. This, of course, gives a long walk to the aft-cabin passengers, though the fore-cabin ones are not allowed to pass through the little gates, which fence off the quarter-deck.

They are paddle boats, and go along very easily. They are clean and airy, and the food, which is prepared when desired, is good and well cooked. There is, also, one general dinner a day. All meals are paid for separately, and are very dear. Two florins, fifty *kreuzers* (4s. 6d. English money) for dinner, without wine or beer. The Vienna beer is, however, very good and cheap,

The Danube between Vienna and Pesth is uninteresting; the shores are flat, with low woods, and here and there a passenger station, with a few houses about it—just such a station as might be looked for in some newly-colonised part, in the backwoods of America.

Hour after hour we ploughed on our monotonous way; but it was midnight before we reached Pesth.

It was of course pitch-dark, and we had to find our way, bag and baggage, over some barges to the Belgrade and Constantinople steamer. Fortunately, we had only our personal luggage with us, and a sailor carried our one portmanteau. Arrived at the steamer, we descended into the ladies' cabin. It was crowded; and we were thankful to take possession of two vacant sofas in the saloon.

Here an old lady reproached us bitterly for being so late; we were due at eight or nine o'clock. All the passengers from Pesth had come on board there and been waiting ever since; it was one o'clock in the morning. What did we mean by it?

We ventured to plead the sand-bank, but she would not accept it as an excuse, and grumbled herself to sleep; and we tried to follow her example, but an aggravating and restless individual would pace up and down the cabin; and when at last he subsided we did sleep. It seemed to us as if it were but for half an hour, for the steward came to lay breakfast at 5 a.m., and eating and drinking began at six.

All that day we steamed at full speed down the river. The sky was cloudless, and the heat intense. The scenery was not more interesting than it had been the day before: the banks just as flat and well wooded. The one peculiarity was the utter air of desolation all around; no smoke from cottage chimneys rose above the low trees; no sign of human life was there. We might have been the first whoever ploughed down that mighty stream or looked on those silent shores. Only one incident broke the monotony of the day.

In the saloon, oppressed with heat and fatigue, sat an elderly man with grey hair and beard, whose purple robes, and gold chain and cross, bespoke him to be some ecclesiastical dignitary of high rank.

We found, upon inquiry, that it was the Archbishop of Karlovitz, the Metropolitan of all Hungary. The name was familiar to us, as connected with the far-famed wine sold by Max Greger. About noon, when the day was at its hottest, we stopped at some wayside station, by a little wooden wharf, and the countrywomen came crowding to the side of the vessel, with baskets of large ripe grapes, of which two handfuls cost but a few copper pieces of Austrian money.

A rush of passengers immediately ensued, anxious to secure some of the delicious fruit before it was all disposed of, and the prelate's chaplain and attendants were amongst the first busy in buying and eating, and taking no thought of their master in the cabin.

There he sat alone, looking at the scene out of the porthole, and evidently longing to make a rush too, but that his dignity forbade. The table in front of our sofa was piled with grapes, and he sighed as he looked at them. We took the gentle hint, and carried some of the best across to where he sat. He accepted them at once, and ate them with all the enjoyment of a schoolboy.

When he had finished them, he rose and came to our table, and bowing gracefully, said, in French, "That he was sure he owed this act of kindness to English courtesy." It sounded something like a sarcasm on the usual manners of the English abroad; for, as a rule, no people on earth are so detestable as the English tourists in the way in which they behave to the inhabitants of the lands they visit.

The archbishop chatted pleasantly on, and seemed very much interested in our errand to the East. He said he felt sure the war could end but in one way: the Serbs were an untrained body of men; the Turks, well-disciplined soldiers. He could wish that the Cross had better defenders in every way against the Crescent.

The shades of evening were just closing in as we reached Semlin, the Austrian town opposite Belgrade, and we hoped to reach our destination before nightfall; but twilight in these Eastern lands is short, and darkness falls suddenly after the sun goes down, and as a long delay occurred here, it was quite dark before we left Semlin.

This delay was caused by some baggage, which had been taken on board at Mohacs, the nearest point to the railway from Csaba, on the road to Russia.

We had been at dinner, when three gentlemen and one lady came on board. Here the word lady by no means implies a lady in conduct, for the person in question was a Russian female medical student. The gentlemen with her were surgeons, on their way to join some ambulance.

The senior of the party wore a shirt-front of black and red oil-cloth, and had his sleeves guarded by deep cuffs of the same—the costume suggesting horrible ideas, but surely it was not necessary to wear it on board a peaceable Austrian steamer. The other two were more quiet and better dressed. The lady wore her hair cut short, and parted on one side; spectacles with gold rims; a black tunic belted in round the waist, and a short black skirt. She smoked cigars, and seemed hail-fellow-well-met, with all her companions.

They brought with them several wooden cases, very narrow and long, which were at once objects of great suspicion to the captain, and certainly looked very much like boxes for holding rifles. After an anxious discussion they had been sealed down, and at Semlin were taken on shore, and a very long parley took place. At last, the cases were left at Semlin, and the party re-embarked in a very crestfallen condition.

It was midnight, therefore, before we reached Belgrade. The plank communicating with the shore was laid, we landed between a line of soldiery, and at last set foot on the shores of Servia.

Chapter 3

Belgrade

Belgrade is a city of which all have read, even before this war, and very few have seen; for, though it is one of the principal halts of the steamers on their way down the Danube to Varna, there is no possible reason why anyone should stop there unless on business.

Its history is, in many respects, the history of Servia, though it has a special one of its own, and has been the scene of many stirring events; but in the present day it must be, in peace time, the dullest of all places, with nothing to do and nothing to see, and no society whatever.

But it was not always so. It was the central point of the long conflict maintained by Hungary and Austria against the Turks; for we must remember that Hungary, for many a long year, was the barrier that held Eastern barbarism in check, and prevented its desolating flood from spreading over Europe.

It must have been a stirring time when Mahomet the Second besieged Belgrade, at the head of his army of 200,000 Mussulmen.

The Turkish fleet lay anchored before it, the land forces surrounded it on every side. Day by day food waxed scarcer, and hope of relief grew fainter, yet the gallant defenders held on; and just when all seemed lost, and surrender imminent, a whisper ran through the beleaguered city,—the fleet that had on board the Crusaders was in sight, they were bearing down on the Turks, and soon they came alongside. Hunyady, their leader, himself led the boarders on the deck of the Turkish admiral's vessel. The conflict was short and sharp, but the blockade was broken; the *Sultan* was compelled to withdraw his army, and Belgrade was saved.

CHAPTER 4

Our Life in Belgrade

We landed on the shores of Servia at midnight, weary with our long journey, bewildered by the strange scene around us. We had been, assured, in England, that all preparations had been made for our arrival; that a surgeon, and a gentleman who was to act as secretary, had preceded us, and were to wait for us in Belgrade; and that a crowd of enthusiastic friends would welcome our coming.

Not a single soul was there. How much we regretted not having accepted the kind offer of the captain of the Austrian steamer, to telegraph for rooms for us to an hotel at Belgrade! It appeared afterwards, that the surgeon had been ordered to Schabatz, quite independently of us, and the secretary had seen the steamer arrive at Semlin, but had not considered it any part of his duty to await her arrival at Belgrade, and that the telegram we had sent from Vienna had never been delivered.

Fortunately, Murray gave the name of one hotel, the Kröne, and enlisting a strong porter, who shouldered our portmanteau, we set off to find it.

We blundered up a long flight of steps, stumbled over rough, uneven ground, and at last found ourselves at the door of an hotel, closely shut up. On this we began to hammer. It was opened by a rough-looking porter, and a slipshod girl descended the stairs, and asked if we were the parties expected.

We really did not quite know, so we took the benefit of the doubt, and said, "Yes." On which, she took us upstairs, and ushered us into a long room, with beds on each side, like an hospital ward, three of which were already occupied. We were marched through that room into another, where were two beds, and nothing more. Servian bedrooms are generally devoid of all toilette apparatus.

We began to take off our wrappers, and to try and make ourselves comfortable, when in rushed the girl again—who turned out to be the daughter of the house—and said we must go out at once. We were not the parties expected. It was an English gentleman.

"Where are we to go?" I asked.

"I don't know, and I don't care," was the reply. "Out of the house somewhere: there's no room for you here."

Upon this, I walked out indignantly into the long room beyond—the sleepers rousing up as I went—and met the English gentleman, who had travelled onboard our ship, and with whom we had had some slight converse.

He said at once that nothing should induce him to turn us out of the room; he could do very well with one of the beds in the long room, and with many thanks I retreated, and we took final possession of the disputed place.

But the girl was spiteful. An English tourist was probable to pay higher than Red Cross nurses, for whom, as for all Red Cross workers, there was a special tariff. So in she came again, whisked off the clean sheets, and replaced them by dirty ones. We were too tired to remonstrate. We wrapped ourselves up in our waterproofs and tried to sleep.

But thought was busy. Here we were, a thousand miles from home, in an unknown land, and not a friend to welcome us; as far as we knew, not a single soul in all the city had ever heard of us. Certainly, we had our letters of introduction—one to the Archbishop Michael, doubtless a dignified and important personage, but not likely to be of much practical use; one to the War Minister—what could he do for us? did he speak anything but Serb?—and one to the agent for Reuter's telegrams. Well, he could telegraph to England that we had arrived, but that was at the moment the most unimportant point of all.

Unable to decide what was best to be done, we resolved to go to sleep, and leave the morning to arrange things for us. And the morning did; for we were awakened by the sound of an English voice in a small room adjoining ours, and, dressing hastily, I rushed out and met an English officer on the stairs.

"Can you tell me," I said, "where I can find Mr. Gordon, our secretary?"

To my delight his answer was a warm shake of the hands, and the words "I am Mr. Gordon. I expected you on Monday."

I explained that we could not get through, and he apologised for not being at the wharf to receive us. He begged us to come down and have some breakfast, and he would go and find Dr. Sandwith, who knew all about our plans, and where our quarters were, and he would take us to the War Office to get our cards and brassards.

We were delighted to find our troubles ended; and I may here explain that this officer was the Mr. Gordon who afterwards joined Dr. Humphrey Sandwith, and did such noble service amongst the Bosnian and Bulgarian refugees on the Drina frontier of Servia.

His pleasant manners, his kindly smile, his frank, open way of speaking, were all most pleasing, and we were highly prepossessed with our young and gallant secretary.

And while breakfast is getting ready, we must just explain what cards and brassards are. Brassards are the white bands with a red cross in the centre, worn round the left arm above the elbow by all Red Cross workers when on active service. They are stamped with the badge of the society to which the workers are attached, and in the cases of the workers of a neutral society being attached to any army of the combatants, they are also stamped with the badge of that army's Red Cross Society. These were used in the Franco-German war, but the cards were a new introduction, as far as regarded ourselves.

In the Franco-German war we had commissions printed on parchment, and filled in with our names, appointing us on the part of the English Aid Society to work with the German Army, which would have made it awkward when the French took Orleans had we worked then under them.

It ought to be left, as it was in Servia, for the society of the land to which workers are sent, to stamp the brassards and give commissions on the presentation of proper references, and then if their services have to be transferred, it is very easily managed.

Neutrals should never be sent with a commission from their own land to any army. They should go as members of a Red Cross Society, and act strictly as neutrals, but subject to the orders of the medical department of the country which they have work in.

The Red Cross organisation of Servia was very good. Ambulances or individuals could not go where they pleased, or work where they pleased, or with whom they pleased.

Their place was assigned to them. There, and there alone, were they entitled to quarters and rations, or could be taken on the staff of any hospital, or form any ambulance; and a card with a red cross on it was given to every worker, with a number and their name, and the place where they were to go, and written on the back were orders for transport (where possible), quarters and rations. These cards were issued from the medical department of the War Office, and were to be returned when service in any place was finished, fresh ones being then given. It was these cards which we were to receive when we went to this department of the War Office after breakfast.

That meal was soon despatched, though eaten out of doors in the shade of the acacia trees, which formed a shady avenue opposite the Kröne, and a cab having been called, we all started off, but the cab had no springs, and the stones were something dreadful to jolt over.

As we were holding on and driving to Dr. Sandwith's hotel, in the fervent hope that it was not far off, his cheery voice greeted us.

He told us that our quarters had been ready ever since Sunday; he would take us to them at once. His warm welcome was most inspiriting, and we gladly started off to the quarters.

A short description of our first home in Belgrade will give a fair idea of a first-class Servian house, but then our kind host and hostess, M. and Madame Dilbert, had passed much time in Austria, and *Madame* also was an Austro-Hungarian, while *Monsieur's* mother had been an Austrian.

In the first place, we must speak of their great kindness and hospitality; we lived there for several days at two different times, as their honoured guests, and were by them introduced to several Serbs of the upper classes. All spoke German, M. Dilbert's charming little daughter Katherine, and her Bavarian governess, French as well.

The house stood nearly in the centre of the Grande Place, an open space, always full of people; it was the heart of the town, and in a street leading out of it was the post-office.

Opposite the house, on the other side of the Place, was the police and transport-office, a low one-storied building, shaded by trees. The sides of the Place were formed by neat houses, one or two of a superior class. All along the upper side, on which stood M. Dilbert's house, ran a neat broad pavement of red tiles or bricks, bordered by granite stones. This had been introduced by M. Dilbert himself, and was a great comfort, for the Place itself was in summer a hopeless space of stones and dust, and in winter an expanse of mud.

The front door was reached by a double flight of some half a dozen steps, and led into a chemist's shop with a laboratory behind.

Here were to be found every kind of medicine and instrument, purchased in England, France, Germany, and Austria.

At the side of the house was a *porte-cochère*, leading into a stone paved yard with a pretty garden behind, and on the left hand was the door of the private house. A broad carpeted staircase led up to a suite of rooms, all opening into each other; the two central ones were the largest. The one to the back was the dining-room, the one to the front the drawing-room; the central window having a balcony overlooking the Place, and commanding a lovely view over the Save, to the Austrian shore.

The rooms had all parqueted floors, brightly polished. In the dining-room was a large round table, a buffet containing the valuable glass and china, shown through the glass doors, a grand-piano, and a long divan running down all one side of the room; but there were comfortable chairs as well. At night it was lighted up by a brilliant lamp hanging from the ceiling, the light toned down by a rose-coloured shade; and when the white cloth was laid, and the plate and glass sparkled on the table, nothing could look more comfortable and home-like.

Coffee, white bread, and butter from Semlin (none is made in Servia), were served at 8.30 a.m. The principal meal—of several courses—took place at one, and supper at eight, also a very substantial meal. Good country wine and excellent beer were handed round, and the cuisine was perfection.

But this is rather anticipating, for it was only ten o'clock in the morning when Dr. Sandwith took us there, and *M.* and *Madame* reproached him for not having looked after our arrival and knocked them up. The Consul-General of England (Mr. White) had been three times to see if we had come.

They made us promise to return to the early dinner, and then Mr. Gordon and ourselves went to the War Office, and were shown into the medical department.

Here we found Dr. Sava Petrovatz, one of the heads of that department, whose special duty it was to superintend the Volunteer and Red Cross parts of the work.

He welcomed us kindly in perfect French, took down our names, gave us our brassards and cards, and said that we were to go to Schabatz on the Save, in the rear of the Army of the Drina. He did not know what work we should find there, but we must write and tell him our opinion about it. We then bowed and withdrew, and went to the post-office to get our letters.

CHAPTER 5

Sketches Taken in Belgrade

Who that visited Belgrade during the war will ever forget "Herr Spooner," the English clerk of the post-office?—that kind, good-natured and practical individual, who was always at everybody's service; he seemed to know all languages, where everybody was, who everybody was, and to be able to give advice on all points, to half a dozen people at once.

This post-office was a primitive place. The English letters were handed over to Mr. Spooner, where he sat, in a sort of cage, except when he was hunting up lost newspapers, or running after somebody's all-important business—never weary, and always ready. On these occasions the plan was to walk into the inner room, when the Serb official in charge would ferret out a pile of letters from all lands and leave you in peace to discover your own. This had its advantages. People had an eligible opportunity of discovering who was in Belgrade, who was expected there, by the letters awaiting their arrival, and, in general, who corresponded with who.

The telegraph-office was upstairs, and the diligence-office, as all public conveyances had been taken up by the government; but no one went by a diligence who could avoid it, and the telegraphs were uncertain in their ways. Even telegrams with answers paid for, produced no result whatever, so that to ensure safe delivery, all who had important telegrams to send, crossed to Semlin and sent them from thence, and even posted letters there in preference to Belgrade.

But telegrams from the actual seat of war seemed to arrive at every hour, or at least were said to do so. They were instantly printed, issued from M. Dilbert's shop as a central position, and sold at a very small charge, for the benefit of the Red Cross Society, of whose committee he was a leading member. Each one at that time announced a glorious victory, or successful skirmish, with so many Turks killed and wounded, that we discovered, that according to a proper and arithmetical calculation, the whole Turkish Army on the Morava must have been annihilated in the course of a week; but the poor people flocked to buy these telegrams, and little crowds assembled at the street corners to hear them read by their fortunate possessors; and our good host believed in them, and great at that time was confidence in ultimate victory.

Ah, we should have to accompany the gallant Servian Army into Bulgaria and possibly on to Constantinople, for the Bulgarians and Bosnians would rise when once the Turks were retreating!

Had we not heard the like before? Had we not seen the false boasting bulletins of the Gambetta Government? Had we not been told how we must follow Aurelles des Paladine's victorious army, as he burst through the iron chains of the German *corps d'armée* that enclosed captive Paris? We knew too well what such telegrams were worth, and we wondered why it is always thought well to deceive the people.

It was only from the English papers that anyone could gather the truth. One correspondent might look more brightly and favourably on Turkish prospects, another on those of Servia, but the substratum of truth was always there.

Here let us gratefully say what unvaried kindness and courtesy we met with from all the English correspondents. That everyone was an honourable, gentlemanly, and truthful man we have every reason to believe, and that they gladly risked even their lives to obtain correct information we know. No men incurred more danger or endured more hardship than they did, or were willing and anxious to do, for that purpose; and the desire to get to the front, expressed and felt by English correspondents, surgeons (and shall we add nurses?) was the wonder of the Servians, whose proclivities lay in an exactly opposite direction. To discover the truth in Belgrade itself was no easy matter.

The air of Belgrade is pure and light, the days sunny, the evenings deliciously calm and cool; but we all agreed "there was something in it that poisoned the springs of truth, charity and goodwill." It must have affected the nervous temperament of those resident there, for it was pervaded by an atmosphere of falsehood and dissension, such as never was known elsewhere. Everybody quarrelled with everybody else, and everybody misunderstood what everybody else said.

The gossip, the scandal, the envy, jealousy and malice, that pervaded all ranks and classes of the natives, even extended to the passing strangers there. You could not meet anyone who had not a wrong to complain of, and the unhappy National Aid Society came in to make confusion worse confounded; but at this time only rumours had reached Belgrade of a proposed gift of 10,000*l*. to Servia, and 10,000*l*. to Turkey, and the poor Serbs were already arranging what hospitals required help, and in what way it could be best expended, strictly on the sick and wounded. This was their most firm and honourable intention; not one sixpence would have passed into the hands of the government, it would have been placed in the care of the Red Cross Committee.

They did not wish for an hospital in Belgrade, nor was it needed. There were many vacant beds. One hospital, which would hold 200 patients, had only 89 in it. The others were in the same condition.

Belgrade was three long days' journey from Alexinatz, where the fighting was expected. It was known and well considered over by Baron Mundy, the talented Austrian Inspector-General of Hospitals and Red Cross work in Servia, and by Drs. Beloni and Sava Petrovatz, the first of whom had a Vienna degree, and the latter a Paris one, that Belgrade was too far from the front, that hospitals should be formed in the immediate rear of each army, with temporary ambulances in the front,—and these places were, Schabatz for the Drina, Tchupria for the Timok, Paratjin and Krushevatz for the Morava, Doïni Milanovatz, and Posharevatz for the Négotin Army.

The line of road from Alexinatz to Semendria had many small towns upon it, only six, eight, and ten hours' distance from the front, and it was here that hospitals were needed; for though the Russians were there, they cared for none but their own wounded, as it was afterwards discovered, and it was on this line that the great English hospital should have been placed.

When Colonel Lloyd-Lindsay came, he refused, as we heard, to give out either money or stores to the Servian Red Cross Committee. Though there were hospitals without chloroform or carbolic, and surgeons praying for instruments for their ambulances, he held on his own obstinate way, and would do nothing but form a hospital at Belgrade. It was said afterwards that a small gift of money was made to the Servian Committee. The poor Serbs thought half a loaf better than no bread; they consented, but could never be expected to feel much gratitude, either to the colonel or the English Society.

Besides, the proceedings of his forerunner, Dr. Laseron, had seriously annoyed them, however politely they might express themselves. His origin (it was reported that he was by birth a German Jew) was not likely to impress them in his favour, and his conduct in going up to the front, with the expressed intention of crossing into the Turkish lines, subjected him to grave suspicions. He went, but returned to Belgrade and telegraphed to England that he was going to Semlin, to get a permission from the Turkish consul-general there to go to Widdin, to inspect what was wanted in the Turkish medical department.

He did not go, however, but returned to England to say what he could have written as well; and then went to Germany and Austria to buy at a dearer rate, carriage included, what he was told and shown that he could buy equally as well, and cheaper in Belgrade.

But at the time we arrived, he had come and gone, and earnest hopes were expressed on all sides that he would not return.

Before we went back to dinner at our kind host's, we paid a visit to the Archbishop Michael, accompanied by Senator Philip Christich, who may be justly called the best of all the Serbs.

He is an elderly man, with snow-white hair. He speaks English, German, and French, all marvellously well; has travelled much, and accompanied the Princess Julia, Prince Michael's widow, to England, when she visited it, some years since. His calm judgment, his moderate sentiments, his learning, and his goodness, are everywhere quoted as a proof that Servia can produce a first-rate man. He was afterwards sent to Constantinople to negotiate the peace, and is now, (1877), the diplomatic representative of Servia there. He has filled the post of prime minister, and his counsels, had he been in power when the war first broke out, might have obviated many of the disasters which ensued.

As the archbishop can only speak Serb, and Russian (we must presume that he is learned in Latin and Greek), it was necessary to have an interpreter, and Herr Christich most kindly took that office upon himself.

The palace is a large, rambling building, with a crowd of ecclesiastics lounging about the stairs and ante-rooms; and though the priests in Belgrade are the best of their class in Servia, they did not give us the idea of being gentlemen or scholars.

We were shown into a large, long room, with a parqueted floor and a few chairs, and presently "His Eminence the Metropolitan of Servia" entered.

He is a short, fair-haired man, about fifty years of age, and, like all Greek priests, his hair and beard were rather long; his eyes were turquoise blue, and his smile pleasant, but the face was not a powerful or intellectual one. It had a soft, sleepy expression. He seemed to be a good-tempered, gentle-minded man, and certainly not a bigot, for he lives in perfect peace and good-will with his Roman *confrère*, the talented and fiery Bishop Strossmeyer, Roman Vicar-Apostolic of Servia, whose palace is in Hungary, not far from the Save, where he keeps up the old state and style of a prince-bishop—so rich, so powerful, so beloved, that were anything to cause a difference between the Vatican and himself, it is said that a million of the Slav people would follow their bishop wherever he chose to lead.

Conversation with Archbishop Michael was, of course, impossible. He spoke at some length, and M. Christich explained that he welcomed us, and gave us his blessing, and that he begged to be of service in every possible way.

We expressed our wish and hope of being useful to his suffering flock, and so the interview ended; and we returned to the Grande Place, and the house of M. Dilbert.

Chapter 6

On the Save

The most romantic-minded of writers could make nothing out of Belgrade. The view from the windows of M. Dilbert's house was far the prettiest thing in the town. The shores of the two rivers, the Save and the Danube, which meet at Belgrade, and flow on in one broad and rapid stream, are here very flat and marshy, and the country around the city barren and dreary.

The old fortress is crumbling to decay, and the lower town is a nest of small streets with one-storied houses. There is a rough dusty piece of ground planted with young trees, and called by courtesy the Park, and the new quarter of the town has long, wide, straight streets, very stony, with glaring white houses on either side at intervals.

The longest street, or rather *boulevard*, runs from the town in a straight line for more than a mile, and ends in the road leading to Semendria.

It is very wide, with a double row of trees on either hand, and very large houses. Here is the palace of Prince Milan, the Russian Embassy, two or three large hotels and *cafés*, and several official residences.

The palace is simply a handsome house, standing a short distance back from the road, with shrubs in front and gardens behind.

Close by in a road at the back was the War Office, a house surrounding a plot of green grass, on three sides fenced off from the road by a high paling, and here various departments of the War Ministry had their offices.

On this road, and on one off it, were two large hospitals. One was the military hospital, the nursing of which was done by Servian ladies, under the superintendence of the wife of the War Minister, Madame Ristich.

She took us round herself, and also showed us a long coach-house or stable, which had been turned into a ward, where were some of the worst cases.

The whole arrangements were certainly not up to our ideas of what an hospital should be, more especially the ward I have specified, and we remarked that the use of disinfectants, either as dressings or for cleansing the wards and purifying the air, seemed totally unknown or neglected.

Madame Ristich was there every day, but she could not be everywhere at one time, nor be there night and day; and what we heard of the nursing of the Servian ladies was certainly not very favourable.

The account of it was given to us by the chief of the Servian medical department, Dr. Beloni. They were not only ignorant, but careless and indifferent, and paid more attention to the surgeons and dressers than to the patients.

M. and Madame Dilbert had accompanied us, and as we were walking homewards, a tall, soldierlike-looking man, came out of a short side street, and asked M. Dilbert to present him to us.

It was Colonel McIver, who was at that time engaged in raising and organising a regiment of cavalry to serve as *Uhlans* in the front.

He invited us to see the camp, and showed us his tent. He was waiting for horses, he told us, and afterwards he had to wait for saddles, so that he did not leave Belgrade for a long time after we did—indeed, their campaign only lasted two months.

Next day we were informed that the hired Government steamer, *Columbus*, would start for Schabatz at 7 a.m. on the following morning, and at that hour we all arrived on the wharf.

There lay the *Columbus*—no steam up, no sign of moving. Mr. Spooner went off to make inquiries, and found that the arrangements were altered. She was not going then. Nobody knew when she was going, as she had been seized by the Austrian Government on a pretext that she was for carrying arms and ammunition, and she was an Austrian ship. We therefore decided to go by the Sissek boat, which stops at Schabatz on her way up the Save.

We went on board her, and took up our places on deck. Eight o'clock came, and she did not move, and it then turned out that we were waiting for General Ranko Alempits, Commander-in-Chief of the Army of the Drina, who had been down to Belgrade to receive a wiping, as rumour ran, for not "going forward"—*i.e.*, exposing his troops to be cut in pieces by the Turks. Such orders resembled those given from the War Ministry of Tours in the late war, and were founded, like them, on what would be the most successful thing to be effected, rather than on what it would be possible to do.

The general was a pleasant-looking man, with a bright blue eye, a fair, pointed moustache, and a merry smile. His red trousers were baggy, after the French style, and his crimson *kepi* worn very much forward.

Colonel McIver, who had come on board with him, introduced us to him, and also presented Mr. Gordon.

Shortly afterwards we cast loose from shore, and steamed up the Save—Servia on the left, Austria on the right. The sun shone brilliantly, the blue waters sparkled in the light, and the shores on either side were green and fresh, the Servian shore being far the most picturesque. No sights or sounds of terror were there, to mar the peace and quiet of the scene.

Just before dinner was announced, Mr. Gordon came to me, and said that the general had requested one of us to go with Mr. Gordon to Badovinsky, the headquarters on the Drina, to inspect the ambulances there.

It was decided that I should go, Louise to remain, as we then supposed, in charge of the hospital at Schabatz, where the English surgeon was; at all events till we could form a correct judgment of the state of affairs there—the number of wounded, and if our services were really required in that place.

It was evident that a visit to the front would enable me to see what probability there was of wounded being sent back from the ambulances in the camp.

It was very hot about noontide. We got into the shade at the dinner-table, and the unlucky mortals who vainly thought they could brave the sun, very soon had to follow our example.

We had hardly finished before we came in sight of what they called Schabatz. We had two correspondents on board the boat—most genial and gentlemanly men; they were, Mr. Bowes, of the *Standard*, who was bound to be Turkish in opinion; and Mr. Brennan, of the *Manchester Guardian*, who was bound to be the reverse.

They had come up to Schabatz, hoping to find their way to the front on the Drina, for the difficulties of getting to the front on the Morava were almost insuperable; only Mr. Forbes, of the *Daily News*, Mr. Villiers, of the *Graphic*, and Mr. Corbould, of the *Illustrated London News*, were there.

The general heard them express this wish, and immediately invited them to headquarters. He had no mysterious plans to conceal. He had to hold the line of the Drina, to keep in check the Turkish Army at

Belina, and at the same time to be in readiness to march forward if that army went to the aid of their fellows on the Morava; so that with this contingency before them, they could not stir.

The invitation was gratefully accepted, and therefore, when we came alongside, we all looked anxiously for some means of conveyance, and especially for the town itself.

We saw only a rough wharf, and what seemed a collection of mud cottages, some half a mile off. One solitary carriage, the general's private conveyance, and a few light waggons, with open sides, a little hay at the bottom, and a ragged pair of ponies in front, were all that were there.

Into one of these we were packed, and the gentlemen arranged themselves in the others. The general departed, leaving his *aide-de-camp*, Captain Alexitch, to escort us to Badovinsky; and we jolted into the town. But the stones of Schabatz exceeded in malignity the stones of Belgrade. Our very teeth chattered with the bumping and the shaking, and we arrived at the hotels in what might be called the main street, breathless and bruised.

Here the English surgeon was standing, together with an Austrian lady, of stern and forbidding appearance, who instantly demanded to see our cards, and asked where we intended to go.

We replied that we were ordered to take charge of the hospital there; to which her rejoinder was, "That she was there: that there were no quarters for us, and very few wounded."

We were, of course, much astonished; and when we had washed off the dust, and got ourselves together again after our shaking, we went with the secretary to the hospital, which had been formed in the Bishop's Palace.

We found many wounded men lying on their beds in the garden, and as the sun was very hot, and the insects very troublesome, and as the men had to be carried up and down a long flight of stairs, we rather doubted if the fatigue was at all compensated for, by any advantage of the open air; but as we heard afterwards that the surgeon in charge did not lose one of his cases, perhaps it was all right.

The inn was decidedly rough, and it may be as well to say here, at once, that the humblest village inn in England would be cleaner than a large Servian one.

Our bedrooms all opened into a corridor, which looked into the yard. Except a small glass window, which opened into the corridor only, there were no other means of light and air. We dined in a small room, with Mr. Gordon, the correspondents, Captain Alexitch, the *aide-de-camp*, and an English tourist whom the general had met on the boat, and invited to accompany the party.

We retired early to our own room, where the furniture consisted of two iron bedsteads with straw mattresses, two chairs, and a table, and here we consulted what was best to be done.

The conduct of the Austrian lady, who shall be nameless, had been so insulting to both of us on our visit to the hospital, and the statement of the surgeon that our services were not required there, so positive, that it was our duty to report this to the War Office, and ask for further directions.

We therefore thought it better that, while I went to the camp on the Drina, Louise should return to Belgrade; that I would telegraph from Badovinsky as to the wisdom of forming an ambulance there, and she would telegraph from Belgrade if the War Office gave us fresh directions—and on this plan we decided. We were to leave at 5 a.m., the boat for Belgrade at seven, so that she would not be long left alone in that dreary place, and so we went to rest till morning.

Chapter 7

The Army of the Drina

At an early hour on the following morning we were up and dressed, and having our coffee and bread in front of the inn, at the tables placed there for the purpose, when Captain Alexitch made his appearance, ready to escort us. This officer was decidedly the most soldierlike and elegant man in the Servian Army.

He had served many years in the Russian Army, and when the news reached him where he was quartered, far away in Siberia, that Servia had drawn the sword against Turkey, he resigned his commission, and travelled eighteen days and nights to reach Belgrade. He had applied for a staff appointment, and certainly no man was better qualified for one; but there was a delay. At present he was extra *aide-de-camp* to General Alempits, and we heard afterwards that he never received any appointment whatever.

The Russians arrived; all commissions, all staff appointments, were given to them, and many Servian officers resigned in disgust, and served as simple volunteers. Amongst them Captain Alexitch, who, at the time we first met him, wore the volunteer dress, and was the only man who ever looked like a gentleman in it.

This wonderful and fearful costume consisted of a loose tunic of brown cloth, drawn in behind with strings. It was served out of the War Office stores, and consequently shapeless and sizeless. The rank was marked on the collar, a patch of red bearing one, two, or three, small five-pointed gold stars, according to rank—sub-lieutenant, lieutenant, or captain. The field officers had their stars on a patch of silver lace, edged with red. The medical and civil departments had theirs on black velvet, for the juniors, and on silver lace, edged with black velvet, for the seniors.

Blue trousers, with a red piping, were worn for juniors, but with a broad red stripe for field officers and the staff.

The generals wore red trousers, and so did their regular *aides-de-camp*, but later on in the autumn the officers gave up this horrible dress, and wore blue coats and French *kepis*, and the staff added huge waving plumes of white feathers. It was a remarkable fact that as things grew worse, the dress improved. At this time the costume was completed by a head-dress called the insurgent cap.

That cap was a thing of horror. It was made of coarse blue cloth, with flaps fastened up, which could turn down over the ears at night, but formed the sides of the cap by day. It was worn with the points before and behind, like a cocked-hat on a very small scale. There was always a tendency to slope the cap to the back of the head, which imparted a dissipated look to the unhappy wearer, combined with an air of utter imbecility; and the average appearance of the men was a cross between a convict and a charity boy. The trousers were always either too long or too short, and therefore were tucked into half-boots to hide all mistakes.

Captain Alexitch, looking his best under these trying circumstances, and further smartened up by a pair of buckskin gloves, the relics of his Russian uniform, had "required" four waggons and plenty of clean hay. In the first went Mr. Brennan and Mr. Bowes, in the second Mr. Gordon and myself, in the third Captain Alexitch and Mr. W———, the English tourist, and in the last Alexis, by profession a barber, but as all his customers were off to the war, by present employment courier to Mr. Gordon, and the hand bags. Louise waved us a farewell, and we started off, but at a funereal pace, for by this time we were aware of the stones, and not till we were fairly out of the town did we break into a jolting trot.

Our destination was Badovinsky, the headquarters of the Army of the Drina, though the camp was some three miles in advance.

In July, General Alempits had fought a successful battle, or rather successfully defended his camp against a Turkish attack, and, driving back the enemy, advanced and entrenched himself on the far side of the Drina.

This river forms the boundary between Servia and Bosnia, and the Turks were driven back into Belina, a Bosnian town, exactly opposite Badovinsky, though quite out of sight, and four or five miles beyond the Drina, which was held down to its junction with the Save, by the right wing of the general's army, amongst whom were the Italian volunteers, a splendid body of men, principally from North Italy, under the command of General Sgarralini, one of Garibaldi's most trusted followers, and one of the Thousand of Marsala.

The Serbs, therefore, had the command of both shores of the Drina, from some miles above Badovinsky and Belina, down to the Save.

This stream might have been of great use had Servia possessed a gunboat of shallow draught, but that in summer it is half-dried up, and no boat could navigate it, except at certain parts.

The country between Schabatz and Badovinsky is very flat and woody; a good broad road leads to the latter place, and any enterprising government could have laid down a line of rails most easily, and at little expense.

This would have saved much time, and even cost, in the transport of troops and stores; but new ideas penetrate but slowly into Servian brains, and so great is their jealousy of foreigners, that they will not adopt their plans, and prefer waggons creeping along a sandy road, to a more speedy transit by steam.

Had Philip Christich been in power, this would not have been the case; but then, his wish all along was for peace. He foresaw how hopeless the struggle would be, yet, once embarked on war, he would have called in every modern appliance to make up for want of numbers and training, and, as it proved, of courage.

And it must be confessed that success imparts confidence, and confidence in victory is the chief ingredient in what we call courage in troops. Defeat after defeat no doubt demoralised the Servian troops in the Morava valley.

To them it seemed, at last, to be flinging away life uselessly, and be it remembered that these Serbs were not isolated members of society, but men with wives and families. Life was dear to them, and not only life but limb, and the power to work for those wives and children, and we must not judge them too harshly.

We English are, by nature, a fighting race. We fight as well under difficulties—even defeat—as in success and victory. We "do not know when we are beaten," but this is not the Servian character; they are a quiet and timid race.

General Alempits' army, however, did not know what defeat meant, and therefore were brave and hopeful.

The government had thought he ought to make a forward move—bold spirits chafed at his inaction; but, surely, later events must have taught them that the defensive was the only safe course for a Servian Army.

The general held his position till the autumnal floods and the swelling of the river drove him out of it. The July battle was the only one fought. A few outpost affairs occurred, but there were no wounded after July, except a few isolated cases.

Our knowledge of what passed on the Drina is, however, very limited, as very little authentic intelligence was ever published about it, and the interest of after months was centred on the struggle in the Morava valley.

Chapter 8

To Badovinsky

We jolted merrily over the level road, the only inconvenience being the dust, when we got used to the shaking.

The way was bordered by hedges, and the country studded with trees, like an English park; in fact, the scenery was very English, but the land was all grass land.

The dust rose in clouds, and the waggons, or, rather, their drivers, tried to slip past each other, so as to be first, and avoid the dust of those behind.

At last the first waggon halted, and we saw the driver go into a field where there was a small haystack, and pull off it a huge armful of hay.

Captain Alexitch came up, and asked what was the matter, and it appeared that Mr. Brennan was suffering fearfully from the jolting of the waggon, and fancied more hay would remedy the evil; but, though it might give temporary ease, a few days proved that there was a serious illness upon him, of which he died at Vienna two or three months afterwards. He was not well enough to leave Belgrade; he felt this, and we understood that he had requested to be superseded, but as yet no relief had come, and he died at the post of duty, as truly as any soldier falls on the battlefield; and England, perhaps, hardly realises how deep a debt of gratitude is due to the brave, faithful, and talented men who have earned for her journals the European fame of being the only ones whose news can be relied on.

We who have witnessed their daring, their dangers, and their hardships, whilst honestly doing their duty, can bear testimony to their endurance and their fidelity.

After this, it may be forgiven that I have to state that on this particular occasion the dust of these correspondents was so dreadful and so annoying, that we let them get well ahead, and our driver turned down a side road, also wide and good. We emerged again on the high road about a mile from Badovinsky, and saw no sign of our companions.

Here we found the high road lined on either side with wooden palings, such as in England enclose private grounds, and standing within them what appeared to be groups of one-storied buildings.

And now an astonishing sight greeted our wondering eyes. A little further on, the broad road was crossed at right angles by one equally broad, and the road up which we were now slowly driving, and the left-hand road that crossed it, were crowded with women, all wearing white cloths on their heads to keep them from the sun. There were "women to right of us, women to left of us," women before us, and women behind us, and not a man or a child among them!

It was Sunday, and Mr, Gordon, with a proper expression of gravity, suggested that service was probably just over, and they were coming out of church. To this theory I objected, on the ground that no church in all Servia, nothing short of St. Paul's in London, could have accommodated, with even standing room, that crowd of white-capped females.

Later on, we heard the explanation of this scene from General Alempits.

We had noticed that sentinels barred the road to the right, and also the one opposite to us, both of which we were told led to the camp.

It seems that on the preceding Sunday the general had given leave for the wives of all the soldiers in camp to pay them a visit there. He expected some five or six hundred, all he imagined who were near enough to come there; but when the day came, it seemed as if the soldiers had borrowed the custom of polygamy from their enemies the Turks, so numerous was the assemblage. They came not in hundreds, but thousands, not only from near but from far, not only wives, but mothers, grandmothers, aunts, sisters, cousins, and sweethearts; all had come, many tramping thirty or forty weary miles to see their dear ones in camp.

The general looked at the crowd that blocked every avenue between the huts of green branches which were the soldiers' shelters, and it struck him:

> Suppose the Turks should make a sally from Belina, what a pretty pickle (to give a free translation of his words) they would all be in. They would cling to the arms of their beloved ones, to keep them out of danger; they would hamper every military movement; they would run in everybody's way, and if the attack were to succeed (and under such circumstances it probably

would), the conqueror would carry off the female flock, or at least all the young and pretty ones, to Belina, and what a catastrophe that would be.

So he resolved to have no more Sunday picnics, and planted sentinels at the roads leading to camp, with orders not to let one woman pass through.

But of this order the women from a distance were not aware, and there they were, some four thousand of them, waiting patiently for the chance of the one particular warrior in whom they were interested, having leave to come across the Drina to Badovinsky; but the general, not wishing to cause jealousy or dissension, refused all leave for that day.

It was a very cheerful scene, there was a well-to-do air about everybody, probably due to the bright colours of the dresses, and the snowy whiteness of the handkerchiefs which, they wore on their heads.

We sat watching them for some minutes, and wondering where we should find General Alempits' headquarters; and whilst waiting, like Mr. Micawber, "for something to turn up," the something came in the shape of Captain Alexitch, and the other waggons.

The captain ordered us to go down the road to the right; we did so, and found ourselves opposite a yard, fenced off from the road by a ragged paling. The churchyard formed one end of it, and the gable end of a one-storied house the other.

Sloping from this wall for about the width of eight feet, was a roof of green boughs supported on fir poles, and making a covered space about six feet in width, and twenty in length, but open at the ends and side. Down this ran a rough deal table about three feet wide, a rude bench was fastened to the wall, just leaving room enough to pass between it and the table, and there was a corresponding bench on the outer side. One chair stood at the top, and was evidently designed for the illustrious guest of the day, whoever it might happen to be.

Several officers were lounging on the benches, smoking and drinking beer, and we discovered, to our astonishment, that this was the headquarters in Badovinsky of General Alempits' army, and the officers who were waiting for their midday meal—the headquarters' staff.

They sprang up to greet us, Captain Alexitch introduced us, and we all became great friends, then and there.

A more pleasant, gentlemanly, kind-hearted set of men I never encountered than those staff-officers.

I never felt the least awkward or constrained at being the only woman there; they did all they could to make me feel that my visit was a pleasure to them, and I believe it was, for till the day that the war ended, that staff never ceased to make every effort to induce us to go back to the army of the Drina. In this rude mess-room we all assembled, wondering what we were to do next.

The chair at the top was assigned to me, as the post of honour; it had an uncertain seat and one short leg, propped up on a stone. As I was trying to glide gracefully into it, it gave way and the leg went down into a hole, which was confusing and spoiled the effect of my endeavour at seating myself in a dignified manner. Two or three officers rushed at the chair and replaced the stone, and I had to sit upon it as best I could; but, except for the honour of the position, I should have preferred the bench at the side, on which, however, I was never allowed to sit.

The wonder what we should do was ended by the appearance of a dusty carriage, in which sat General Alempits, himself also very dusty, as were the ragged horses and the old harness. On seeing us he stopped, told us that he had been in camp and had rather expected us to come out there. I could have said that I was ready to start at 5 a.m., the time appointed, but the gentlemen could not be got together till 6.30 a.m.; this secret, however, I did not reveal.

The general then told Captain Alexitch to take us into the camp after our early dinner, and show us all that there was to be seen. I then took leave for a short time, and we were glad to retreat into the shade of our branch-roofed mess-room and refresh ourselves with beer and biscuits.

CHAPTER 9

Headquarters in Badovinsky

The next thing was to settle ourselves in our quarters. A young officer summoned the secretary and myself, mounted us into a waggon, jumped up by the side of the driver, and rattled us full speed down the road beyond the mess-room (luckily there were no stones), dashed in at an open gate in a very high paling, and deposited us at the door of a low, whitewashed house, which stood in the midst, of what in England would have been a garden, but here was only a field. Other but smaller houses stood at various distances around.

The central house, like so many others, not only in Badovinsky, but in various parts of Servia, is used as the general refectory for all, and the sleeping apartments of the heads of the family. The married sons and daughters live in the smaller ones.

All Badovinsky is built on this principle, and therefore stands on a space of ground as large as an English country town, though in number of houses and population it is but a village. The room into which we were shown was large and low-roofed, with a tile floor, and divans round it, covered with rugs and cushions; in the centre was a square four-legged table.

Here slept three Bosnian women, refugees, and here the secretary and myself were intended to sleep. This we discovered from Alexis, who acted as our interpreter, and, as we found afterwards, it is a Servian custom for men and women to sleep in the same room like the Easterns; they only take off their upper garments; they just let a little water from a tap dribble over their hands, which they rub over their faces, and their ablutions are done. At intervals they take a bath in the tank, which almost every house possesses, or in the nearest pool or stream; but I fear the intervals are long ones.

As those are not our English habits, the secretary and myself looked at each other in ludicrous bewilderment, and at last both burst into a fit of hearty laughter. He suggested that he would go to the quarter-master, and see about my having other quarters; that as it was fearfully hot, I had better rest there and wash off the dust of the road, and he would come back or send Alexis, as soon as possible. Off they went, and then arrived seven or eight women, who stood in a row, and stared solemnly at me. It seemed that the family had given shelter to some Bosnian refugees, or rather that they had been quartered upon them by the government; a small sum being paid for each. They were all well-dressed and exhibited no signs of poverty or distress, though they were refugees.

We hardly understand in England what is the position of Bulgarian and Bosnian refugees.

We cannot for a moment compare their sufferings with those of the poor people in France, who fled before the German invasion, or the ruin brought upon them by the destruction, in many cases, of their homes. A Bosnian, Bulgarian, or Servian cottage, in the country, is simply a large one-storied hut, divided off by partitions, built not of stone or brick, but clay, whitewashed over.

The furniture is of the simplest kind, an iron pot is the principal kitchen utensil, used for stewing meat; there are no beds, and no tables or chairs; plates and glasses are unknown; the family all eat out of the same dish, and have drinking cups. These, of course, are the poorest and humblest of all. There are better houses; but in no place, except Belgrade, is anything like real European comfort known.

Therefore, a family fleeing before the Turks had only to pack up a very small cartload of goods, which they were always able to do, and leave a house worth about 30*s*. of English money to its fate.

No doubt to have to leave home and wander forth without know-ing where to go—to fly before a cruel and savage enemy, young and old, sick and well, all involved in one common misery—is indeed a wretched thing; but in these cases it does not represent such a money amount of loss as it would otherwise do; and it always seems strange to us, how much more money was asked for from England to remedy this evil, than was asked for to repair the ruined houses, the wrecked farmyards, the destroyed furniture and clothes, of the poor peasantry of France, many of whom, to this day, have not been able to replace their goods and chattels.

But it is a well-known fact, that an object of charity to be intensely interesting, should be at a great distance, and if on the verge of civilisa-tion so much the better, and this certainly has been the case with the

Bulgarian and Bosnian refugee funds.

But *revenons a nos moutons*; there stood the women perfectly silent and still, but smiling blandly at me.

I began a series of pantomimic signs, to intimate that I wanted water (my Serbish was in its infancy then).

They stared harder still, and then consulted together. At last a bright idea struck one of them. She went and fetched a soup plate and a decanter of water; it was plain that washing in a room was not a process familiar to them; the pump in the yard was the usual resource.

I produced soap and a towel from my dressing-bag. (We always carried these necessary articles of *toilette* about with us.) Upon this the women sat down on the ground in a row, just where they had stood, and prepared to enjoy the novel exhibition.

As I used the soap, and rubbed my face with the towel, and brushed my hair, they broke into the broadest of grins, and showed their white teeth, and when the process was finished they rose, and, each one advancing, patted me on the shoulder and said "*Dobra*" (very good).

Just then, back came the quartermaster's *aide-de-camp*.

Mr. W—— and the secretary were to have their room, a special clause being inserted in the verbal contract that the three Bosnian ladies were to be elsewhere accommodated with sleeping quarters. So, I remounted the waggon, and was rattled up the road past the mess-room, then a few yards down the road by which we had arrived, and shown into another central house standing in a green space, and shaded by grand old trees.

Here I was shown into a half-darkened room, for the blazing of that August sun was more than could be borne. In this room a large pair of boots with spurs stood in one corner, tobacco and pipes were on the table, and dusty great-coats hanging up.

I wondered what this new arrangement might be, but I soon found out that two good-natured Servian officers had vacated the room for me, and slept outside under the shade of a tree. They had their reward—the nights were superb, and they had far the best of it.

I made up my bed on a broad divan, with a rug, a cloak, and a clean towel pinned over a dirty cushion by way of pillow, and then sallied out back to the mess-room to the early dinner, which I found just about to begin. That dinner was in itself a curiosity, and a fair type of camp life upcountry in Servia.

Half the table was covered with a dirty cloth, of a red and purple pattern; the other half had none; and the effort seemed to be to get places at the cloth end of the table: this was like being "above the salt."

I took the head of the table, as requested, and again that unlucky chair went down on one side, and was again righted by united efforts, and on a larger stone; and this being accomplished, dinner began.

The cooking was something too atrocious. There was soup, perfectly tasteless and all grease, and the meat out of it all fibre, and with no sauce; after this, a dish of meat, done up with *"paprikos"* (red *capsicums*), and so hot that it was uneatable, except to seasoned palates. But there was very fair beer; and with the black bread, made of Indian corn meal, we contrived to eke out a good dinner.

There were no knives and forks; everyone had their own—generally a clasp-knife and a small pocket fork; and I was also so provided.

It happened that, the day being very hot, one of the officers—a superbly-made and handsome man of about thirty, years of age, opened his coat, and having no waistcoat underneath, showed a spotless shirt of snowy white.

Captain Alexitch gently reproved him for doing this in a lady's presence.

To my amazement, his answer was, as he bowed courteously to me, "This is not the first time *Mademoiselle* has seen me in my shirt."

"What do you mean?" I said.

"You do not remember me, then?"

"Not at all."

"Yet I was some time under your care and that of your friend, and had it not been for that I should not be here now. It was in your ambulance at Orleans."

After this explanation, remembrances of him began to dawn upon me. We finally identified the very room and bed, where he had lain for five long weeks, and of course we became great friends. He was a young Prussian, of good family and fortune, who, not deterred by the remembrance of his wounds, had volunteered to join the Servian Army.

We chatted on pleasantly, not over our dessert, but over our dirty table. The Prussian praised our Orleans ambulance, and told tales of the great war, as he called it; and the other officers declared that to the army of the Drina we must and should go, in case they were wounded.

At three o'clock, when the noontide heat had somewhat decreased, waggons came up, under the command of the transport captain; and, escorted by Captain Alexitch and Major Pallacruska, the general's military secretary, we started for the camp.

CHAPTER 10

The Camp on the Drina

The sun was still shining brightly as we dashed down a sandy road, with hedges on each side, and then came into a belt of pines, beyond which was a sandy shore, bordering a narrow and shallow stream, which summer heat and drought had contracted from its winter width, as the sandy expanses on either side bore witness.

"The Drina," said our guide; "the boundary of Servia. On the other side is Bosnia."

The stream was here crossed by two temporary wooden bridges, that could easily be destroyed in case of necessity. One was reserved for the passage of officers, the other was for general traffic and heavy waggons.

We crossed by the traffic bridge, and found ourselves driving through sundry fortifications of turf, past rifle-pits, *lunettes*, *têtes du pont*, and lines.

Through these we found our way, and came to a broad avenue. Here, on either side, were many huts of boughs, the dwelling-places of the troops. These huts were grouped together, each regiment occupying a group, and each group had its little chapel, a hut of boughs, like all the rest, but open in front, so that the priest and the tiny sanctuary, which enclosed the altar (as is always the case in the churches of the Greek rite), could be seen by all outside.

It was Sunday, and the sound of solemn chanting rose upon the still air, from men kneeling in and before the little chapels. There was a sense of sadness in hearing it. Who might live to join in those chants when Sunday came round again?

We need not have felt this. The general was too wise to risk his men in open field against the well-trained Turkish troops, and was content to hold his own, and detain a large *corps d'armée* to prevent an advance into Bosnia. If they attacked, he was fully able to defend his position; but even in that case there might have been much loss of life.

The men looked rough and ready. Few had any regular uniform, except the brown tunic and insurgent cap. The trousers were of all shapes and colours, and their boots and shoes of divers kinds. Some had new rifles, but most of them had old ones, and many of them were very old-fashioned muzzleloaders.

We passed down the broad avenue, and came to an open space bordered by trees. Here a small canvas tent was pitched, and there was also a large hut of green boughs, with a table in the centre that would hold twenty or thirty men, and rude benches on either side of it.

This was the camp headquarters' mess-room, and was so far more comfortable than ours, that the sides were closed in as well as the roof.

Hot coffee, strong and thick, was ready for us, red wine of the country, and the usual corn bread.

General Alempits' second in command was sitting here, a colonel with an unspellable name, a fine soldierlike man, who spoke perfect French. When coffee was finished, he proposed that we should walk towards the part of the camp which faced Belina, where our waggons would meet us; and we started off, the colonel walking with me, Captain Alexitch, Major Pallacruska, and several other officers accompanying the gentlemen.

We went by the huts of several regiments and their chapels, where service was going on, and the officers uncovered as they passed. We came at last to a rather larger chapel, which the colonel told me was for the soldiers of his faith; he was a Roman Catholic. There were not many, so there was but one chapel for them; but perfect freedom of conscience was not only allowed, but enforced. There were many Jews serving in the army; they shared all the privileges accorded to Christians by the government, with the one exception of not being permitted to settle in the interior. As the Jews are not an agricultural people, this was not felt as a hardship in reality.

They much preferred Belgrade, but it has been made into a grievance by some of their co-religionists in other countries, and nominally it is so; yet strangely enough the Jews in Servia, as a body, neither resent nor regret this law, and live in perfect peace and friendship with their fellow-citizens.

A Jewish gentleman told me this himself, and I have reason to believe it, for we saw a Jew most hospitably received and most kindly treated at M. Dilbert's house, and also by the officials of the War Office-; indeed, he was so perpetually up and down at M. Dilbert's, with whom he was in a sort of temporary partnership for the sale of surgical instruments, that we all gave him the name of "*der Ewige Juden*," which is the German name for the Wandering Jew of old legend.

Walking still farther on, we came to the green banks which had been thrown up, and formed the front lines of the camp. One or two forts stood isolated on the level ground beyond, with rifle-pits between them and the lines. Into one of these forts, which were of earthwork, we were taken, and, standing on the ramparts, looked over the flat land in front, with nothing between us and the Turks in Belina but the outposts.

In front all trees and shrubs had been cleared away for a space of half a mile, then came a fringe of low shrub bordering a shallow streamlet, and beyond the shrubs on the other side we caught the gleam of a gilded minaret. It was that of the mosque in Belina.

The outposts were crouching among the brushwoods of this bank, and we were well within cannon range; but all was calm and still, the sun shone, the birds sang, a soft luminous haze veiled the distant sun; that one bright speck of gold seemed to burn against the deep blue sky.

It was strange to think that there, close by, in the street below that minaret, the Turkish troops were passing up and down, ready to muster and march out at a moment's notice; for Belina was the headquarters of the Turkish Army on the Drina; and yet all was as quiet and silent as on an English Sunday at home.

We sat on the bank enjoying the scene and the fresh air, and discussing affairs in general.

I asked the colonel if the troops were not a very mixed race—not only in respect of religion, but of nationality.

"It is quite true," he answered. "We have here Wallachians, Bulgarians, Bosnians, and Servians proper. We have Jews, Mussulmen, Latin and Greek Catholics, Protestants of all denominations, and people who have no recognised faith; all are subject alike to military service."

"I have heard," I said, "that the Latin Catholics are not heart and soul in the Servian cause—that they dread the ascendency of the Greek Church."

"So, they say in other countries that do not know us as we are," he answered; "and there is certainly a feeling of that sort in Bosnia, where there are many more Latin Catholics than here. Bosnia has not done what she might; she might have given assistance if she would, but she has held aloof. It is useless saying that she could not rise—we know she could; but she has tamely submitted to the cruelties inflicted upon her. The men might have joined in, even if the women and children were refugees, but they are taking charity over in Hungary, and not striking a blow for freedom. But as to religious differences, the laws make no distinction here, and none is made. Did you hear that grand chant rising from the chapel?"

"I did," I answered, "and it seemed to me to be the same from both the Greek and Latin chapels."

"It was the same," he said. "That was the war-song of Servia, and the refrain is, '*For the Cross of Christ and for Fatherland.*' Well, I am a Latin Catholic; that chapel was a Greek one; but our war-song is the same—we remember nothing else. *There!*" (and, as he spoke, he sprang on the ramparts and pointed with his drawn sword)—"*there*, behind us are our homes, our wives, our children, all that men hold dear. *There!*" (and he pointed towards Belina)—"*there* is the hated foe, we remember nothing but that; and we fight side by side in the faith of the Cross."

Both were silent for some moments. In such enthusiasm, in such grand faith, there was something too solemn for words.

The officers then came around us, and told us tales of the July battle.

Amongst them were these incidents of Eastern warfare:—

The Turks, when they occupied Belina as headquarters, broke into and ravaged the Greek church, and took from it the large cross. Crucifixes are not used in the Greek churches. Then they came on to the assault of the lines, carrying it in front of them, and when they came near they held it up, crying out,—"*You cannot fire upon your Christ, you cannot, you dare not, fire upon your Christ!*"

The Servians did not fire, but a forlorn hope, as it might be called, rushed forward—a hand-to-hand fight ensued. The Turks were disordered by the sudden and unexpected attack and fell back, the cross was captured and carried in triumph into the entrenchments, and the guns opened fire and completed the rout of the Turks.

I saw the cross, placed on high, over the chapel of the headquarters.

At another point of the attack a *dervish* led the way—a *dervish* is a sort of monk or priest, eminent for asceticism and sanctity—and he advanced well in front of the Turkish line, twirling on high a long stick with a brass knob at the top, exactly like those which drum-majors use when they march at the head of the band.

He began to shout loudly—"*Allah* comes! *Allah* comes! Oh, *infidels* and unbelievers, flee before him!"

But the *infidels* in question were by no means inclined to flee, and one special *infidel*, who was particularly irritated by the *dervish's* injunction, dashed at the *dervish* and cut him down, then returned twirling the stick in humble imitation of its late owner.

He stuck the stick on the top of the entrenchments, and defied the Turks in general, and all the *dervishes* in particular, to come and take it back; but the invitation was not accepted, and the stick was there on the day I visited the camp, and it was lent to me to hold in my hand as a glorious trophy.

After this, being all in good spirits and in a mood to enjoy ourselves, it entered into the heads of the adventurous correspondents, the *aides-de-camp*, the officers in general, the secretary and myself, that a drive between the outposts and the entrenchments would enable us to look back and have a good view of the lines, from the same point of view as the Turks from the minaret at Belina, for the land was so level and so low that they were not visible beyond the brushwood on the little stream, except from a height.

The sun was sinking in a golden haze; it would be difficult to see us from Belina, the watchman on the minaret was probably dozing, and if we were seen it would be still more difficult to hit us, and so away we went.

The scent of the marsh flowers was strong and sweet; mist was rising all around; the Turks were asleep; the lines looked picturesque in the setting sun, with the sentinels pacing up and down, and the cannon peering out here and there; and had it not been for a suspicion of malaria, our drive would have been most delightful.

We passed the outlying redoubts and re-entered the lines far to the right, then through the camp, across the bridge, past the sandy shore and fir-wood, and so back to the mess-room and our supper.

Chapter 11

A Dinner in Bosnia

After supper we all strolled about in the moonlight, and the secretary and Mr. W—— accompanied me home. I went to bed by moonlight, and, in spite of the divan being very hard, I slept soundly, and it was broad daylight when I woke.

With some difficulty I made some women whom I saw in the courtyard understand that I wanted water, and at last they brought it, and when the rough toilette was finished, I started off in search of breakfast.

I found Mr. Brennan and Mr. Bowes, and we began our hot coffee and black bread. Very soon afterwards arrived Captain Alexitch and Major Pallacruska, bringing a kind invitation from the general to dine with himself and Madame Alempits in camp.

Of course, we joyfully accepted, for, truth to say, in the intervals of our assembling around the mess-table, nothing could be duller than Badovinsky.

The gentlemen smoked and slept; I slept and did not smoke. There was nothing to see, and nothing to do; no books, no newspapers.

In fact, except in the house of M. Christich, I never saw any books in any language in all Servia, except a few magazines in German, with plates of the fashions, and even they had not penetrated to Badovinsky.

All the wounded then there were assembled in one ambulance, in the only place in all the village capable of receiving more than half a dozen at a time, and this one Madame Alempits had expressed a wish to show me herself; so it was a matter of etiquette not to go there till I went with her.

At 10 a.m. we started for camp to see all that we had not seen.

Our friend the colonel in command met us on the plateau, where the mess-room was.

They first took us to see the artillery. The guns were not very large, but new, and said to be very effective.

The gunners were of the regular army, and presented a most respectable appearance. Their commander was a tall, fine man, who had served in the Russian artillery, and knew what he was about.

Then we went to see the volunteers of the first class.

The first class are, of course, the best men of the reserve, young and well-trained, but their uniforms were of many sizes, and various colours, which they attributed to the slowness with which the clothing department issued the stores; but the truth was, there was nothing in store. Every article had to be made, and of course that is a slow process, though there were sewing-machines in use at Belgrade.

After this we went to the camp of the Italian Legion. General Sgarralini had not arrived at that time. They were temporarily commanded by some other officer, and I met there Captain Ceretti Celsi. As I could speak Italian, we entered at once into conversation; besides, we knew mutual friends.

Mr. Bowes and myself had wandered on ahead with Major Pallacruska, and when the rest of the party arrived, they found us installed in the commander's leafy tent, drinking coffee, and watching the interesting ceremony of presenting medals to the men who had distinguished themselves in the July battle.

They had been struck off after that affair for distribution to all who distinguished themselves in battle then and afterwards.

They were silver, about the size of a shillings suspended from a ribbon of the Servian colours, which are a tricolour of red, white, and blue, like the French tricolour; only in the Serbish one the red and blue come together with the white at the side, though the ribbon from which the cross of the Takova, their highest honour, is suspended, has the crimson in the centre, and a narrow band of white on each side, edged with a band of blue. The motto on the medal was, "For Valour."

Later on in the war a gold medal was given for valour, much larger than the silver, and hung from a crimson ribbon; but these silver medals were the first honours distributed for valour in this war.

When the distribution was over, I went with Captain Celsi and Mr. Gordon to see the huts where lay the sick of the Italian Legion. They had no wounded there.

The poor fellows were suffering from diarrhoea, low fever, and dysentery, the effect of cold, exposure, damp, and malaria. We promised to send some quinine and flannel for belts.

The officers then begged for quinine and flannel belts for the rest of the legion, and though I believe that they were sent afterwards by a gentleman, at that time connected with a society in London, I could not feel that it was a rightful part of Red Cross work to keep soldiers well; only to tend them when sick, and cure them if possible; but to keep soldiers in health is to add to the fighting power of an army, and is not either a neutral or charitable work.

To cure them, so that they can rejoin their corps, may seem but a narrow distinction, but wars now-a-days, (1877), are so short and sharp, that if a man is ill enough to be sent back from his little regimental hospital to the rear, he will probably not be strong enough to rejoin his regiment for active service in the field for two or three months.

I strongly urged the transfer of all the sick to the hospital at Schabatz, as they could not, I felt assured, recover in such a bad air as that on the Drina.

This was carried out a few days afterwards. About sixty sick were sent from the camp to Schabatz.

It was now time to go to the headquarters' messroom, and we strolled back there.

Just as we arrived, the general and Madame Alempits drove up. I accompanied her to the general's tent, occupied in his absence by the colonel, and we sat there chatting for half an hour. Madame Alempits was a ladylike woman, about forty years of age; she spoke perfect French, and was very lively and intelligent.

Presently dinner was announced; the general entered the tent, and offered his arm to take me in to dinner. Madame Alempits followed with the colonel. The long table in the mess-room was covered with a clean white cloth at the upper end; plates, glasses, knives and forks of all sorts and sizes, down each side. The mess-cook had exerted himself to do honour to the great occasion, and besides the usual soup and stewed meat, we had roast turkey and roast pig, done after the most approved fashion, in a coating of clay, and baked in a hole covered up with hot wood ashes.

The general poured me out a glass of red wine, and called to Major Pallacruska to fill it up with water. The major did so, struck his hand sharply on the top of the glass, and presented it to me, with the contents effervescing like soda-water.

The general laughed at my astonishment, and asked me to taste the wine. It tasted just like soda-water; and seeing the water being poured out of jugs in great profusion, I asked how it was possible to bring such quantities of soda-water so long a journey, so as to be able to have so much of it.

He then explained that close by was a spring, the water of which was indeed natural soda-water, and that several of these existed in Servia.

Now, some speculative individual might make a fortune by buying up the land just where that spring rises, and sending off the water in casks, or jars, or bottles to the cities where soda-water is so much in request.

Anyone in Belgrade could give the desired information. Truly the natural treasures of Servia are unknown and unexplored.

Dinner passed over very pleasantly, followed as usual by strong black coffee; healths were drunk, ours of course amongst the number, and toasts were given. I will not betray the name of the gentleman whose sympathies ought properly to have been all Turkish, and yet who was so overpowered by the frank and kindly treatment of the Servian officers and the hospitality of the general, that he actually made an eloquent speech, wishing him and the cause he so nobly defended all success. Being afterwards "chaffed" about it, he tried to blush, and protested it was a mere after-dinner *façon de parler*, "and the soda-water was strong."

No, I will not betray the secrets of that pleasant dinner in Bosnia.

And speaking of Bosnia, I may just say here, that the idea of annexing Bosnia to Servia is a most fallacious one. The Bosnians will not have it, and the Servians admit that it can only be done by force.

We once saw a new paper, called the *Oriental Star*, professing to be the organ of the League in aid of the Christians in Turkey, and for a paper which is supposed to be an authority in Slavonic matters it makes the queerest mistakes. The writer of some of the articles has evidently never been in Servia.

There in the first number (*vide* page 3) is the cool proposal that "Turkish Croatia, Bosnia, Herzegovina, and Northern Albania" should be added to Servia!

Imagine gallant and then successful Herzegovina and its spirited prince being annexed to humbled and beaten Servia, with the reproach of cowardice resting on her armies! Not one of these provinces would consent; and more especially if success were any test, Servia at that time should have been annexed to Herzegovina.

The writer does not understand that a positive dislike of each other exists between all those provinces, and only force could unite them in a galling and easily broken bond.

The Servian wish is that every State should be independent; with a central council, composed of representatives from every province, under a president elected by the council.

This is an idea that we heard discussed and advocated by men in high position, wise and calm judging, who well knew their country's strength and weakness, and most earnestly desired her welfare and progress—men of independence, who scorned Russian pre-eminence or visionary ambition, and whose wisdom and moderation may be relied upon.

Each State would thus retain its internal independence and laws, and a mutual bond of sympathy and alliance would unite all and strengthen all for no one is strong enough to stand alone; but this is just what (as they said) Russia would not like—a powerful and independent group of States, a barrier to her progress to the Danube.

Dinner over, we returned to Badovinsky, and lounged about and slept till supper.

Mr. Brennan was very poorly, and we were anxious that he should return to Schabatz; but as the Belgrade steamer was not due, that day or next, he thought it useless, and did not like to separate himself from his most kind friend and attendant, Mr. Bowes. No brother could have been kinder, no woman more gentle, than he was to the sufferer.

Mr. Gordon and myself had looked at one or two houses for an ambulance, but they were too small for any practical purpose, and I said that I felt assured from what I had seen and heard, that there never would be enough wounded on the Drina to make it worthwhile establishing an English hospital at Badovinsky. The few there might be could well be sent to Schabatz, where there was plenty of room for them; the weather was lovely and transport easy, for in Servia the summer is hot and fine, and not till the weather breaks up, in the late autumn, is there any danger of rain or cold.

After supper we strolled about in the brilliant moonlight.

Mr. Gordon told me that at daybreak next morning they were all going to the camp, and I had better come too, for there was to be a "reconnaissance" in force, which would probably draw the Turks, and if so there might be wounded.

"I humbly decline the expedition," I said; "I am sure, from what I heard, that it is only undertaken for the benefit of the correspondents, that they may have something to write about the camp on the Drina. If you have wounded, send them straight back and I will look after them."

"Then mind you wake up early, at least," he answered, laughing,

"*Mon ami*," I said, "it must be more than those popguns, four miles off, to wake me up. I slept through the firing from Mont Valerien, on the Prussian lines, by Versailles."

Mr. Brennan was so ill that evening that he went home early and resolved not to go out next morning; but Mr. Bowes, always active, bright and cheerful, volunteered to go and do duty for both, and I went home, feeling that the whole affair was no business of mine, and once more slept soundly till morning.

Chapter 12

A Servian Ambulance

Next morning, I went to the mess-room, and found Mr. Brennan sitting there. He seemed sad and despondent, and expressed himself as feeling very ill, and quite unfit for work. He did not know how he could bear the journey back, and wished he could find some Hunyady water, which, he said, always did him good.

I tried to cheer and amuse him, and to make him take his bread and coffee and an egg, which I found could be had. We chatted over mutual reminiscences of the Franco-German war; wondered how our friends were getting on, and if there was really a "scrimmage" at the front.

Mr. Brennan thought he had heard desultory firing, and hoped Mr. Bowes would take care of himself. I suggested that I fully believed no one would get hurt.

At last he proposed our going to see if we could buy some Hunyady water. There was a bare possibility of some having been sent to Badovinsky for the use of the staff.

We went to the commissariat department; we found our way into every house that looked as if anything had ever been sold there, but all in vain; and whilst pursuing our researches, the party returned in high spirits.

They had sallied forth; the Turks had not descried them. Mr. Gordon and Mr. W—— had actually ridden on, close to Belina, and the sentinels did see them at last, and began to fire. Their enjoyment at the bullets whizzing about was perfectly ludicrous; they were like two big schoolboys out for a frolic.

They declared that several Turks were killed, but no one seemed clear upon the point. One poor Serb, however, was wounded in the leg; and now I regretted not having been there; for there was no surgeon, and all the combined intelligence of the party only arrived at the brilliant idea of putting on a tourniquet—which was not wanted—as tightly as possible below the wound, which was in the leg; thus causing exquisite pain, and being perfectly useless. I fear that he suffered long, for I heard many weeks afterwards that he died at Schabatz.

Of what use this skirmish could be it is impossible to say. I do not pretend to understand military manoeuvres, though we have seen two or three things which we felt were great mistakes, and they proved to be so.

It was dearly paid for by the loss of one life; whoever or whatever the poor fellow might be, he was "somebody's darling," and somebody may be mourning that day's work even now.

While the warriors retired to wash off the dust, smoke the pipe of peace, and drink to their exploits in native beer, I went to the house of Madame Alempits, and found her in the cheerful little room which was at once drawing-room, dining-room, and bedroom.

Two small camp beds served as chairs and sofa; a table was in the centre, and actually a closed washing-stand, with a bit of glass hung above it.

Madame Alempits laughingly pointed out what she called the luxury of the room. She had brought up the "furniture" from their house at Belgrade, which was a large and well-furnished one.

We went together to the ambulance. It had been a farmyard and grain-store.

It was surrounded on three sides by a two-storied erection. The lower part was open to the yard, and had been stalls for cattle; the upper was entered by ladders, and was a kind of gallery, enclosed by thick wicker-work. There were no windows, light and air being only admitted through the wicker-work. The roof was thatched. It was so narrow that the sick and wounded were laid along it, and we could hardly pass.

In the centre of the yard were three tents—one for stores, one for patients, and one for the surgeons and medicines.

The large tent had a double row of beds— one row down the centre, one down the sides.

The men looked clean, but very hot. The sun blazed down on the tents. There was no ventilation, and the poor fellows were brushing away the flies with branches of green boughs.

The only nurses were a widow lady—very young and very pretty—and her maid.

She came in whilst we were standing there, and kissed Madame

Alempits' hand, then went round the beds.

I watched her, and soon discovered that she knew nothing of nursing, and her maid still less. Besides, if she was—as I was told she was—superintendent of the ambulance, why were many things as I found them if she had ever seen an ambulance before?

I noticed that Madame Alempits behaved very coolly to her, and appeared anxious that the ambulance should be broken up.

In this I could honestly aid her. I pointed out that the want of air and light in the upper gallery was a fatal objection to its being used as a ward; that the heat was far too great for the tents, and the means of ventilation and cleanliness deficient; that there were not enough attendants for so many patients; that their diets were scanty, ill-prepared, and not well chosen; that to mix sick and wounded together was a great mistake; and that I saw no possibility of remedying this defect here.

The pretty widow resented these remarks, and sent for the head doctor, who took her part, and declared there the ambulance must be, and there the patients should be.

Madame Alempits and myself bowed and departed, but she begged me to come that afternoon, and give in the report to the general. She quite agreed in all that I had said, and trusted that even if the ambulance were continued, the present inmates, and the sick in camp, would be sent down to Schabatz or Belgrade.

I may just mention here, that this was done three days afterwards, and the ambulance closed, and that the presence of the pretty widow there had been a source of great trouble and scandal, which the staff were only too glad to get rid of.

After dinner, Mr. Bowes told me that he must go down to Schabatz that night, and kindly asked me if I would like to go too. I willingly assented. All my errand there was done, and it simply remained to give in my report to the general and say farewell, but Mr. Brennan was so ill, that he decided on waiting at Badovinsky that night, and going down at foot-pace next day.

It was therefore arranged that we should start at five o'clock, when the heat of the sun was over, and that at 4 p.m. we should call on the general and his wife.

Mr. Gordon took a stroll in the shade with me, and said that the general had given him the command of a couple of hundred men as captain of transport.

"Transport of what?" I asked.

"Wounded," he said, gravely.

At this I laughed very much; I knew from what I heard that the general did not intend to attack, and much doubted if he would be attacked. There was no reason why it should be done at the risk of great loss of life. The real point of attack was Kragojevatz, the ancient capital of Servia, and its arsenal, on the way to Belgrade; and even the capture of Schabatz, between which and Badovinsky was a mountain ridge, difficult to cross and very easy to defend, was not a matter of great consequence.

This was the opinion of all the best judges, and even that if a battle did ensue, it was not probable there would be such a number of wounded as to render a transport corps of two hundred necessary.

Mr. Gordon did not see this, so we agreed to differ, and I said that if we could get a suitable building in Schabatz, and the War Office permitted it, we would form an hospital at Schabatz.

The War Office did not permit, for telegraph orders met me at Schabatz that night, ordering us not to work at Schabatz—but this is anticipating.

However, as women are very fond of saying, "I told you so," I may add that there never was a battle on the Drina. There were a few skirmishes, and half a score of wounded. There were also a good many sick, but all were sent by the usual way to Schabatz.

CHAPTER 13

The Return to Schabatz

At four o'clock, Mr. Bowes and myself went to call on General and Madame Alempits. Coffee was brought in, and, with it, honey in glasses. This seems to be the Servian mode of saying "welcome." I was about; to refuse the honey, when Mr. Bowes silently telegraphed to me to take it, and he afterwards explained it to me.

The general asked me if there was any house in Schabatz fit for an ambulance; I said there was one, and he replied that he would telegraph to place it at our service.

I gave him my verbal report as to the Badovinsky ambulance, and he said that the sick and wounded should be sent down to Schabatz.

After thanking him for his great kindness, we took our leave and went to look out for our waggon and horses.

We found them ready, a rough waggon with plenty of hay, and a pair of ponies, ragged, but up to their work.

Off we went amidst a cloud of dust and voices of lamentation of kind friends of the staff.

Badovinsky was soon lost in the closing evening light.

What a quaint peculiar drive that was!

Dashing past dark silent woods, halting for a moment where some wood fire lighted by the roadside, marked the spot where a hut of boughs with a table outside, took the place of a refreshment booth for the many passengers to and from the camp.

Here and there came out women in white headdresses, who offered us coffee, and would take no money, till we resorted to the cunning device of giving it to the "bairns." Then on again, with no sound or sign of life, except the rattle of our own wheels, the moonlight casting ink-black shadows on the road, while we, the solitary travellers, were recalling people we had met—brilliant wits gone from amongst us, kindly hearts that had ceased to beat, sweet voices silenced for ever—recalled, amidst a golden mist of remembrance of days in Paris, and hours passed under "the branching limes" of Hyde Park, in the merry month of May.

And this was so far away, and times were so changed, and we were in a half-civilised land; and what was to be the end of it all no one knew!

It was dark when we reached Schabatz, and were greeted by the firing of isolated rockets; fires were burning in the main street, and the population, dressed in all their best clothes, were parading up and down, admiring the imposing spectacle of a few dip candles arranged in the window-sills of the inns, the *Prefecture*, and the best houses.

"What is this fearful amount of dissipation about?" Mr. Bowes inquired.

I could give no satisfactory answer, but as we drove up to the inn, the waiter greeted us with the intelligence that it was the prince's *fête*.

A *fête* on the scale of the province and the prince, I thought, unless theoretical ideas are to count.

Mr. Bowes ordered supper, and, this over, retired to write his letters.

I found the room we had occupied kept for us, and was glad to sleep off the fatigue of the drive. I do not think that anyone can appreciate what that fatigue is, till they have tried a Servian waggon amidst the fearful dust of a Servian road.

Next morning, I went to see the surgeon in charge. The Austrian lady and himself were dressing the wounded, and asked me to go round with them. I suggested that a good many were well enough to send as convalescents to Belgrade, and the surgeon offered to show me the building he thought would suit us; he had received a telegram from Badovinsky about it.

He showed me the building. Mr. Bowes and Mr. W——, who had come down from Badovinsky, were with me; and, on my return to the hotel, we all decided that it was utterly impossible to work in Schabatz.

I will not enter into further details on the point in question. I took the advice of kind-hearted, judicious, and honourable English gentlemen, and when Louise arrived the next day at noon, I found that she brought final orders from the War Minister to return to Belgrade, and proceed to Doïni Milanovitch, at the other extreme end of Servia, on the Danube.

Mr. Brennan came down from Badovinsky that evening in charge of Mr. Gordon. His illness pressed heavily upon him. Louise, who arrived from Belgrade with a chest of medicines for the camp on the Drina, and the orders before mentioned, quite agreed with all the others that he ought to go home to England; for she, who had not seen him for some days, could trace more alteration than anyone else did in his look and manner.

She had brought the chest because it was dangerous to send such valuable goods alone; and she knew that she would meet us in Schabatz, and that we should know the way to send it on straight.

The voyage down was not as gay as the voyage up. Illness on the one hand, disappointment on the other, are not ingredients of cheerfulness. We had hoped to get to work at once, but now delay must ensue. Well, our intentions were honest and unselfish—to do the greatest possible good wherever the War-Office thought it could best be done, and it mattered little where or how.

Belgrade was reached at last, and the hospitable house in the Grande Place.

We have no other remembrance of Schabatz, but of the stoniest, dustiest, dreariest place on earth: abroad street, with one-storied houses on either side, and sundry small shops and drinking-houses of somewhat better appearance.

It stood in a flat plain. Other towns in Servia might be as small, and dull, and dusty; but, at all events, they had the charm of lovely scenery around them.

Schabatz stood in a cheerless plain; yet it is one of the principal towns in Servia, and an important port on the Save.

Belgrade looked as usual, blue and bright—that is, the sky and the rivers blue, and the whole town white in the strong sunlight.

The city was very full; the Russian invasion had not yet commenced; but there were many English tourists.

I think if tourists who come merely from curiosity, or to write a letter to the papers, or to make a speech to their constituents, could have an idea how much they are in the way of the workers in a land which is the seat of war—how utterly useless they are, and how much all the officials, polite as they may be, wish them a thousand miles away—they might have the good sense, and the good feeling, to pass their holidays elsewhere.

It was most unlucky, but the beginning of the war of 1870-71, and up to Sedan, was in the holiday time of the English tourists, and they swarmed over the early battlefields of France, glass in eye, pipe in mouth, hunting for relics, and criticising past military events. They did not come in the hour of need, in the bitter winter, with even the little personal help that would have been welcome.

It was just the same in Servia. All the summer, up to the battle of Alexinatz—which has been justly called the Sedan of Servia—they came in crowds. They brought letters of introduction, and the poor officials, wishing to be polite and to enlist their sympathies, were obliged to find them horses and quarters upcountry.

They did not come later on, and it was as well, since every vehicle was occupied with sick or wounded soldiers on the retreat from Paratjin to save their lives.

No! their summer holiday was over, they were sitting over blazing fires, holding up glasses of ruby wine to see how it sparkled in the light, laughing over their three days' adventures in that out-of-the-way land, giving themselves out as authorities on all that concerned it, and being looked up to as oracles.

One gentleman, who shall be nameless, simply got as far as Belgrade, and then went to the North of England, and gave lectures on "Servia and the Servian War."

Those who had to work in hunger and cold, trying to save the lives so wasted in this unequal contest, prising every drop of wine, looking on every egg as a treasure, that might help to strengthen some weak frame; those who passed days and nights on the battlefield, gallant unselfish fellows, who had put aside every dream of home comforts for the sake of the wounded out there, ay, even those who bore hardship cheerfully, that the truth might reach England in the newspapers—*these* men, and these alone, know what Servia is, and what that war was.

And the volunteers who fought with her troops know too, but soldiers are not often penmen, and it is left to civilians to record the events of that brief but eventful campaign.

CHAPTER 14

A Great Mistake

The great excitement at Belgrade at this time was the coming of Colonel Lloyd-Lindsay with the 10,000*l*. voted to Servia by the Committee of the National Aid Society.

As far as we could make out the story at this distance, Sir Edmund Lechmere—a member of the Order, or, as I think they now call themselves, the Guild of St. John—a most excellent and energetic man, had called his friends together, advertised in the papers, collected some 2000*l*, and sent out some clever surgeons under Mr. McKellar, an old friend of ours in the Franco-Prussian War.

They were Messrs. Attwood, Boyd, Sandwith, Hume, and Gimlet—six in all—some qualified surgeons, and all young men of eminence as young men in their profession. That they were all gentlemen, in every sense of the word, we can bear witness to.

But letters appeared in the papers asking why the National Aid Society, with a balance in hand of over 80,000*l*., did not come forward.

The excuse made was the same as was made, when aid was asked of them for the wounded during the war in Spain, and this excuse was that, by their rules, they could not give relief in cases of civil war or rebellion against the lawful ruler of a realm.

So much pressure was at last brought to bear upon them that they yielded. A meeting took place, and Sir Edmund Lechmere consented to merge his Society and its funds into those of the National Aid Society, on condition of some of their committee being placed on the committee of the National Society.

The whole and sole mischief of this was, that in the National Society all power is centred in one man, Lloyd-Lindsay. The St. John's committee were reduced to mere cyphers.

However, 20,000*l*. was voted, 10,000*l*. to Turkey and 10,000*l*. to Servia. Some of it was expended on stores and instruments, and the colonel started for Belgrade, accompanied by Mr. McCormac, of St. Thomas's, as inspector and surgeon-in-chief, several surgeons, a secretary, an *aide-de-camp*, a valet, and a courier—at least, this was the suite with which it was said he arrived in Belgrade.

But now the question was on all sides, Where is the English lord—when will he come? And the day after our return from Schabatz he did come.

His entry into Servia had better be given in the words of one of her most learned and accomplished men, Herr Meissner, a professor of science, and librarian of the National Library and Museum at Belgrade.

It was published in the *Daily News* of October 28th, 1876, after the colonel's celebrated speech at Reading, and is as follows:—

> Sir,—The speech of Colonel Lloyd-Lindsay has attracted some attention here, as he was in Belgrade some weeks ago on behalf of your Red Cross Society; otherwise, the remarks on the proclivities of so small a politician would not have been noticed. Acting on the advice of our friend, Dr. Sandwith, our government sent a deputation to the steamer to bid the colonel welcome. I was one of that deputation, and you may judge my surprise when he at once attacked our government and our policy to me, in reply to my courteous welcome.
>
> In addition to this act of astonishing bad taste, he soon filled the air with sundry very ill-natured remarks concerning the Servian Government and people, some of which can be quoted if necessary. It was with a sense of relief that we saw him depart for the more congenial atmosphere of Constantinople; for at one time the policy of refusing hospital aid so offered was seriously discussed.
>
> We thought, however, that the colonel did not, in the matter above referred to, correctly represent the English Red Cross Society. Your special correspondent has correctly criticised the strange arrangements for the relief of the wounded made by Colonel Lindsay, but we hope and trust the English Red Cross Society will be represented here in future by some gentleman who does not so openly manifest unfriendly sentiments towards us.
>
> I have the honour to be, Sir,
> Your obedient servant,

Belgrade, Oct. 21st, 1876.

Joseph Meissner,
Professor and Librarian at the
National Library, Belgrade.

Very severe articles on the National Aid Society also appeared in the same journal, of the dates of September 13th, 14th, and 15th, with several others.

We have no wish whatever to state anything on our own account, as we were not in Belgrade at the time of the extravagant expenditure and luxury of the Katherine Hospital, as the hospital formed by the National Society was called; but it was the talk of all Belgrade. When we came back in October, we saw at the War Office a table of ambulances, patients received, discharged, or dead, most beautifully arranged, so as to show the whole at one glance, and the deaths were marked by crosses in blue; the predominance of blue in the column devoted to the Katherine Hospital was remarkable.

Let no one imagine this was from want of skill or care; it was simply attributable to the distance of the hospital from the front.

The wounded were half dead when they got there, and in the colonel's report he says:—

> To take upon itself the establishment of reserve hospitals and ambulances, had been held to be no part of the duty which a neutral Society should undertake. This principle had as far as possible guided the conduct of the Society in the East, and it had undoubtedly brought its agents into some unpopularity, more especially in Servia, where a disposition had been shown to cast upon the English Aid Society duties which might perfectly well have been performed by the government, had they not been solicitous to economise their financial resources to carry on the war.

A more unjust and prejudiced paragraph was never written. In the first place, did not this very Society establish an hospital at Bingen, on the Rhine, and largely aid one at Darmstadt, both far enough away from the seat of war, in 1870-71? In the next, Herr Meissner's letter will fully account for the unpopularity in Servia, which the colonel admits was the fact. And in the last place, the Servian medical department exerted themselves in every possible way, to help their own wounded; and if the government, or rather the War Ministry, could not grant them large sums to meet extraordinary pressure, it must be remembered that Servia is a poor country, but not a bankrupt beggar like Turkey. Turkey, according to the colonel's own account, availed herself largely of English help. There were hospitals at Sofia, and a reserve hospital in the Turkish rear, besides an ambulance in the front.

In Servia there were five surgeons in front, and the Belgrade Hospital in the rear. In Turkey, the Society took over and paid three English surgeons, "who had previously been in the pay of the Turkish Government," besides having four surgeons of their own there.

In Servia, they took over no English surgeons in the pay of the Servian Government, though there were several ready and willing to serve at the rate of 20s. a day, instead of about 15s. a month paid after the war; but they did take over Sir Edmund Lechmere's surgeons, and paid them instead of his doing so. They supplied Mr. Black of the Ottoman Bank, at Adrianople, with funds for the assistance of the hospital there; also in Constantinople, they left money with Lady Elliot, while the sum of money left with Consul-General White, for the current expenses of the Belgrade Hospital, represents all left in Servia, to be given by what the colonel calls "local means of distribution."

These facts will speak for themselves.

In the face of the opinion about reserve hospitals, one as we know was formed at Belgrade, where it was not wanted or wished for, and one of the objects was, as the colonel calmly says, "to establish an hospital after which other hospitals in Servia might be modelled."

Who was to establish these hospitals? Was it possible or wise to introduce English luxury into this primitive country?—to initiate men into habits which they could never carry out. The Belgrade Hospital was no model of anything practicable in Servia; and surely Turkey is not so far ahead in civilisation that she required no tuition on this subject! At all events, no remark implying such censure is made in this report published on October 15th, 1876, in the *Times* and *Standard*, and probably in all the other papers. It is worth reading as a curiosity. One paragraph more deserves attention.

> Mr. McCormac inspected *all* the Turkish military hospitals, and left with them various medical stores.

> He did not inspect all the Servian ones, nor leave stores with them.

It is always painful to have to criticise a work of charity badly done, but it is the duty of those who were on the spot, and saw the working of the whole thing, to point out what may serve as a warning for the future, and in the face of present events, when the National Aid Society may have to come forward to strengthen the hands of our own government, to ask people seriously to consider, shall this blundering continue? Shall our money be spent at the caprice of one man, uselessly, as compared with what it might have done, and to rise up and say, "We will have a voice in the distribution of what we have given."

Very few words will conclude this tale as far as the Battle of Alexinatz. Reports came down from the front that a great battle was expected, and Colonel Lloyd-Lindsay applied for permission to go on there with surgeons and stores.

Still trusting in English honour, if not in English goodwill, the passes were given, and he went on as fast as government post-horses could carry him.

They arrived at Alexinatz while the battle was going on, but one waggon of stores was lost.

A young surgeon, who had been placed on it to guard the property, got tired of his lonely position and went into the front carriage. The next thing was, the waggon and horses were missing—we heard of their fate afterwards; and as the drivers carried off the stores to the Servian Army before Négotin, no great harm was done by "this local means of distribution," though it assuredly was not intended by the colonel.

But Alexinatz was reached at last, and here the surgeons did good service to the wounded brought off the field.

They found there Mr. McKellar and his gallant band, and the colonel commenced his amiable conduct towards them by reprimanding them for wearing Servian uniforms, without which they would not have been allowed to go to the front; and indeed, as they had been sent by the Order of St. John to help the Servians, they had accepted rank in the Servian Army.

It is not to be supposed they had time to change their dress, though they were informed that they had been taken over by the National Society.

They went off to the field and worked under fire.

What the colonel did during the day does not appear—he probably watched the battle; but a florid account appeared in one paper of Mr. McCormac attending to the wounded till he was up to his elbows in blood (which seems incredible for so skilled a surgeon), and having to be "washed at the pump." The objection to this part of the story is that there was no pump there!

Evening came on; all was lost, and a hasty retreat had to be made, but there was plenty of time to carry off all the wounded. The colonel was assured that there was time for him to eat his dinner, and that he had better do so, and not create a panic; however, he prepared to set off at once as fast as he could go, and he probably left the second waggon behind him.

The surgeons waited to the last, and then only retreated, in imminent peril of being cut off by the enemy, to Rashan, a few miles in the rear; and there they stayed, hard worked and more than half starved, while their chief, who should have waited to see what could be done for the retreating wounded and his noble surgeons, dashed all the way back to Belgrade ready and anxious to start by the steamer for Widdin in the Turkish lines.

At Belgrade other store chests had been left on the wharf, awaiting orders. On the colonel's return, he ordered these chests to be shipped on board the steamer.

Smarting under the news of the defeat, the porters on the wharf refused, and made remarks, which it was as well the colonel did not understand.

Mr. Spooner exerted all his influence, worked hard for hours, and at last induced the porters to get the chests on board the steamer, in time to allow the colonel and his own surgeons who had returned with him to leave that day. He, his staff, and all his chests, started for Widdin, and were not followed by "the blessings of a grateful people."

The colonel had come straight from the front, and gone straight into Turkish lines, just what his predecessor, Dr. Laseron, had wanted to do. Was not this enough, combined with his past conduct, to raise suspicion in Servian minds? Let the truthful and far-seeing correspondent of the *Daily News*, Archibald Forbes, answer that question.

The following paragraph is taken from his letter to the *Daily News*:—

> It is represented that Colonel Lloyd-Lindsay came to Belgrade, and that he penetrated through Servia to the frontier, where the fighting was raging, charged with an exceptional and an almost sacred function, as chief of the Red Cross Association of England. Coming in this capacity there were no secrets from him, the Servian military position in all its weakness, and in all its peculiarities, lay patent before him, as the embodiment of English charity to the unfortunates of the war. But it is urged that this exceptional function of his should have closed his mouth

against the public utterances of strictures, which may be true or may be calumnious, but to find material for the framing of which was not his errand to Servia.

It is in a sentence charged against Colonel Lindsay, that he has used for political, if not party purposes, opportunities which were afforded him, as the representative of a cause to which politics and parties are alike foreign; and that his public comments on the Servian soldiers, of whose conduct in the field he had only the experience of a few hours, and that at a distance, amount to something to which, under the circumstances, the hard word of *espionage* must be applied.

And it was so. A still harder and plainer word was used when darker days and a more disastrous defeat came on. Still the question was asked, "What did that English lord tell the Turks?"

His conduct threw a cloud over the English name in Servia, and it would never have been redeemed from that cloud of shame and mistrust, had it not been for the enduring and faithful service of Sir Edmund Lechmere's surgeons, and the devoted efforts of such men as Dr. Humphrey Sandwith, and Dr. Ziemann of Manchester.

Service under the Red Cross in Servia is so inextricably mixed up with this gentleman's proceedings, that no apology is needed for showing how great a failure he made of the work there.

CHAPTER 15

A Wrong Letter of Introduction

The weather in Belgrade at this time was lovely, but very hot, and we anxiously awaited our signal to go to Doïni Milanovatz. Our orders from the War Office were to await the arrival of our head surgeon and physician, Dr. Walter Leckie, and then to proceed, taking with us, if possible, one more surgeon or dresser.

A letter had informed us of the approaching arrival of a young medical student; we of course gave in his name, and he was appointed as second to Dr. Leckie.

As we were all sitting in the drawing-room at Herr Dilbert's, discussing the coming of the "English lord," who was reported to have arrived by the Vienna steamer very early in the morning; a young English "*Herr*" was announced, and in came a very young, fair man, accompanied by an interpreter, who explained that he was Mr. S——, whom we were expecting. He had come in the same steamer with Lloyd-Lindsay, but an odd adventure had detained him from seeking us out earlier in the day; at lead; this was his version.

Onboard the boat was a gentleman, Mr. Salusbury, coming to join the Servian Army. Some lady friend of his in London, whose history was a little behindhand, had given him a letter to "Kara Georgevitch," and no sooner had he and Mr. S —— landed than they inquired the way to the house of this individual.

Our young friend, Mr. S——, informed us that he translated for Mr. Salusbury—why or how we never could tell, for he spoke no language but his own, except a few stammering words—and, between them both, and asking for Kara Georgevitch, they found themselves safely lodged in the hands of the police.

Kara Georgevitch is to the reigning family of Servia exactly what the young Pretender was to the House of Hanover, and to bring letters to him was treason of the deepest dye. The very sound of his name is like shaking a red rag before a bull. Mr. Salusbury was immediately placed under arrest.

Mr. S—— had letters to the War Minister and the archbishop, and was looked upon by the stern chief of the police as an innocent accomplice, an object certainly of suspicion, but not of actual imprisonment. He was liberated under surveillance, and made his way back to the post-office, where he had already called for letters, and there found help from Mr. Spooner, who went to the chief and explained the state of the case.

Mr. Salusbury had actually brought the letter, believing Kara Georgevitch to be the reigning prince; but he had come to fight for the cause, not the man, and was equally glad to offer his sword to Prince Milan.

After a little persuasion, he was liberated; but our friend was disgusted to find the letters he had just posted lying open on the table in the police-office.

Not that the police could have been the wiser for the perusal of their contents; for it was a singular proof of Servian dullness of apprehension (and was named as such by several of the high-class men of Belgrade) that in this office—from whence all passes were issued, all post-horses obtained, where all heavy baggage was deposited in the owner's absence—not one of the officials could speak anything but Serb. It had always been so; so few strangers were in Belgrade, no passes used, no post-horses wanted in peace time, except by natives, that this arrangement did very well. It did not strike whoever was at the head of that department of affairs, that in war time it must be altered or enlarged; and if it did, here came in that Servian jealousy of foreigners, that bigoted reluctance to go forward in the path of progress, which has hindered all along the development of that country's resources.

Mr. S—— had come with the interpreter, who spoke very bad English, to ask for his orders. We told him that he was to accompany us to Doïni Milanovatz; that we had received a telegram from Dr. Walter Leckie, saying he was at Vienna, and coming on in a few days, and had sent an answer to beg him to start by the first boat.

He then went with us to the War Office, and was presented to Dr. Sava Petrovatz. On the way there he told us another doctor had come with him from London to join us.

This was named to the head inspector, who shook his head, and said that one doctor and a dresser would be quite enough. Was not this Herr S——, whose name was down as assistant to the ambulance?—

he was to go, but certainly not Dr. Costello.

Also, there was at Doïni, in charge of the wounded already there, a Servian physician, who had studied in Paris, and spoke perfect French, and therefore no one else was needed.

Mr. S—— had his card and brassard given to him; and on our return we met Dr. Costello, to whom we explained the state of the case.

He was very much disappointed, and at first inclined to blame us, till we explained that the post he came to fill had been taken up by Dr. Leckie days before.

He said the office people in London had told him he was to work with us. To which the answer was, that they appeared utterly ignorant, or studiously disregardful, of Servian rules and regulations, that we had no power one way or another, and that he had better go to the War Office, and get put on some other ambulance.

He took this advice a day or two afterwards, and ultimately went to Krushevatz, close to the frontier by Djunis; but to the last, when we parted at Jacobina, during the wretched retreat from Paratjin, we always remained good friends.

Mr. S—— also had come in the same steamer with the "English lord," and amused us much with an account of his proceedings.

He, his *aide-de-camp*, and the surgeons, were much too grand to dine at the public table; so when the *table d'hôte* was served, they had a table to themselves at the upper end of the saloon.

They associated with no one, and spoke to no one; thus, losing a valuable opportunity of acquiring information as to the land they were going to.

And it so happened that there were some persons on board, who, from their official positions, could have been of great service to them; but these came on shore disgusted with the high and mighty exclusiveness of "the English lord" and his party, and with the contemptuous way in which they treated other Red Cross workers on board.

Our secretary, now transport captain, had returned to the Drina, with the promise of rejoining us as soon as possible—a promise, to our sorrow, unfulfilled; and yet at Doïni, as it turned out, there would have been nothing for him to do.

We had orders to go on now that we had one gentleman with us, and our doctor should be sent on as soon as he arrived. The *Deligrad*, the one war-steamer which Servia possessed, was to go and fetch some Russians from Kladonitza, opposite Orsova, and would drop us *en route*; but her departure was so uncertain that we thought it better to start by the Austrian steamer, so as not to lose any more time.

These steamers once stopped at Doïni Milanovatz; but since the war all traffic with the Servian shore had ceased, and the nearest point on the Austrian shore was Drenkova, from whence carts could be taken to Svenitza, exactly opposite Doïni, and there the Danube could be crossed in small boats.

There were wounded already there from the battle near Saitchar, the accounts of their condition were anything but satisfactory, and more fighting was expected in that quarter, between the Servian Army near Négotin and the Turks in Saitchar; it was therefore well to get to Doïni as soon as possible, and we arranged to start next evening by the Austrian steamer.

We went down to the wharf at the time when the steamer was expected from Pesth, but as usual she was late.

Many Servian friends had accompanied us, and while we were all laughing and chatting together on the wharf, we were most insolently addressed by a person who proclaimed himself a "Member of the Council of the League in Aid of the Christians in Turkey," and who defied us to leave Dr. Costello behind; demanding in the name of the Society that he should be taken on, or that I should give him 10*l*. out of the funds which had been subscribed in answer to our appeal.

This I declined to do without proper authority, and referred the angry individual to the War Office, and the medical department; but he grew more and more noisy. Poor Dr. Costello stood by, silent and ashamed—as he told me afterwards—and so bad was the Member of the Council's conduct, that the Servian gentleman with us asked his name. It was duly reported, and he left Belgrade very shortly afterwards, without going upcountry at all.

He came out as a great authority on Servian matters on his return to England, and we infinitely enjoyed the advertisement which announced his doings.

It grew so late that we begged our friends to go home; at last, most unwillingly, they consented.

We tried to doze on the hard boards of the waiting-room on the wharf, and it was one o'clock in the morning before the vessel arrived, and the passengers began to pour on shore.

Amongst them, to our delight, was Dr. Leckie, who praised us enthusiastically for coming to meet him at that hour of night, or rather morning, till we explained that we were off, and gave him his directions as to where to go, and whom to see, and he promised to follow by the next steamer.

At last all our heavy baggage and ourselves were fairly on board, and we started downstream for Drenkova.

Chapter 16

Once More on the Danube

The steamer was very crowded, and the heat of the ladies' cabin below quite unbearable. We therefore slept as usual in the saloon, it was cooler and fresher there, and we had not a long journey before us.

On the 31st August, 1876, about 9 a.m., we reached Drenkova and landed. We immediately secured three waggons to transport ourselves and our baggage to Svenitza, and were about to get into them when, to our horror, we saw our great chest, the bale of clothes, and the smaller medicine chest, carried off to a warehouse and shut up there, while the men quietly locked the door, and strolled away.

We had engaged an *infirmier*, or hospital attendant at Belgrade, named Milan, or Milano, after the prince.

His father was a Serb, his mother an Italian, and he spoke both languages equally well, besides understanding German and French, when he was spoken to in those tongues.

He was a black-eyed, fresh-coloured, handsome fellow, of about twenty-three. He had been a volunteer, and slightly wounded in some of the earlier engagements; and, being liable to serve in the second reserve, was very anxious to get some employment which would prevent his being called upon to go to the front again.

He had obtained proper leave to be attached to the English Ambulance, and made himself very useful as our attendant, though his erratic behaviour to the world at large, and his absurd way of going on, induced us to name him Flibbertigibbet.

On this occasion he flew into the post and telegraph office, and demanded what all this was about. A stolid Austrian official said that the baggage would not pass without a special permit.

"How is this to be obtained?" I asked.

The answer was that I might telegraph at my own expense to the Consul at Orsova. He could give leave, and probably would.

I instantly begged them to send off a telegram, and paid a florin for it, which I verily believe was too much. I also represented that the baggage had been passed from Austria into Servia once, when it came from Vienna to Belgrade; that it had never been opened, as they might see; and that therefore this delay was absurd.

But they stuck to their point. The chest might have been opened and arms put in. There must be a formal leave.

There was no help for it, so we sat on the steps of a rough inn, and waited.

Drenkova is a small, dull village, consisting of a group of houses, clustered under the cliff, being very hot and very dusty.

Hour after hour slipped away. I bothered the officials at every half-hour, and they actually telegraphed on their own account, to ask why no answer had been sent. The reply came instantly—Consul had left his office and gone home, was asleep, and not likely to be back before 4 p.m.

Then we consulted together, made severe remarks on consuls absent from duty from eleven till four, and wondered what we should do. I refused to leave the chests so full of valuable instruments and medicines, even if I had to sleep at Drenkova.

And so, it was settled. Mr. S—— was to escort Louise to Domi, a telegram being sent to the Captain of the Town announcing their coming, and I would follow with Milano, if I could extricate the baggage from its difficulties, in time to do the distance to Svenitza before dark, the road being dangerous then.

I looked at the driver of the waggon that was to start first. He had demanded a florin on account, and it seemed to me that he had expended that florin in drink, but Milano assured us that it was fully accounted for by the fact that he was a gipsy and his manners peculiar.

Off they went, and when they got about two miles from Drenkova, the driver, half asleep, let the ponies (for horses they could not be called) swerve to one side, and the waggon was all but over the side of the road, where the bank rose some twenty feet above the shore of the river. Mr. S—— pulled sharply at the reins, and they just escaped. The driver crossed himself, and resigned the reins to Mr. S——. Afterwards he contented himself with selling farthing-worths of tobacco to all the people he passed on the road.

Just here the scenery is most lovely; hills covered with wood come sheer down into the Danube, here and there retreating, and leaving space enough for a few cottages and a church, with a little space of sandy beach and brown rock before them, and the river breaking in white ripples upon the shore.

All the scene—fold after fold of forest-crowned mountains, beaches of yellow sand, blue sparkling water, and quiet villages sleeping in the sunshine—was most beautiful.

But after such a narrow escape our friends were in no mood for admiring scenery, however charming, besides, they were naturally anxious as to the fate of myself and the baggage. Their progress, owing to the trading propensities of the ex-driver, was a slow one, but they reached Svenitza at last.

Meantime, I had hardly waved them a farewell before the chief of the Customs, who was really a very good-natured man, came out in evident delight.

The consul had woke up, or been awakened by repeated telegrams, and the answer had come, "Let the baggage pass with a guard to the frontier."

The guard appeared in the shape of a quiet, elderly Austrian soldier. I was to pay him two florins for his guardianship, and one florin for his return fare. To this I willingly agreed.

Milano had secured two waggons, both with gipsy drivers. In one the huge chest, the little chest, and the bale were deposited; in the other, Milano, myself, and the soldier.

All this was quickly arranged, and we dashed out of Drenkova at a hard-gallop.

We gave the sentinel tobacco, and he smoked and told us tales of his life at this out-of-the-way place. Our boy driver begged a little, and dropping the reins devoted himself to the full enjoyment of his pipe. The horses trotted along, and as the road ran by the side of the Danube, following its windings, with the cliffs on one side and the river on the other, they could not well go wrong.

This road was part of the superb military road made by the Hungarians, which extends for miles and miles, between Svenitza and Orsova, where it runs through the Pass of Kazan. The way has been blasted out of the rocks. It is a splendid piece of military engineering.

We met with no accidents; the waggon with the chests bumped along with its heavy weight full speed, and we kept it well in front, so as never to lose sight of it. The consequence was that we did not lose our stores, and the best advice to be given to all travellers is, never lose sight of your baggage, even if it is registered; just give a glance to see that it is on the trucks for the train you are going by.

Svenitza was reached at last, a duplicate of Drenkova, but larger, and with a very broad beach, for at this time the Danube was very low—indeed it had been so all the year.

A company of Austrian soldiers were on evening parade in the little street, with their tight blue pantaloons, and their black cloth gaiters over them, and their old-fashioned shakos, broad at the top.

But a pleasanter sight by far was Louise's bright face, beaming from the top of a rickety flight of steps which led into a little inn, and Mr. S———, red cross on his cap and brassard on his arm, who came running up the street to meet us.

Two Austrian officers stood smiling by. They were Hungarians and Slavs, and had a kindly sympathy with Servia and her helpers. They laughed at my arriving under arrest, as they called it, and objurgated the stupidity of the Drenkova officials.

Milano ran off to secure boats, and we all strolled down to the shore. The river was deep and wide, and we were anxious to land at Doïni Milanovatz before sunset. We saw it across the stream far in the distance.

The river was fortunately very smooth. The boats were broad and flat-bottomed, and though they looked small for so rapid a stream, the Austrian officers assured us that such boats crossed to and fro every day; so, we embarked—the heavy chests in one boat, Mr. S——— and the smaller baggage in another, with Milano; and ourselves in the third.

The Austrians accompanied us to the shore, and stood there watching us long after we were fairly afloat and crossing the Danube.

CHAPTER 17

Our Country Town

Fortunately, the Danube on that particular evening was as calm and still as some little inland lake.

The hills closed in all around; the narrow entrance from Drenkova, the still narrower exit by the Pass of Kazan, were not visible; it was in fact a wide landlocked sheet of water, with a green island at the upper end, Svenitza on the Hungarian side, and Doïni Milanovatz on the Servian shore.

The hills receded at this part of the river so that a broad space of level ground lay between them and the water, further increased by a muddy shore, from which the river had receded, leaving exposed the ragged-looking roots of some old willows that bordered a sort of walk by the edge.

The stream ran fast and strong, and we had to pull up it a long way, to prevent being swept down below the landing-place; but, as we neared it, we espied several gentlemen in good European clothing, grouped under the willows and watching our slow progress—the huge medicine chest, with its large red cross, presenting an imposing appearance in the centre of the baggage boat.

We decided upon it that these were the officials of the town to whom we had telegraphed from Drenkova, and we were not mistaken.

As these gentlemen were the principal inhabitants of the place, they offer a very fair type of the average Servian of the higher ranks, and therefore deserve a short description.

First came the captain of the town, an office of importance during the war; his business was that of finding quarters, ordering rations to be served, storing government baggage, receiving stores, procuring transport to the front, or elsewhere, sending off all official telegrams, and acting in general as military magistrate. In peace he was a sort of mayor.

He was a grizzly man, about sixty years of age, in a mis-fitting tunic and blue insurgent cap. He spoke and understood no language but Serb; was bitterly prejudiced against all foreigners, and always acting on the defensive. He required to be cunningly dealt with, for much depended on keeping him in good humour. Such was Der Herr "Capitan," as he was called, in a jumble of German and Roumanian *patois*.

Next in importance was an individual whose title, literally translated, was that of "Master of the Magazine."

His office was simply that of chief commissary, for at Doïni were landed all the flour and wine for the army lying between Doïni and Négotin, and barring the advance of the Turks from Saitchar.

The Master of the Magazine was a sickly, delicate-looking man from Belgrade; he spoke French and German, was very quiet and gentlemanly, and had been to "Bucharest," that test of polish and education! He was in some government office in the capital, and had been sent to do duty here, which office he carried out in a lounging style, which contrasted with the fever and bustle of the *capitan*. He was a splendid chess-player, and was by far the most intellectual and amusing of our Doïni friends.

Then came the post-master, a Serb, who spoke German, and was always quiet and obliging. He was also a chess-player, and thoroughly versed in the art of telegraphy; he was therefore in charge also of that department. He was a resident, and his wife had gone to Belgrade at the time of the battle by Saitchar. He was a tall, dark, sallow man, who smoked and slept half his days away.

The fourth was also a Serb, who spoke perfect German. He was the agent of the Austrian Lloyd's, but a resident proprietor, having one of the best houses in the town and a beautiful vineyard in the neighbourhood.

He was quite a character in his way—a confirmed hypochondriac. There was always something amiss with him that required medicine, and he was never so happy as when he was dosing himself or being dosed by some of us.

He was always most kind and polite to us, but had a perfect detestation of England, and used to hold long arguments with our doctors on politics. Sometimes he was cheerful and sociable, sometimes oppressed with gloom. That was on the days when he was suffering from what he called "your English spleen." He was a well-educated and intelligent man, and had travelled as far as Pesth, and of course Bucharest. He was an old bachelor, but engaged to be married to a lady in Belgrade; and when we knew what Doïni was, we pitied the dull and cheerless life she must have there with a husband afflicted with the spleen.

Last of all was our young and gay sub-surgeon, the son of an ex-minister, a youth of some twenty-five years, recalled from his studies in Paris to serve; in the volunteer forces, and "exiled here!" as he piteously expressed it. His delight at, our arrival was most unfeigned, for we found a few days afterwards that he took advantage of our presence to get leave for a fortnight to Belgrade, and he never returned to Doïni.

He had a great affection for cigars and sipping *raki*, in the absence of absinthe, and an equal aversion to anything like work. He was a short, stout, dark man, looking older than he was, always pleasant as long as he was not asked to do a hand's turn of work, but always willing to give his advice, and then retire to a *cafané*, or small drinking house, and leave it to be carried out or not as we thought best.

These were the gentlemen who assisted us out of our boat, gave us a kindly welcome to Doïni, and informed us that our quarters were ready, and that they had prepared supper for us.

A guard was put on the heavy baggage, the rest was carried to our quarters, in charge of Milano, and we began a slow progress across the rough grass fields, up the dusty road, and so into the main street of the town.

It may be as well to describe that town, before speaking of our life in it.

It is one of the largest provincial towns in Servia, and life there is a true type of Servian middle-class life.

It consists of one long street, lying parallel with the Danube; on either side are one-storied houses, the roof in many cases projecting over the side walk. Two or three two-storied houses have just been built, but they are looked on as innovations. In the midst of the street, on the left-hand side going up it, is the church, a whitewashed building, standing detached in a yard, divided from the street by open palings.

It had been newly done up, and was in the interior gorgeous with *fresco* and gilding—the *frescoes* on the "Royal Gates," as the doors are called which shut in the sanctuary, being very fair specimens of Austrian art. It belonged to the Orthodox Greek Church. Farther on the street was crossed by a narrow stream, now dried up to a mere thread of water, but it was a mountain stream, and very full and rapid in the rainy season.

It was traversed by a strong wooden bridge, and beyond that was an open space, in the centre of which was an old-fashioned well, from which was drawn in buckets all the drinking water used in Doïni by man and beast.

A long low range of buildings formed the back of the Place; these were the stables for the post and military transport horses. At one end a room built off, and divided into two, was the post and telegraph-office, at the other end the two rooms were those appointed as quarters to the Master of the Magazine and the Serb military doctor. The post-master had his residence elsewhere, for a few scattered houses and cottages were to be found on the outskirts of the one street, both on the sides towards the hills and the river.

The street continued beyond the bridge, and ended in a gateway, which was the boundary of the town. The view over the Danube from here was very lovely, and the village cemetery was on the slope of the land towards the river, about half a mile from the gate. The rule of extramural interment is strictly observed all over Servia.

In this town of 2,000 inhabitants there was no decent inn, no library, no place of public resort, no means of instruction or amusement, no books, no newspapers—no way of getting away from it but by a heavy diligence, twice a week, over the hills, by way of Maidenpek to Belgrade and the Danube. Steamers plied twice a week up and down the river, but since the war these had ceased to call at Doïni.

A very few of the inhabitants spoke broken German; they were the shopkeepers—for there were two or three rude stores, where a jumble of everything was sold.

Caviare, made from the roes of the sturgeon caught in the Danube, is the only produce of Doïni, except, of course, pigs.

Such are the provincial towns, of Servia.

Literature, art, and science are at their lowest ebb, and years must pass before they can take even a low place among the highly-educated Western nations.

The war crushed out hope and ambition together, and has thrown them back fifty years, for it has taught them not to rely upon themselves, and to distrust all others.

It may be remarked here what a bigoted jealousy of foreigners and their ways exists in Servia. The people do not desire contact with other nations, and very few care to learn any language but their own.

We even heard a distinguished general declare that he was proud to say he knew no word of anything but Serb, and that unless we asked in Serb for wine, we should only have water. Luckily, *vino* is not hard to learn or remember. This general fought against our troops in the Crimea, with the Russians, and has the highest respect for them. He has a Russian wife, who speaks both German and French, and has a quiet contempt for the Serbs, which she shares in common with all of the "Ruski" race. But the general knew the words "good wife" in every European language.

This jealousy of foreigners may account for the fact that most of the officials, with whom strangers had to deal, spoke no language but their own, which much increased the difficulty of working with them.

Nor would it be worthwhile to study a language very difficult to learn, and very harsh to listen to, used only in one small province, and which has no modern literature to make it worthwhile to spend even a week in the study.

This is proved by the fact that at the theatre in Belgrade, where nothing is allowed to be acted that is not written in Serb, and of Serbish origin, there is never an audience; for those who do not understand Serb do not go, of course; and those who do, declare there is not a drama that will bear sitting out.

It is time, however, to return to our life at Doïni Milanovatz, and our daily intercourse with the people of this town, so near to the Wallachian frontier.

CHAPTER 18

Our Doctor and the Ambulance

The officials and ourselves made a solemn progress through the town and over the bridge. Our young surgeon, or rather medical student, Mr. S——, looked remarkably as if he were in charge between two of our new friends.

The people came to their doors and looked sleepily at us, and the sudden night came down as we arrived at the door of a long, low house, and entered a large dark room, which served as a *café* to that part of the village.

We crossed this and found ourselves in a sort of farmyard; on the left hand, the building was divided into three rooms. Opposite to us were two more, beyond them a space where coffee was roasted, fowls plucked, and quarrels carried on; beyond this again the kitchen, which actually had a hot stove.

This side of the yard was completed by a cow-house, a stable, and a piggery.

Turning the corner and facing the left-hand side was a covered gallery for the storing of forage, corn, and pumpkins, which are the winter food of the cattle and pigs.

Underneath was the place where all washing of clothes was carried on, and two small rooms with broken windows, now occupied by some Bulgarian refugees.

The yard was completed by a heap of firewood and odds and ends of all sorts, separated from the road by high wooden palings, and a wide gateway for the entrance of carts, which was just at the end of the long *café*.

Two of the left-hand rooms and the two opposite the *café* were allotted to us. The only bedsteads in the town had been pressed into our service, and, with the white sheets and counterpanes, they looked clean and cheerful.

Having deposited our baggage, we returned through the town to another *café* where the supper was provided.

It consisted of soup, *paprikash*, or meat stewed with *capsicums*, and hashed ducks. Good red wine was served with it.

The red wine of Négotin is a capital sort of claret. Like the wine of Karlovitz in Hungary, the grapes from which it is made grow on a stony soil. It is a deep red colour, brilliantly clear, slightly bitter, full-bodied, and mixes well with water. It contains much iron, and is not only a pleasant, but a highly medicinal drink. It is a capital tonic, and we have often said that much of the health and strength we enjoyed in Servia (except when attacked by special disease) was due to the iron in the good red wine of Négotin.

It costs three *francs* a bottle at Belgrade, but, of course, much less in the provinces. It keeps for years; we drank some of 1864, and very fine it was; but the *Préfet* of Négotin told us that, as yet, they had failed to enable the wine to bear transmission to other countries. But he fully hoped to do so ere long, and then let Karlovitz look to its laurels!

In spite of our fatigue our sleep was not as undisturbed as it might have been, for we were not alone in our room; armies of fleas attended upon us, till we rose and slaughtered the foe wholesale. In the morning, coffee and black bread made their appearance in the *café*, to which eggs were added, and then came the boxes. These we unpacked and made all ready for coming contingencies, and then came the Servian surgeon, and we proceeded to inspect the wounded then in ambulance.

This ambulance was simply another *café* opposite.

The large brick-floored room opened from the street; out of it was another, also looking to the street, and behind, several smaller rooms. The rough cooking was done in the yard.

In the brick-floored room lay some twenty poor wretches, still in their filthy bloodstained clothes, though it was nearly a month since they were wounded.

Straw was littered down on each side of the room, and kept in its place by a fir pole laid at the edge, leaving a path in between. There was no division between the men; they lay about two feet apart, dirty, flushed, feverish, and infested by huge and hideous flies, which they tried to brush away with withered branches of lime trees.

"Three hopeless cases here," said Herr M———, in French.

The other room was in just as bad a plight, and here were two or three more "hopeless cases." We looked at the wounds, and fancied our doctor who was coming would not think so; but we said nothing, and even listened calmly to Herr M——'s proposal for a cruel and useless operation, which certainly the poor subject of it could not have survived.

It could not be done till Dr. Leckie arrived, for we had the letter placing Herr M—— under his orders, and we knew that he would never consent to it.

The orderlies, or hospital attendants, lounging about were the most dirty, helpless creatures imaginable. Several of them wore no shoes or stockings. If they could have understood our terse and forcible English, as we spoke to each other, they would have read their coming doom in the words, "but they go as soon as he comes."

The day passed on, a rude supper-dinner was served, and we tried to sleep under difficulties as before. So next day we devoted to "cleaning up" our rooms and that one reserved for the doctor.

We turned out all the furniture; we pressed a woman into our service, a Bulgarian refugee, and we all rubbed and scrubbed and splashed about carbolic and water, till we felt clean, and the rooms smelt so at least.

This lively exercise tired us out, and, as the morrow was Sunday, we resolved to rest.

We were sitting in the sun about noontime, when two gentlemen came through the *café* into the yard. It was our doctor and another assistant.

Milano flew off to buy some chickens, which were slaughtered before our eyes in the yard, and made as much of a banquet as he could.

Chickens were one *franc* fifty *cents* a pair, ducks two *francs*, and a goose two *francs*.

We sat and discussed affairs, and agreed on the improbability of our having many wounded. It did not seem likely that the Turkish commander would attack the Serbs under Colonel Medvodviski.

To force the mountain pass from Saitchar, by way of Négotin to Doïni, would be a heavy undertaking, and the possession of Doïni utterly useless. It was not on the way to Belgrade, or anywhere else, and if there was fighting, it would more probably be on the other side of Saitchar, where the road to Tchupria, or Paratjin, might be attacked and defended; but then the wounded Serbs would fall back on those places, and, as no quarter was given, assuredly we should have no wounded Turks. But events in war are uncertain and capricious.

By the time we had remodelled the ambulance here, and looked after the wounded, we should see what other work was likely to present itself; and the officials in Belgrade certainly believed in heavy fighting, for they had sent a Russian ambulance to Posharevatz to take up their place on the right rear of the Servian position on this side of Servia, whilst we had been sent to occupy the left—the Roumanian ambulance at Posharevatz being sent to Tchupria to act as a field ambulance in case, of need, as it had no nurses with them.

Dr. Leckie was as horrified as we were at the state in which he found the wounded, and on the Monday morning, went to see another house nearly opposite the church, where were also wounded.

These he had removed to the first house, and we set to work to clean the second.

One room was so bad that it was necessary to fumigate it Mr. G——, the new assistant, therefore prepared the oxide of manganese.

But two Serb women who were leaning on their brooms, by way of scrubbing the floor of the front room, were seized with an idea that this was a species of incantation to drive away the evil one, and, dropping their brooms and neglecting their pails, attended upon the supposed ceremony, enlightened as to its various processes by the veracious and mischievous Milano.

Dr. Leckie stood by, laughing, and Mr. G—— put on a supernaturally severe look.

At last the sulphuric acid was poured on, the fumes began to rise, the door was shut, and the women, led by Milano, crept slowly and cautiously to peep through the keyhole, and see the departure of the devil.

Of course, they saw nothing but the vapour, which made them cough and sniff, and they highly enjoyed the whole thing. After that the town at large believed enormously in the great English doctor, who had come so far over the seas, with such wonderful medicines, that even the evil spirits must depart when he "smoked" them out.

If oxide of manganese and sulphuric acid could indeed drive out evil spirits, such as too often infest more civilised lands than Servia, what a run there would be on the chemist's stores!

A little fumigation might be usefully applied to many a diplomatic conference, for instance; and if this had been the case at Constantinople, we might not now be spectators of a savage and useless war.

Two days sufficed to make this house ready, but we had to wait several more for the trestles.

We could not get beds, but there were plenty of mattress cases; these we had washed in carbolic and water, very weak of course; and we also used Hartin's crimson salts, which we found the best form of permanganate of potash, when mixed largely with water. All the blankets and bed linen were washed in this, and Dr. Leckie ordered trestles and planks, on which to lay the beds.

This is a much cleaner plan than laying them on the floor; there is a free draught of air under them, and it is easy to wash and sweep beneath; besides that, it is much better for the surgeons and nurses not to have to stoop down so low as when men lie on the floor.

And while we were waiting for our trestles, Dr. Leckie had to arrange a difficulty about these said wounded, who, it appears, were the property—so to speak—of an ignorant Serb surgeon, who had fled with them from Négotin, and this most incompetent old gentleman refused to give over his wretched victims till he got orders from Belgrade.

And these orders he actually refused to apply for. We had the order to take charge of all wounded; he alleged that this was not retrospective. The young Serb surgeon stormed; till the wounded were given over to us, he could not get away, and each day as it passed rendered the state of some of the poor fellows more and more desperate,

He very nearly tore his hair, declaring it was most unfair that we should begin with such a deathrate; five or six must die. But what could be done?

We all answered that we were willing to run that risk, and try to save their lives; and Dr. Leckie, aided by the Master of the Magazine, the post-master, and the young Serb, took it upon himself to telegraph to Belgrade, to supersede the old Négotin doctor.

The reason this man was so unwilling to go was, that when he left, he must naturally return to Négotin, and Négotin was in the front, a place much to be avoided in the opinion of all Serbs.

The answer came at once; our troublesome friend was superseded then and there, and we arranged for the transfer of the wounded next day to our ambulance.

CHAPTER 19

Our Sick and Wounded

Needless to say that the 8th of September was a fine day. We had not had a drop of rain while in Servia—always a cloudless sky and a brilliant sun.

Everything was ready. The new house looked, and was, beautifully clean and sweet.

Dinner was served round early; and at three o'clock the order was given, and every man who could walk started for the English hospital on foot.

Whilst I awaited the comers at the door of the new house, Louise led the procession over the bridge, bearing a green-lined parasol over her head, through which the gleams of sunlight produced the effect of a cool green halo.

Occasionally she waved it in front of the advancing column, not to cheer them on, but to keep them back; for, in their anxiety to arrive at their quarters, some would have outstripped their weaker comrades, and those who hobbled on crutches.

Behind them were the stretchers, carried by the orderlies, with the very severely wounded. We had only three of these stretchers, and a surgeon walked by each, to regulate the pace of the bearers, and watch the sufferers.

As they arrived at the door of the English hospital, I pointed out to each man the bed he was to occupy. By each one was a spittoon, with sand in it, for the Serbs have the bad habit of spitting about the floors.

All the men were made to take off their coats, and lie down properly on their new clean beds, and they looked around them in wonder and delight.

The very severely wounded—our "hopeless cases"—were put apart, completely undressed by the orderlies, and clean shirts put on, *for the first time for weeks.*

The stretchers went and came two or three times, and with the last came a miserable object of pity—a boy scorched out of almost all resemblance to humanity, and utterly deprived of sense.

That very morning a soldier, coming with despatches from the army to Doïni, had found him in a wood, and knew nothing more about him than that he supposed the boy had escaped from the Turks, when they took and burnt a village near Négotin, some few nights before.

Of course, a bed was found for him, and his fearful burns were dressed. He must have been some time in the wood, from the stage in which the burns were, and from his starved appearance.

Like all the rest, he thoroughly enjoyed the soup and good red wine we served out; and we decided that he was not a "born natural," but his senses were weakened by fear and pain.

We had selected two of the Négotin men as *infirmiers*, Nicolas and Alexis. They were very steady and very teachable, and gladly adopted and enforced our ways.

Alexis was especially intelligent. He had been *infirmier* at the civil hospital at Négotin, and was so pleased with what he learned from us, that he declared he felt quite competent to go and study medicine at Bucharest, which was his most earnest desire.

Both these men spoke good German, and are to be heard of at Négotin from the *préfet*. They would be invaluable to any hospital or ambulance forming in Roumania, or elsewhere, having had English training, and acted as dressers under an English surgeon.

We left directions that no "*raki*," that strong and pernicious spirit, should be allowed inside the house, except by medical order; and though at first this was a privation, it was cheerfully borne.

The poor neglected wretches had been in the habit of sending out to buy "*raki*." We had even seen some in the *café* of our quarters. Now no man might leave the place without permission, and no one enter it, except on business. Also, every man was to have water and soap night and morning; and we gave out combs for their hair.

Never was tuition in civilisation, sooner or better appreciated.

These men, who had never been accustomed to lie in a bed, or undress at night, or wash themselves, except once a week, at once adopted the new ways, and delighted in them.

We were astonished when we went early next morning, to find, instead of a set of dirty, sullen, wretched-looking objects, clean, smart-looking, cheerful men.

Nicolas, it seemed, was a barber by trade, and had been requested to exercise his art on the unkempt heads of the patients. They had all been cut and shaved at their own request, and, after the fashion of our doctor, had retained no facial adornment but neat, well-trimmed moustaches. The difference was wonderful, and we rewarded their effort at meeting us half-way, with boiled eggs and red wine.

A system of extra diet was introduced.

The usual breakfast, soup and meat, was handed round at 5 a.m. Some were too ill to be able to eat this, and hitherto had gone on as best they could, too often supplying the place of food with sips of "*raki.*"

Now at ten commenced a distribution of eggs, wine, bread, soap, and mutton chops, according to the medical order for each man. One old man of seventy, with a fearful wound, was allowed a little "*raki,*" because he had been used to it all his life and missed it; but he was strictly allowanced.

About one o'clock, after the morning visit of the surgeons, they had dinner: soup, *paprikash*, and haricot beans; and now, by our orders, fresh vegetables: cabbages, onions, potatoes—anything for a change—and plenty of good ripe grapes. Fresh vegetable food is most important in all these cases, and in general easy to be procured.

Draughts of quinine and other tonics were also served round, because epidemic fever was in the town, and it was necessary to guard against it. At four o'clock, soup, eggs, wine, and chops were again given to those who required it. At seven came supper—bread, milk, and fruit. Coffee was not given out in the rations, nor did the men care for it.

The government rations for each man were, half a pound of meat a day, a few haricot beans, a couple of onions, some *capsicums*, a pint of bad wine, and a loaf of black bread. The bone and gristle (fat there was none) were counted in the weight.

We made requisitions on the Captain of the Town for good wine, fresh vegetables, eggs, milk, grapes, coffee, sugar and bread.

The men *did* live upon their rations in hospital, but did not thrive upon them; even the "hopeless cases" cheered up under the new system, and a few days showed wonderful improvement in all of them.

It will be seen that we introduced no luxuries, only the simple principles of cleanliness and good food. Nicolas and Alexis used to say, and I believe it was true, that never more would our sixty patients of Doïni relapse into semi-barbarism.

The idle luxury of the Katherine Hospital at Belgrade, not then however opened, was a state of things abnormal to their life. The habits of the English hospital at Doïni, were simply those which could be, and I feel assured would be, adopted in the homes of our patients.

The cooking was done in an outhouse; the mutton chops were fried by being put in a flat earthen pot with a wooden handle, which was stuck into the hottest part of the red wood ashes, and the effect was capital. When the chops were brought into the wards, so savoury was the smell, that men for whom they were not ordered would sit up in bed, and beg that we would ask the kind doctor to let them have some too—a request never refused.

We perfectly understood the men, and they understood us. They are very sharp at a language of signs. We picked up a little Serbish, and they picked up a little German, and we got on capitally.

We had brought out a bandage machine and brown calico, and we made bandages of the required size and length.

This is much better than bringing out sacks of bandages, which are sure to be either too long or too short, or too wide or too narrow, and go to waste.

The laundry was organised, disinfectants put in the water, and the linen kept always clean and sweet.

There was not the slightest smell in that hospital, any more than there is in a London drawing-room.

The windows were kept open at the top, the floors were well washed, every dressing thrown into proper receptacles, and taken away as soon as replaced. There was nothing that could have offended the eye, ear, or nose of the most fastidious, if they came when work was over, and it always was over by noon, except on special occasions.

We also received from the military clothing department at Belgrade a number of capital dressing-gowns of strong linen, blue and white striped, and in these those who could walk, were allowed to sit in the sunny yard, and later on to walk abroad accompanied by an orderly.

The work of an hospital when once fairly established, and all things going on in a groove, is monotonous to relate, though very interesting to those actually engaged in it; and our fights with the Captain of the Town kept us in a constant state of amusement He would give no extras. "What did the men want beds for? They were always accustomed to sleep on the floor, it was good enough for them. Eggs, indeed! sugar! coffee! wine! they should have none of them, the town could not afford it." A little telegram from Belgrade instigated by our doctor, woke him up, and we got the eggs and wine, but the vegetables and mutton we had to buy, and coffee and sugar were not actually necessary.

It may be as well to say here, that *not one death* occurred. Our hopeless cases are alive and walking about.

Our doctor's surgery was conservative, and therefore we had but one capital operation, and that answered admirably. The Serbs have a great objection to losing a limb, even to save life. They have a superstition that if a man goes to his grave with one leg, he will rise in the day of judgment and exist in all eternity with only one leg. But few could be argued into consent.

Our doctor sent for the Captain of the Town and the Master of the Magazine, and in their presence the wounded men gave consent to the operation.

We were, therefore, especially glad that all went off well. The officials were present on the important occasion, and viewed the scene in horror and awe. At last the captain bolted; he could stand it no longer, and predicted the instant death of the sufferer.

When he found afterwards how well he was doing, and heard from himself that he felt nothing (for the chloroform had done its work well), the captain conceived a high opinion of English skill and care, and came to beg some medicine for his wife; but he grumbled and economised to the last.

I trust this chapter will not be found tedious.

The work at Doïni was quiet and monotonous, and yet I think its effect will endure in Servia, after the far harder and more exciting work of Paratjin has passed into a terrible episode in the history of this war.

CHAPTER 20

Life Upcountry in Servia

We had of course a life apart from the hospital. Our first thoughts and cares were given to that, but wounded men, unless in very severe cases, do not want being attended to all day, and especially in Servia, where they slept, as did all the town, from 1 to 4 p.m., and again from sunset to sunrise.

This was their custom, and it is so much better when dealing with foreign wounded to adopt as many of their national habits as possible, and, above all, to prevent them from sinking into nervous, fanciful invalids, by avoiding invalid ways as far as practicable.

It is a great secret to keep the men in a cheerful, hopeful, helpful state, to make them do as much as possible for themselves, by way of employing their minds: and when once regular hours and regular meals are introduced, everything runs on a groove.

But our life outside the hospital was to a certain degree devoted to keeping things in that groove.

In this our doctor was invaluable. He spoke French, German, Spanish, and a little Italian; he had travelled everywhere; he had served with the Chilian Army as chief physician; he had dealt with all sorts of officials, and with every class of men; and, besides a thorough knowledge of his profession, he was an accomplished gentleman.

Of the two assistants there is not very much to say. Mr. S—— left us very soon. He went down the Danube in an open boat, and actually arrived safely at Orsova. Mr. Gordon was recalled to London by business, some time before we left Doïni.

Indeed, after the first, there was no work for them. After extra diets for the hospital, extra diets for ourselves were a consideration. We have heard since of chests sent with other ambulances, which contained "medical comforts," and these comforts were not medicines; but we had none of these. Milano and Nicolas hunted about, and found chickens and ducks, but the chickens were only skin and bone, and the ducks as hard as boards.

No one could live on the rations provided, and we had to do the best we could.

The people of the quarters were most uncivil when the landlord was away. He was a captain in the army before Négotin, and not often at home, and his son was the most ill-conditioned cur that ever stepped.

He practised a series of petty annoyances, which at last ended in our complaining of him to the Captain of the Town. He had been at Paratjin, in the telegraph office, but this was too near the Turks to please him; he got leave of absence, and on the score of sickness contrived to remain at home.

He was ordered to leave Doïni, and go to Tchupria, nearer still to the Turks, on one side at least, and departed, weeping and bewailing his fate.

The reason of all this was, that the people did not like giving up their rooms as quarters. The government did not pay as much as private individuals, but at last they found that no more private individuals came by that way, and when we did depart, were very grieved to lose us.

But not one soul in all the place gave any help or sympathy to *their own wounded*. They charged for everything used in the hospital at an exorbitant rate, and yet all the town was being doctored and physicked by us for nothing.

An epidemic of low fever and diphtheria was raging. The place must always be a fever-stricken hole; but it was rather worse than usual at this time, owing to the number of refugees camped in the meadows outside the town.

Every refugee was allowed quarters and a trifling sum per day; but, during the fine weather, they preferred camping out.

They had escaped from Bulgaria, Bosnia, and the frontiers of Servia, with all their goods and chattels, even their cocks and hens. They were comfortably dressed, and showed no signs of poverty or starvation.

The distress existing among the refugees in Servia was greatly exaggerated. Government did its duty well by them.

The Bulgarians were a very quiet, grateful people, and used to come with presents of good fresh milk, and ripe grapes, in return for "medicine and attendance."

The people came out of their houses as we went past down the street, and laid their little children before us. We never went without quinine and *ipecacuanha* with us, and Dr. Leckie administered the doses in the streets, for it was sometimes impossible, and even dangerous, to enter a very small hut, with fever and diphtheria in it, and the patients were brought to the door.

The mortality was very great at first, but we got it under at last, by the use of enormous quantities of quinine.

It was no wonder there should be fever. The interiors of the houses are very dirty. There are no beds, only divans with rugs; no means of cleanliness and decency; no drainage, no abundance of water, at least to use in washing.

The food is inferior in quality, and, except *paprikos*, very little fresh vegetable is used.

The clothes are worn for months—at least the undergarments—and it is very unpleasant to approach too near to a party of even well-dressed women.

On Sunday every one came out in their best, and there was a grand service in the church at ten o'clock a.m.

The women wore jackets of silk, satin, or velvet, most beautifully embroidered with gold and silver. These jackets were usually of some gay colour—pink, sky-blue, peach colour, violet, crimson, and a few black; while brides wore white, and used their jackets long afterwards. They cost from 6*l*. to 8*l*., 10*l*., or even 12*l*. of English money.

A shirt of soft white cambric muslin, usually worked in what is called satin-stitch, was worn underneath, and a skirt of silk of various colours, not always harmonising well with the jacket. The hair was braided close around the head, over a crimson cloth skull-cap; unmarried women had a natural flower, usually red or crimson, over one ear. This was a sign that they were single. Married women wore silver pins with large heads.

When a flock of these women went fluttering up and down the street in the sunshine on a Sunday morning, they looked like a bed of flowers.

Sometimes they put gay handkerchiefs over their heads, sometimes white ones. They were, as a rule, very good-looking, when under five-and-thirty, with black hair and eyes, and rich ruddy complexions, but age very early, and then are excessively hideous, yellow, and wrinkled.

They are an easy-going, good-tempered, indolent, ignorant set of people, not given to strong emotions or impulses of any sort.

Most of the men were away at the war; all who got leave were always coming home and staying there. We were pestered with applications to take on helpers in the ambulance, which would have prevented their being sent back to the front.

One young man, an ex-innkeeper at Négotin, was really very useful to us, and we did retain him. In his gratitude he kept us supplied with jars of really very fine Négotin wine from his own vineyards. He wrote the hospital reports in Serbish, as he spoke that and German perfectly, but then he had been educated at Bucharest!

It is probable if we ever went to Bucharest that we should find it a second-rate Eastern place, but at present we look upon it in the light of a combined Athens and Paris, where learning and fashion have arrived at an unheard-of height; where study by day, and elegant dissipation by night, render it a city of delight.

Perhaps it is as well that we should never be undeceived.

Almost every day, at first, funerals came down the street to go to the cemetery.

The procession usually consisted of half a dozen dirty little boys in red cassocks and white surplices, straggling all about the road, and carrying little banners or pictures; then a priest, dirtier still, his long hair hanging over his vestments, if a ragged sort of cloak of indistinguishable hues could be called a vestment. Behind him came the body on a bier, carried by men, not on their shoulders, but suspended from short leather loops in their hands. It was open, and the body was left fully in view, with white muslin folded over it.

The coffin, its lid, and a wooden or iron cross to stick on the grave, carried by an attendant, closed the procession; unless a crowd of women, and a man or two, coming along irregularly in the rear, could be called part of it.

From this motley assemblage rose up a sound of most discordant and lugubrious chanting.

We followed one funeral to the cemetery—it was that of a child.

It stopped at the gate which marked the boundary of the town. The bier was set down, and the priest, facing the people, chanted a prayer or two.

We came up here with them and looked at the little bier. The child was about four or five years old. She had died of diphtheria; the remedies were applied too late to save, and there she lay in her little white dress, with a wreath of white flowers on her fair hair, and but for the pale waxy look on her face, she might have been sleeping.

The scene was most picturesque—the vine-clad hills, the rushing river, the blue mountains, the long, grey road winding away to the barrier of hills, the weeping women grouped around the bier, the sad, solemn chant in which the priest, for the child, bade an eternal farewell to home, and the intense sunlight that threw a golden light all around.

When the chant was finished, the procession passed on from the town, with its stir of life, to the silent graveyard. They quickened their pace, and trotted on as fast as they could till they came to the gate of the cemetery.

Here a singular scene took place. The mourning mothers who were walking behind broke off, and each one flung herself on some little grave, weeping bitterly, and kissing the new earth that covered her own babe, laid to rest but a few days before. Sobs and shrieks rose on the air as we passed on to the grave prepared for this last little victim of dirt and epidemic.

A short service was hurried over; the small coffin was brought forward; the body was taken off the bier and laid in it. The priest poured some red wine on it, which stained the pure white robe, and placed bread, salt, and some small pieces of copper money beside it. Two or three women flung themselves on the coffin, and passionately kissed the little dead face, with shrieks and sobs, till the priest ordered them away; the coffin was lowered into the shallow grave, the lid just put on, and the priest, taking a spade, shovelled some earth upon it. The attendants filled in the grave; one stuck the little blue painted cross in the mound above it, and all was over.

The women recovered their cheerfulness in a most surprising way, leading us to believe all their shrieking and howling was part of the orthodox ceremony; and we walked back to the gate, where we found a table laid out with wine, *raki*, cakes, and fruit, of which everyone was expected to take a little. This is what is called the death-feast, and is always provided at every funeral.

The meaning of the wine poured on the coffin was, they told me, to consecrate the body, but as for the bread, salt, and money, I should be sorry to believe that the explanation given by two or three of the people separately from each other could be true. They all said it was to provide for the journey to the next world.

If so, it is a strange remnant of pagan customs; and the death penny—that was to pay Charon for the passage over the Styx.

The lower orders do believe that it is for this purpose, whatever may be its real meaning, and we must hope that this strange idea is only popular ignorance, and misunderstanding of some ecclesiastical custom with a Christian meaning to it.

One of these long-haired priests, or popes, as they are called, was a patient of ours. A dirtier, more idle, more selfish creature never trod the earth. He was a refugee from near Saitchar, with his wife and child. They were in poor circumstances, but not worse than usual, nor worse than they were likely to be in, when every farthing that came to this young man was spent on *raki* in some small *cafané*.

Like all the other popes (and we had several in Doïni besides the pope of the parish), he was no better born or educated than the peasants around him. He could read the service by heart, but knew nothing of Greek beyond that.

His poor little wife was suffering from *erysipelas*, and his babe from starvation, for he was too idle to prepare its food, while his wife was unable to do so.

We sent food and medicine; they seemed to do no good, and Dr. Walter Leckie suggested that we might try the effect of seeing them taken ourselves. We did this, and improvement soon set in, but it was disgusting to see the dirty, effeminate-looking fellow smoking and drinking with his fellow popes, as dirty and ignorant as himself, in every little low *cafané* in Doïni, while the poor wives were starving at home.

They ought to have been especially careful of their wives, for the Greek priests are only allowed to marry once. Most assuredly, the Greek Church is seen to the worst advantage in Servia, where it seems to be but an idle, superstitious form of belief, or rather ceremony, producing no effect on the lives of the people,

A very High Churchman wrote to us, expressing his sympathies with "their brother Christians," and, like many of the Ritualistic party, hoping for union between the Greek and Anglican Churches.

Our answer was, that without entering upon any doctrinal points as to whether the Greek and Anglican Churches believed the same things, or were right or wrong in their belief, one thing we could say—looking at the energy and activity of the English Church, and the high character and scholarly tone of its ministers—"Never try to link a living body to a dead one."

The church services were but poorly attended, and the congregation consisted almost entirely of women, who stood all the time at the back of the church; the very few men present standing in stall seats by the side walls, up as far as to the royal gates.

Louise asked one man, "Why he and his friends did not go to

church?"

His answer was, "Why should we? God was present everywhere. The women only go to church to look at each other. We stay in the *café*; God is there just as much as in church."

We never saw a trace of any religious practices anywhere—no one ever went to pray in the church, though it was always open; and when at one time orders came to fit it up as an ambulance, the people actually preferred it to our taking up the large *café* (where we had supped on the night of our arrival) for that purpose.

We suggested that this would put a stop to all religious services; they seemed to look on that as a matter of profound indifference. It was the proper and respectable thing for the women to go to church on a Sunday morning. If they could not do so, for want of a church, why there was an end of it.

It is to be feared that religion is with these people a mere matter of form and ceremony, not a vital principle.

Every day came frantic telegrams about taking up the church as I have said, fitting up the old ambulance from which we had removed the men, and getting ready for 200 wounded. The beds came, or rather the mattress-cases, and were filled with clean straw. All the carpenters in the town were making trestles and planks; sheets, blankets, pillow-cases, everything, were sent. We went hard to work and got fifty beds ready in three days, and then paused to take breath and wondered where the wounded were to come from.

It appeared afterwards that there was an intention to try and retake Saitchar, but even then it would have been nearer to send the wounded to Tchupria.

Day after day we waited, but no wounded came, and only two or three events broke the quiet monotony of daily duty.

Chapter 21

The Préfet of Négotin

Our *préfet* deserves a chapter to himself, not only for his kindness to us, but also for his personal qualities; but, at all events, he shall take the first place in one.

The days passed on with cloudless skies and intense heat. The wounded got better and better, and the Captain of the Town worse and worse in his temper.

One bright morning, Milano rushed in just as we had returned from the ambulance—"*Signora, signora*, the Préfet of Négotin is here!"

"Run, Milano," was the answer. "We left the hospital all right, but just see that all the *infirmiers* are at their posts."

"Shall the men have clean shirt? Shall we put green boughs in the rooms?" he asked.

"Not at all; the men had all clean shirts two days ago. Let him see the hospital just as it is."

Certainly, there was not time for any adornments, had any been needed, for as we entered the hospital, we saw a very small crowd of our own officials surrounding a tall, handsome, gentlemanly man, who, on seeing us, uncovered his head and bowed low. The Servian surgeon had joyfully departed to the dissipations of Belgrade, so Dr. Walter Leckie had to do the honours, and we found that the *préfet* had passed sixteen years in a diplomatic appointment at Bucharest; and most assuredly had profited by it, for he was not only a man of intelligence and education, and of enlarged ideas, but of polished manners.

The Serbs are very quick at catching up improvements of any sort, when once they can be roused out of their national and constitutional indolence; and contact with other nations more busy and bustling than themselves, is the remedy for this.

The *préfet* having saluted us in perfect French, and thanked us for coming, entered the wards, spoke in Serb to every man, and inspected everything.

He then turned to Dr. Leckie, and expressed his high approbation of all he saw and heard, saying that no hospital in Belgrade was as good or as well-managed.

Considering how rough and ready this one was, it was great praise, and it is to be hoped not undeserved.

He then wished to visit our quarters, and we all paraded in a body down the street and over the bridge. First, we went to see the horse hospital, behind the old house we had just prepared for fresh wounded.

Here were half a dozen wounded horses, all rapidly getting better, under the charge of a Servian trooper; then through the house with its vacant beds, and so across the street to our quarters.

It was fortunate that only a few days before we had hoisted the Union Jack and the Red Cross over the ambulance, and they brightened up the street with a blaze of colour; also we had two small flags of the same kind tied to the top of the pump in the yard.

The *préfet* saluted the flag, and made some pretty speech about how proud we ought to be of it, and then came into the room where were all the stores. We produced the instruments and the rarest medicines. He examined all, and took the greatest interest in them.

Amongst our stores were some bottles of strong smelling salts, a parting present brought by our kind friend. Major de Winton, from Mrs. Bell, of Oxford Street.

The *préfet* took up one and smelt it. "It was most delicious I most refreshing! Such things could not be had here!"

Of course, we presented it to him, and one also to those nearest to him. Suddenly we saw the Captain of the Town looking gloomy and injured. We instantly offered another bottle. He beamed brightly, and nearly stifled himself sniffing at it.

After this, our doctor held a long conference with the *préfet*, which ended in his making an order on the captain, to supply us with everything we required.

He told us that he much regretted he could not ask us to come to Négotin, where there was a good civil hospital, which we could have taken up; but it was too near the Turks. It was his duty to remain there till he was actually driven out of it; but he had brought all the archives into Doïni, as he fully expected an attack, and could not imagine why the Turks did not come on.

And that was an unanswered question all through the war.

The *préfet* also took special notice of the burnt boy. He was gradually recovering the power of speech and connected thought, and we had picked up his history from his answers to the questions of the *infirmiers*, and from Négotin people, who had come into Doïni.

The Turks had invaded and burnt a village near Saitchar. In the flight from the village this boy had strayed, and been forgotten. He had either fallen into the fire in his fright and efforts to escape, or been thrown in by the Turks, as some said. But no one had seen this done: and it seemed improbable that the Turks should not have finished killing the boy, if half of what was said of their cruelties was true.

His people were known, but were believed to have escaped over the hills to Maidenpek and Belgrade, and the *préfet* promised to institute strict inquiries about them.

A few days after that we bought him a suit of clothes. He had been dressed before in what we had by us, but was now well enough to wear a jacket.

The *préfets* in Servia appear to occupy a position something like a lord-lieutenant and county magistrate in England. They are universal referees and rulers, and looked up to as the direct representatives of government. They are therefore selected from amongst the first men in Servia, and the Préfet of Négotin was indeed a most superior man; but, from what we heard, we judged that he was in reality by far the best specimen of all the *préfets*, and filled his responsible post not only with dignity, but courage.

He took the same view that we did—that now, at all events, there was not much chance of wounded being sent to Doïni; and we all resolved to ask to be removed as soon as our present wounded needed no further care.

The following Sunday we took an afternoon holiday, and, borrowing the boat belonging to the Austrian Lloyd's Company, we started for Svenitza, Dr. Walter Leckie and the Serb translator, our friend of the vineyard, accompanying us.

We were rowed over the calm river to the sunny shore beyond, and here the Austrian Custom-house officials met us, and being easily convinced that we had no contraband goods with us, let us pass up the rugged path into the street.

We strolled about, but there was nothing to see; the church was shut, and there was hardly anybody but a few Austrian soldiers.

The gentlemen strolled on to see an encampment of gipsies, where they declared, when they came back, that they had seen the loveliest Gitana imagination could conceive, and begged us to go directly and get a glimpse of her; but the sun was hot and the road was dusty, and we preferred the cool shade of the little village inn, with its rude wooden balcony looking on the Danube, and our Servian home on the other shore nestling under the hills.

The Austrian officers whom we had met before came and chatted with us. They were, as we have said, Slavs by birth from Austro-Hungary, and had strong sympathies with Servia.

From them we first heard of Lloyd-Lindsay's lost baggage—how it had been taken by the driver to the camp before Négotin and given to the Serbs—and they thoroughly enjoyed the story. They had been at Drenkova, when Lloyd-Lindsay passed on his way to Widdin, and they asked who was the great, tall, fair man in a white cap who was with him. We identified him as Mr. McCormac, and the Austrians agreed that it must be so, because he looked like a civilian, not a soldier.

As the sun was setting, we re-crossed the river, feeling all the better for even this change of air and scene.

The town was full of rumours at this time of the perilous position of the Turkish Army, which was said to be surrounded by the Russian and Servian forces, and would shortly be compelled to surrender. Then came the report of an armistice having been arranged; but it never was clearly known in this part of Servia whether there was any truth in it or not.

However, that might be, certain it is that the government steamer, *Deligrad*, came to Doïni two days after the Sunday on which we made our expedition into Hungary. She brought bedding and stores for us—amongst other things a large cask of good red wine.

We went down to the shore of the river, which was just by the cemetery, for the river was so low that the usual wharf was impossible, and there we saw the wine—red wine of Négotin for hospital use.

The Master of the Magazine ordered it to be taken to the hospital and placed under our charge, but the Captain of the Town ordered it to be taken to his house, and he would issue every day as much as might be required.

The Master of the Magazine had only to submit, but that wine underwent a singular change between the shore, the captain's house, and the hospital.

When the quantity demanded was sent down, it was a thin, sour, white wine! We remonstrated, but all in vain. The patients, accustomed to good wine, could and would not drink this poor, acid stuff, which would have done them no good, and we had to buy wine for them.

We reported it afterwards at headquarters, and heard, as we fully expected, that the wine we had asked for, Négotin, had been sent, and that doubtless it had been changed in the captain's cellar. This is but one specimen of the heartless indifference with which the people of the country treated their wounded, and defeated the efforts of the Belgrade officials, whose honest endeavours to carry out every plan suggested by competent persons, to supply everything in their power, and help in every way, deserves all praise. The wounded got better and better every day, and most of them could walk out. Not one was in a dangerous state. The hospital had been kept clear of fever, and was the healthiest house in the town.

It was the doctor and ourselves who suffered from intermittent attacks of malarious fever that gradually sapped the strength.

Dr. Leckie and Louise were far the worst, and at times were really ill.

It was proposed that, next time the *Deligrad* came on her way to Orsova, Dr. Leckie should go on leave for twenty-four hours to see the splendid Pass of Kazan; and a few days later she arrived again, and he went down the river in her.

The following day we walked to the shore to meet him on his return and report all well in the hospital, which he had left under our charge, when, to our surprise, as the *Deligrad* steamed slowly up against the stream, we saw that her decks were crowded, and that she had two huge river barges in tow, also crowded with men.

They were Russians, to the number of 2,000 in all, and were all coming as ambulance attendants!

A more shallow, idle pretext for sending armed men into any country was never invented, and no one believed in it. The Russian ambulances had their full staff already; and these were soldiers on leave of absence from their regiments, wearing their Russian uniforms, and under officers also in uniform.

In all this there was a want of truth and an amount of underhand dealing unworthy of so great a country as Russia.

The captain of the *Deligrad* came on shore to see the hospital, and was much pleased with it. He suggested that he was soon coming to fetch some more Russians, and that we had better take advantage of that to go and see the Pass of Kazan ourselves.

We thanked him for his kindness, and said we would gladly accept his invitation, as we should then see the whole Servian shore on the Danube.

CHAPTER 22

Wine and Caviare

The weather continued very hot, and the grapes were ripening fast. September is, in Servia, the month of the grape harvest, and as we were anxious to see a vineyard, the gentleman whom we have called the Austrian Lloyd's agent invited us all to row a couple of miles up the river, and visit the one he had, on the slope of the hills that closed in the upper part of the lake-like basin, on whose shores stood Doïni and Svenitza.

One fine afternoon therefore we started—our doctor, the young Serb translator, the agent, ourselves, and the custom-house officer, a quiet inoffensive Serb.

We pulled along close to the shore, to avoid the current; but the stream is very strong, and presently one of the boatmen landed, and was joined by two others, who had come by land to that spot.

A stout rope was tied to the masthead, and we were towed by these men. Every now and then the bushes grew very thick along the shore. The men forced their way through them; the rope caught here and there, pulling the boat very much on one side; but as no one seemed to concern themselves about it, we concluded that it was all right.

We passed an island covered with trees, and in the centre an old church. The island was small and uninhabited, and the agent told us that the church was all that remained of old Doïni.

Prince Milosch, the grandfather of Prince Milan, had removed the site of the village lower down, on the shore of the river A new and larger church was built; the houses clustered round it, and he gave it the name of Milanovatz, after himself.

If it were not for malaria, there are spots on the Servian shore of the Danube where lovely bathing villages could be built. There is good shooting on the hills; capital fishing in the river; splendid scenery and innumerable excursions either by boat, or horse, or carriage.

But the climate spoils all; and, as the malaria arises from the mud left by the receding Danube, no cultivation can cure this defect.

At last we arrived at the back of the island, and landed on the broken yet sandy shore.

The whole hillside was covered with vines belonging to different proprietors. A narrow pathway alone marked the division of property.

There seemed to be miles of these vines, all in full fruit. They grew low, not more than two or three feet from the ground, and were bending down with the weight of the grapes.

There were very few white grapes, and these were in taste and size very inferior to the black ones, which might have borne comparison with our hothouse grapes.

As this was a visit of inspection, to see if the fruit was ready for harvest, we walked all over our friend's vineyard, and tasted grapes from many vines. They were not all of the same kind or goodness, and he said that it made no difference when they were pressed; all, except the white, were equally good for wine.

A few plum-trees were scattered about, bearing a rich crop of ripe fruit— a small blue plum, with yellow flesh and not very much flavour—and we also found a few plants of scarlet-runners. We gathered all the beans we could find—green vegetables were a greater treat than fruit; but we thankfully accepted a basket of grapes for ourselves, and one for the hospital.

We rowed back quickly downstream, and reached home as the mists were rising from the river.

Our friend's vineyard produced, on an average, thirty very large casks of good wine, and twenty of inferior quality.

The good wine sold at eight *ducats* a cask—a *ducat* is twelve Austrian *gulden*, about 4*l*. 10*s*. in English money. The inferior wine was only worth six *ducats*. He sold all that he did not require for his own use, and regretted that the wine would not travel farther than Belgrade, where it went by land in ox-waggons.

Next day, as we were walking home from the hospital, we saw a woman taking a very small baby into the church, and, discovering that this was a christening, we followed in.

There was no one but the priest, a woman with a refugee baby, and two other women to act as godmothers, in their Sunday dresses. The ceremony was an elaborate one, all chanted by the priest alone in a very monotonous tone. The party walked three times round a table in the centre of the baptistery, the font being in one corner; and finally the child was entirely stripped, and held by the nurse over the font, while the priest poured warm water all over it, and repeatedly made the sign of the cross.

On another occasion we saw a churching.

Probably it was that of the mother of the child.

The woman went up and knelt in front of the royal screen, the priest chanting from a lectern some long prayer or psalm. The mother was accompanied by the nurse and the baby, and at a certain part of the ceremony she took it from the nurse, and laid it at the foot of various pictures successively, which represented the Annunciation, the Presentation in the Temple, the Dispute with the Doctors, and several other incidents in the life of our Lord.

This ended the ceremony. Neither this nor the baptism seemed to create the smallest interest in any one concerned in them, and were gone through as necessary formalities, rather than as connected with any heartfelt religion.

But the strangest thing of all was the death-feast in the churchyard.

The Sunday before we left Doïni, we saw in this said churchyard a large table laid out, and covered with a white cloth, on which were placed red and white wine, "*raki*," grapes, plums, small loaves of bread, and a large cake with a lighted candle stuck in the midst of it.

Everyone who passed by was requested to enter, and eat and drink, and the table was perpetually replenished from a *café* close by. There was no funeral going on, and all the world was in gay clothing.

We asked Nicolas, our *infirmier*, what it was all about, and he pointed out to us three or four women, who were presiding, and who were laughing and talking with their friends and acquaintances.

He said that these women's husbands had never been heard of since the battle before Saitchar on the 18th of July.

A proper time had now elapsed, and as the Turks gave no quarter, it was to be concluded that they were dead; though if it were so, or if and when they were buried, no one knew. Still, the death-feast must be held, and that once done, they were legally dead, and their wives widows.

What complications might arise if they did happen to return, we did not inquire. It was not probable. No quarter was given on either side, neither by Turk, nor Serb, nor Russian, which certainly simplified matters in a savage way that Christian nations should never have adopted; for be it remembered that the Serbs had no personal wrongs against the Turks, and that at that time Russia had not openly declared war against the Porte.

In the course of the next week the fishermen of Doïni brought in a number of huge sturgeon, which were laid side by side on an open space near the bridge, and cut open. The roes were taken out, and the flesh cut into large pieces.

The roes were made into caviare, the flesh pressed down for oil, to burn in the lamps in winter time; for in the long days the people go to bed and get up with the sun.

The caviare made here is not considered quite so good as the Russian caviare; it is better when quite fresh, but is not well prepared to keep.

It is made very simply. The roes are washed in clean water and salt, then broken up by the hand, and salt and oil kneaded into them, but without breaking the little globules of the roe. It is then packed in small wooden pails, in which it is sent to Belgrade and elsewhere; but when it is used it will not keep unless fresh oil is poured on the surface.

It travels to Paris, and even England, well-sealed down. In Servia it is served on a small plate, with slices of lemon, red pepper made from *capsicums*, and chopped onion.

The Russians in Belgrade consumed enormous quantities of it, as a *bonne bouche* before breakfast or dinner.

In Doïni a small tub, containing two *okers*, about four pounds and a half, can be bought for a *ducat* (12*s*.). In Belgrade the same quantity costs about 30*s*.; in Pesth, about 2*l*.; in Vienna, 3*l*.; in Paris, 5*l*. We took a couple of small tubs to Belgrade, as presents to some kind friends, and even there they were regarded as of great value.

A tub will last a long time, as but little is used at once. Doïni is the chief place on the Danube for making caviare: but the process of cutting up the flesh and kneading the roe is a dirty and disgusting one.

It was strange to see the poor people buying and carrying away a few pounds of the fish, from which to get oil: but this was the first of the sturgeon fishing. Later in the autumn more sturgeon, and even larger ones, were caught, though some of these weighed over forty pounds, and the flesh was too coarse to eat.

Even in Servia caviare is a luxury, but it is not appreciated by the natives; it requires a Bucharest education for that!

CHAPTER 23

The Pass of Kazan

Our days at Doïni Milanovatz were numbered—our patients so far well, that they required nothing farther than ordinary care. A Russian surgeon and his wife from Posharevatz, where the hospital had too large a staff, were to replace us, and we were wanted elsewhere.

But we waited for the *Deligrad*, it would be so much the better and cheaper way of returning to Belgrade.

The weather got hotter and hotter, and the town sleepier and sleepier. Every one slept between one and four, and at that hour the church bell rang, all woke up, and life resumed its usual course.

We grew very anxious to depart, but to go by the way we came cost so much—we had to pay a heavy sum to come; we were not inclined to pay another to leave.

And here it may be well to say a few words to all who think that Red Cross service costs nothing. The theory is, "you will have quarters and rations;" the practice, that you rarely find quarters, and no sane person could dream of living on the rations; even the men do not do it, and in war time you have to pay high for everything.

At last the *Deligrad* arrived, quite suddenly; we did not hear of it till she had been an hour anchored off the town.

We discovered afterwards that the officials did not wish us to go, and fancied that if we missed our passage by the *Deligrad*, we should stay there and the "Russians" would not come.

When the *Deligrad* had passed before, every Russian had worn a brassard and come as an ambulance attendant. Even the quiet sleepy Serbs woke up to the fact that 2,000 men could not be required to reinforce the ambulances in Servia, and accordingly distrusted and disliked the newcomers.

But I happened to go into the post-office and saw the engineer. He told me the *Deligrad* was there and would be off in half an hour, and I hurried home.

We were all packed up, but Milano had to rush about and find men to carry our baggage; the heavy chests were to be taken on board on our return.

Dr. Walter Leckie volunteered to see to all this, and was to accompany the baggage on board.

We paid a hasty farewell to those of our patients who remained—few in number now, and able to get about, except one old man with a broken thigh, a civilian, who had fallen from a cart, and one young fellow whose wound was still troublesome and would be so for months.

Then we hurried to the shore, hot and breathless, only to see the *Deligrad* dropping down into the main stream.

Luckily there was a fishing-boat there, and into this we scrambled, our hand baggage being thrown in afterwards, and the captain slacked the engines.

Arrived at the side, how to get up was the question! Louise solved the mystery by boldly putting her knee on some projecting point on the steamer's side, and being pushed up behind, and hauled up in front, succeeded in landing herself on the deck. Loud applause from the bystanders on the shore. Encouraged by this, I followed her example and found myself also safe on deck. Our baggage followed, and in another minute we were off.

The captain welcomed us warmly, and wondered why we were so late. I explained that no notice had been given us as promised of his arrival, and he shrugged his shoulders and laughed.

He took us to a seat in the fore-part of the vessel, and sat down by us to explain the superb scenery as we passed.

We looked back at Doïni sleeping in the sunshine, and wondered why Prince Milosch had planted his new town on that swamp, instead of the hill above, where the zigzag road wound up to Maidenpek.

We had often heard of Maidenpek, but never seen it. It was a mining town, and when the war broke out, most of the English miners left, and the best had come down and gone over to Austria, only a few days before.

The mine there appears to have been worked by some English companies and never to have been a success. Why, was never clearly explained, for there was ore there.

Soon the river bent round the high Hungarian bank, and we lost sight of Doïni, but the rocks seemed to close the passage in front.

A superb military road runs at the base of the rocks, and just where the defile of Kazan begins are the ruins of a castle, with a road coming down to the river, guarded by three towers one above another, climbing as it were up the hillside.

By some authorities they are said to be of Roman origin, but they have a decidedly mediaeval appearance.

We now approached the defile, whose very name Kazan, or "cauldron," tells how fiercely runs the mighty stream confined within such narrow barriers.

The river turns suddenly to the left, and rushes on between white rocks, streaked with red, stupendous limestone rocks rising sheer from the river on either side, barring out every gleam of sunshine from the river, and turning its bright waters into a dark-blue steel colour, while eagles were whirling above the crests of the mountains. The scene was almost awful in its grandeur.

There were the upper Iron Grates; the lower ones are below Orsova, and are only formed by the river falling over rocks between flat shores.

The captain pointed out to us, on the left-hand side, an apparently inaccessible cavern, called the Cave of the Veterans, where in 1692 an Austrian general, with 700 men, defended himself for three months against a Turkish Army, and only surrendered from want of food; and here too, in 1728, Major Von Stein and his gallant comrades entrenched themselves, and held out with, let us hope, better success; but no one seemed to know what became of them. The entrance of this cave is small, and a loopholed wall of masonry half conceals it.

The pass here is only 200 yards wide, but it is fifty yards deep, and the stream runs fearfully fast. Little boats keep close under the rocks to avoid the current, but the steamers keep in the centre.

The navigation is very dangerous, and the captain left us here to superintend it. There were five men at the wheel, for there are many sunken rocks in the way, and some lift their brown glistening heads above water; but there is not footing for a goat on the mountain side, so sheer do the grand rocks come down into the river.

The captain had told us to look out a little farther on, and see the traces left of the old Roman road on the Servian or right-hand shore of the river.

What a work was that! What a monument of Roman ingenuity and Roman perseverance!

This road was probably a towing-path, but also served as a military way. It followed the windings of the rocky shore, taking advantage of every accidental circumstance; creeping along the level where the rocks receded a little, and then, hewn out of the rock itself, a narrow road from two to six feet wide; but then came a part where this could not be done without blasting—a process unknown to the ancients.

The great mountains came down straight into the river, and the road must pass along them. How could this be done?

Very simply, but very effectually—the forests in the land where the mountains sloped down to the inland plains afforded abundance of material, and a wooden gallery was built over the rushing stream. A wooden shelf was put up against the rocks; it rested partly on props, partly on a narrow ledge hewn out of the rock itself.

The beams were inserted into sockets cut in the rock, and thus the width of the road was doubled as the props leant outwards. It was covered in above, and the ledge and the sockets that held the upper and lower props are still to be seen.

This road was fifty miles in length, including the part before and after the Iron Gates, but this portion was considered so wonderful that a coin was struck to commemorate it.

On the column of Trajan at Rome, where his victories in Dacia are perpetuated in marble, one part of the sculptured bas-relief represents the Roman soldiers busily engaged in hewing wood, and shaping it into beams and planks. It has been supposed that this refers to the galleys made and launched on the Danube, but many think that the fact of this wondrous wooden road has been too much lost sight of, and that this represents the wood being fashioned for the props, floor, and roof.

We leave this to the Society of Antiquaries to decide. It might form an amusing subject of discussion.

The defile now grew narrower still. We could see no way out of it. Here it was only 120 yards wide, and the course of the river more rapid still.

Just as the pass ends, we saw the rock on the Servian side, which had been chipped flat into a tablet with an inscription in honour of Trajan.

The tablet bears figures of *genii*, their wings supporting an eagle, which eagle supports a dolphin in the centre.

The inscription is as follows, in bold Roman letters:—

IMP. CAESAR D NERVAE FILIUS NERVA.
TRAJANUS. GERM. PONT MAXIMUS.

The slab is very much blackened by the smoke of fires lighted by the fishermen who congregate at this spot, for close by is a deep pool under the steep shore where fish abound.

Here the river again made a sudden bend. We rushed out of the dark defile into bright sunshine; the river widened into another broad lake-like basin, with low, flat shores.

On the Hungarian side—the left-hand—stood the town of Orsova; on the Servian, or right-hand side, was the small village of Kladonitza, and here we cast anchor, to await the arrival of the Russian volunteers.

Chapter 24
Servia and Roumania

We stood on the deck of the *Deligrad* and looked at the scene around us.

On the left bank was Orsova sleeping in the sunlight; and built as it is along the river, it presents the appearance of a large town.

It stands surrounded by hills, the last spurs of the Carpathians, and contains about 1,000 inhabitants.

The natives still wear a costume resembling that of the captive Dacian kings on the Arch of Constantine, at Rome, and the women wear red leather boots.

There is an Austrian garrison, police-office, and custom-house here, but nothing worth seeing.

About sixteen miles from Orsova are the ancient baths of Mehadia, still much frequented in summer time.

There are several large boarding-houses, a military hospital, and a casino with *table d'hôte* and billiard-rooms, all belonging to government. Every price is regulated by a tariff.

These baths were known to the Romans as the Baths of Hercules; the springs which furnish them rise in the mountains, which hem in the narrow gorge in which they are found. There are twenty-two springs; some are tonic, some sedative, some stimulating, some relaxing, and some are sulphurous,

A few words may be added here as to the country below Orsova, on the left bank, as it may become of vital importance in the present struggle between Russia and Turkey.

Two miles farther down is New Orsova, placed on an island which has a ruined Turkish fort. It was being repaired, and there was a small garrison there at the time we visited Kladonitza.

This is the last picturesque point of the river, which now winds through the immense plains of Wallachia and Bulgaria.

An hour and a half below Orsova are the Lower Iron Gates, where the Danube glides over a plateau of rock, and then forms two falls with broken water between. There is a practicable passage on the left-hand side, dangerous at low water, but easy when the river is high.

Then comes Skela Gladova, a poor village, where passengers are transferred into the large Constantinople boats from the smaller ones, which bring them from Drenkova, and which alone could pass the Upper and Lower Iron Gates.

Some hours' journey below this again is Kalafat, on the Roumanian shore, and a little lower down, Widdin, on the Bulgarian side, in full possession of the Turks.

Twelve hours farther on is Rustchuk in Bulgaria, and Guirjevo in Roumania, opposite to each other, and both armed to the teeth.

It is here that the Russians were expected to cross the Danube; but the stream "runs deep and strong," the Bulgarian shore is well guarded, and a fearful loss of life must ensue, ere that "silver streak" is passed.

It was from Rustchuk that in 1854 Omer Pasha, aided by English officers, crossed the Danube at the head of 45,000 men.

And now for the Servian shore; for a few words will show the enormous importance of the action Servia might take.

All along the Roumanian shore Turkey faces the Russian troops, wherever they may be, except for a few short miles where Servia faces her, and the Russians, if Servia permits them to pass, can cross the Danube unopposed.

Out steamer was anchored at Kladonitza, on the Servian shore; and a few miles beyond is Klodovo, the Serb Gladova. Just opposite is Tchernatz, in Roumania, the terminus on the Danube of the railroad from Bucharest, the port of which is Turn Severin. Then comes Bras Palanka, a small village; and lastly, Radojevatz, the last village in Servia, for here the Timok falls into the Danube, having formed the boundary between Servia and Bulgaria in possession of the Turks.

If Servia permit, it is within this small space that the Russian Armies could cross, and coming by Négotin could pursue their way by Tchupria and Paratjin and Alexinatz, up the broad main-road, and so enter Bulgaria at Nish Nissa, fairly on their way to Constantinople by land.

It was to Klodovo that the carts were sent to fetch the volunteers from Tchernatz and Turn Severin.

Kladonitza was a small village, placed where the cliffs receded far from the shore.

The river was so low that we had between us and the village a broad expanse of sand and hardened mud. Just opposite the ship was a rude *cafané*, near which two gipsies were playing on the violin in a most spirited way.

We had found on board, Nicolas, one of our *infirmiers*, who had obtained leave of absence to go to Belgrade, and fetch his sister-in-law, who was on her way back to Klodovo.

We told him, as soon as he had seen his sister safe into one of the country carts that were going to Klodovo to fetch the Russians, to come back to us, as we did not know whether we should stay on board the ship, or whether we should get him to find a room for us in Kladonitza, or whether the ship might not start that night.

The captain said that if the Russians arrived in time, he should certainly go as far as Doïni, and anchor for the night, but if not, the navigation between Doïni and Belgrade was too dangerous in the dark, and if this was the case, we might sleep on board ship, and he would do the best he could to keep the small state-cabin for us, or we could, if they arrived in time, land at Doïni, and rejoin the ship at 6 a.m.; but if he could not start from Kladonitza before next day, he felt assured that the ship would be crowded with Russians, and we should be more comfortable ashore.

Presently we saw the carts coming, each bringing eight or ten men. The privates were to go in barges, which were now attached to the ship by long towing ropes. The officers were to be on the *Deligrad*,

And, sure enough, these said officers began to crowd on board, and invaded even the sanctum of the little state-cabin with rugs and pillows and tea-kettles (*samovar* is, I believe, the proper name).

In vain did the captain and the steward declare that this cabin was reserved for ladies; in vain did the captain order them out. As long as there was a foot of spare room, these men could not see why they should not occupy it as well as the ladies.

We found afterwards that this was the Russian habit; but to us English, and to the Austrian captain (for he was half an Austrian, and educated there), and to the quiet Serbs, it was an extraordinary and unheard-of proceeding.

At every moment now, the carts came in with fresh soldiers; and the adjutant, a weather-beaten, courteous little officer, of the 9th Cavalry, told the captain that the whole 2,000 at Gladova could not be brought in before midnight.

The official letters state that only 5,000 Russians were in Servia.

At this very time the Battle of Alexinatz had been fought, and there was a large Russian force there.

Two thousand "ambulance" men had been sent by the *Deligrad*, a few days before this, and now here were 2,000, and 3,000 more were waiting for conveyance, and came a few days later. This makes 7,000, without the Russians then on the Morava.

Their own estimate was that about 9,000 were there, but 3,000 of these were counted as "ambulance," and never served a day in one, but went armed to the front.

We have no wish whatever to speak unkindly of any one, but simply to give a true picture of what we ourselves saw and heard; and if we seem to speak evil of the Russians we met, let our readers judge for themselves if we have not reason to do so; and further, if these men are not a fair specimen of the Russian Army at large.

They were "volunteers;" some certainly were so—peasants from the Ukraine and the Don, and officers who had been excused Siberia if they would form a sort of forlorn hope in Servia; but no man came without leave from the Russian Government, and provided with money by the Panslavic Committee.

The rest were also "volunteers," but consisted of drafts from various regiments, led by their own officers who had received leave of absence, while their pay continued. The soldiers and officers wore the uniform of their respective regiments, the number of which was on their caps and shoulder-straps, and wore the same dress through the war.

The Russians have one great fault, an inordinate love of drink, while the Turks are a most sober people. If, therefore, the Turks commit cruelties from a savage and uncivilised disposition, the Russians commit them from a drunken, brutal one, and their civilisation is about on a par.

A truer sentence was never spoken than "*Grattez les Russes, et vous trouverez les Tartares.*"

Beneath the varnish of St. Petersburg lies the rough material of savage descent.

We found it impossible to remain on board, and Nicolas ran into the town and secured us a bedroom; he then came to fetch us, and escorted us to the "hotel." We entered a huge, dark kitchen, crowded with Russians. who invited us to sit down and drink, an offer we declined, and were taken up a rickety wooden stair into a long, wide corridor, on which opened many bedrooms, with many beds in each. One, however, had only two beds in it, and here Nicolas installed us, telling us to keep the door well locked, while he ran back to the ship to fetch our suppers, and brought up some red wine from below.

He soon returned, and waited downstairs till we had finished, then brought us a jug of water, a basin and a rough towel, informed us that he should sleep on the kitchen-table below, and would call us at 5 a.m., and with this assurance and entire confidence in Nicolas's fidelity and steadiness, we went to bed in hopes of a good night's rest.

Chapter 25

The Russians on the Danube

We had *hoped* to pass a quiet night, but how were our hopes deceived! Up to midnight the carts came rattling in from Klodovo, each bringing its load of noisy, drunken men.

Then the gipsy fiddlers played away most indefatigably, while the Russians alternately sang hymns and danced, and shouted warlike songs, and at last, when they ceased from mere fatigue, and the officers came to their rooms upstairs, a violent quarrel broke out, swords were drawn and clashed together, and finally the contending parties fell against the door with such violence, that we started up fully expecting it would give way and they would fall into the room.

We bestowed, not our benedictions upon them, and assured them that we considered them "dreadful;" and whether they had stunned themselves by the fall, or were affected by our English appeal, they grew quiet and ceased to howl about the "Cross" and the holy cause.

There never was a phrase so sickening to us as that of the "holy cause," when we saw the men who used it. It was a profanation of a great and high idea that was sad to hear, and we learned to dislike the very sound.

When at last there was comparative silence we slept, as it seemed, for an hour, till Nicolas tapped at the door, and advised us to dress at once, and go onboard the *Deligrad*, where we could get our morning coffee better than in the inn.

We followed his advice, and went to the shore. There lay the *Deligrad*; but the plank was withdrawn. No one could go on board.

So great was now the crowd assembling on the shore, so eager was everyone to go in the ship, and not on the barges, that the captain had wisely ordered communication with the shore to be cut off till all was ready, and he could superintend the embarkation.

At present he was either sleeping or dressing himself in his uniform, and was not visible. There was nothing for it but to sit on some boxes of biscuits or flour, and watch the scene around.

It was a lovely morning; the mists on the Danube were dispersing before the rising sun, and these mists are very dense during the summer season.

Picturesque groups were assembled on the shore—rough, wild-looking men, but evidently well disciplined, for at the word of command they fell into line, and stood there patiently.

A little shop was open, and there were sold small hot cakes of Indian corn, with which we tried to stay our hunger; but they were not very eatable; though Nicolas, as a proof of their goodness, pointed to the rush made to buy them.

Meantime, surreptitious attempts were made to get on board the steamer by sundry Russians. A few succeeded by getting into a boat, and climbing up the anchor chains.

One ambitious youth dropped his sword into the river, and commenced a loud lamentation at the loss of a sword which had been three hundred years in the family—the sword of his great-great-great-grandfather's father!—and now to lose it, just as it was about to become additionally glorious by the slaughter of the *infidel* Turks!

This was the burden of his wail as he tried to fish it up in vain, and we were irresistibly reminded of the famous "*Voici le sabre de mon père!*" At last a native volunteered to dive for it, and divesting himself of his upper garment, appeared in a shirt and long linen drawers, and, shaking back his hair, plunged into the water, or rather mud, and commenced groping for the lost weapon. Again, and again he came up for air, looking like a negro, and at last popped up with a shout of triumph, the sword in his hand, and scrambled on shore.

A roar of laughter greeted his appearance, as he stood shaking himself, looking like a black statue; and the Russian, having rewarded him, devoted himself to cleaning his sword, which had fallen out of its leather sheath.

There were many swords of this kind amongst the Russians—broad, straight blades, with beautifully inlaid and worked handles, and their sheaths of crimson leather, embroidered in gold and silver.

And now appeared a gorgeous group—a Circassian prince and his staff, who was going to Belgrade, with 500 men, to offer his sword to Prince Milan.

He had travelled very far from his home near Persia, where he was lord of all around.

He was a fine young man, with olive complexion, black hair and eyes, and a small moustache. He wore a superb cap, of the shape of a busby, of the very finest white Astrachan fur, with a pale-blue bag hanging from it. His coat was of the same rich fur, with the fur inside just peeping out all around; dark blue trousers, tucked into black boots, and a gold sword-belt, from which hung a sword blazing with jewels. Over his shoulders was flung a short *bournous*, of the shape called "*bashilik*," short, with a hood, and very long ends to throw over to the back: this was of pale blue. A row of cartridge tubes was arranged on the breast of the coat on either side, black, tipped with silver, and in shape exactly resembling a pair of Pandean pipes. White kid gloves completed the costume, which, it was to be presumed, was full dress.

His staff also wore the national costume, but the colour of the *bashiliks* varied according to taste. Some were crimson, some white, worn over dark tunics, some blue, and one was a pale mauve, and one a splendid royal purple.

The Russian officers wore their uniforms—most of them were in green; but the adjutant, and a few others in dark-blue coats, all had crimson facings.

One volunteer was a gentleman from Moscow. He spoke perfect French and English; his mother was English, and he was by far the best of the party. He was a handsome man, portly and stately, with a grey cloth coat, lined with grey Astrachan, and a busby of grey Astrachan. He, too, had an ancestral sword.

Presently we spied our old friend, the Préfet of Négotin, who greeted us warmly; and the plank of communication being now laid, we went on board together, followed by a rush of everybody; and while we were struggling for coffee, or rather encouraging Nicolas to struggle for us, a general free fight came on to turn the intruders out.

The *préfet* told us he had been ordered to come to Kladonitza, to superintend the arrangements made for the Russians; that 3,000 more were on their way, but would march to the Morava by way of Négotin, and he had to find quarters, rations, and forage for them all along the march.

Négotin, it may as well be remarked here, is a large town, with a prefecture, a college, a gymnasium, an hospital, two churches, and a capital hotel. Under the *préfet*, with his Bucharest training, and his naturally refined mind and high education, Négotin is going fast forward in the ways of improvement, and promises to be one of the best towns in Servia.

When all the intruders were expelled, the *préfet* took leave of us and went on shore. No one else was allowed to come on board, except a file of men, who went backward and forward with the loaves of bread and the meat destined for the mid-day meal of the soldiers. This consisted of small skinny sheep, roasted whole.

By this time the sun was well up, and the day getting on. We were very anxious to start, for never having gone upstream before, we thought that we should arrive at Belgrade that night, even if it did take an hour or two more than going down.

But still, when the plank of communication was withdrawn, and all the soldiers had been marched on to the barges, though steam was up and all was ready, we did not start, and the prince and his staff crowded together at the stem of the vessel.

We mounted on to the table, which was a fixture on the deck, and saw our friend the *préfet* talking earnestly to a boyish-looking man with long fair hair, parted in the middle, and falling behind his ears, dressed in a black gown that came down to his feet, exactly like an Ulster, a small felt hat on his head, and a purple *merino* scarf twisted round his neck. He was dressed so exactly like a lady of the present day in winter costume, that the evening before we had taken him for a woman.

The *préfet* walked with him a little way down the shore, where, exactly opposite to the first barge, which was of course in the centre, between the ship and the second barge, we now discovered a table with a cloth thrown over and a pair of lighted candles upon it.

Our young friend threw off his hat, Ulster and wrapper, a gorgeous vestment was thrown over him, something between a cope and a chasuble, and he emerged a full-blown Greek priest.

A religious service now commenced, while every man on the barges and on the ship bared his head. A low monotonous chant and responses went on for some minutes, while the priest and the other officials stood round the improvised altar.

At last it was finished, and then the priest advanced to the edge of the shore, preceded by acolytes bearing large silver vases full of holy water.

The priest himself had a bunch of green twigs in his hand. He came as close to the barges and the ship as possible, and dipping the twig brush in the holy water, flung showers of it against the ship.

The soldiers leaned forward stretching over the bulwarks, trying to catch stray drops as they held out their bands and caps, and when they succeeded, they made a succession of crosses on brow and breast. The priest walked slowly along, still sprinkling as he went, and then back again, till he thought everyone had caught a drop. At last all the holy water was finished, the plank was once more put across from the ship to the shore, the last stragglers—the priest included—came on board, the plank was finally withdrawn, the rope cast loose, and the steamer dropped off into the river, the tow-ropes tightened as the barges fell in behind, and we were fairly started.

Then arose wild shouts of joy and exultation, some small cannon on the shore fired at intervals of half a minute, the Servian flag was hoisted, and floated from the masthead.

The *préfet* waved his hat enthusiastically to the soldiery, then tucked it under his arm, and kissed both hands to Louise and myself.

The officers and soldiers sang a grand solemn hymn, "*God preserve the Emperor.*" It echoed over the broad, calm river, and we saw the Austrian guard at Orsova running, muskets in hand, to the shore.

We began to plough our way up stream, the white foam flying from our bows, the heavy barges plunging on behind; still the solemn hymn went on, the guns fired, the *préfet* alternately waved his hat and kissed his hands till the shore grew distant; the huge rocks closed in. The sunshine was hidden, the hymn died down, we were once more in the Pass of Kazan, and the *Deligrad* steamed steadily on her way, with 2,000 Russians on board her, and the barges in tow, on their way to Belgrade and the front in the Morava Valley.

CHAPTER 26

A Day with the Russians

The wind blew coldly through the pass, and in spite of their furs, the prince and his staff wrapped themselves up in gay-coloured blankets, and the chill shadows of the defile suggested to the Russian and Circassian officers the necessity of "something to drink" to keep up their spirits.

This something to drink came in the shape of wine and spirits, brought by a smart Serb lad, who demanded payment for every bottle as he put it on the table, and informed us—*sotto voce* in German—that he knew the fellows: before they got twenty miles they would be so drunk that they would forget all about payment, and knock him down if he reminded them of it.

A large cask of "*raki*" had been laid in by the steward on speculation, for everyone paid for what they had on board, and a very good speculation it was.

Singing and drinking went on indefatigably; first we had a hymn, then a drinking-song, during which glasses were clashed together, and wine flung about.

Then a fair, good-looking Circassian went and fetched his accordion, and commenced singing comic songs. The engineer of the ship, who was standing by us, gave us a clue to the subject of the song, and so expressive was the young fellow's face and manner, that we could follow him. He sang capitally, had a good voice, and was evidently well-trained. Presently he struck up a bold, martial air, with a chorus to every verse, "Rusky will! Rusky will! Hourah!"—which "Hourah" is something between an English cheer and a shriek, and was in this case given so fiercely that the rocks rang again.

We caught the words Tchernaya, Alma, Inkermann, and just as a fourth verse was beginning with the word "Balaclava," the captain came down from the bridge, and, walking up to the prince, told him that song must not go on.

Silence fell on the assembly; more wine was ordered, and sentimental songs were the order of the day—a most dolorous one, given by the prince, being interrupted half-way by "the boy" demanding a florin for the bottle of wine from which the prince was filling the glasses all around to drink the health of some fair but absent Circassian.

We were curious enough to ask the engineer what the song was which the captain put a stop to, and he gave us a verbal translation of it, of which I venture to give a rough, free rendering, to exhibit the amiable feelings of the Russian volunteers towards the allies of their country; but never did they for one moment disguise their hatred of England and the English. In that at least they were perfectly truthful and candid, and this song was, we found, not one written for the occasion, not one sung by a certain regiment, or a certain set of men, but a song common everywhere, at least in the provinces, though it is probable that it may not have been heard in St. Petersburg or Moscow.

Russian War-Song.

What nation draws the unsullied brand
To guard and save the insulted land?
Avenging thus the degraded past,
Our day of triumph comes at last.
Who shall remember Tchernaya's hour,
And trample on Italian power?
Rusky will! Rusky will! Hourah!

Who shall remember Alma's height,
That day of dark and desperate fight?
The tricolour has fallen since then;
We'll tread it in the dust again;
We will its gaudy colours rend.
And leave "Fair France" without a friend.
Rusky will! Rusky will! Hourah!

There stands aloof a nation strong—
England—who wrought us bitter wrong!
But vengeance comes, and, man for man.
We'll claim the dead of Inkermann;
We will erase the scroll of shame,
And write in fire our honoured name.
Rusky will! Rusky will! Hourah!

We were excessively amused at this song of vague threats, but also much obliged to the gallant captain for putting a stop to it, simply on the ground that the "Hourah!" was perfectly ear-splitting.

So, the morning wore on. At last we came out from the pass into the brilliant sunshine, and, rounding a point, saw Doïni Milanovatz once more.

As we neared it, we saw a group on the shore—Dr. Leckie, Milano, the Master of the Magazine, the Captain of the Town, the post-master, our interpreter, and several others with bullock waggons containing the heavy baggage.

The steamer slacked, and our doctor and Milano came on board; the Captain of the Town was following, when he was called back, and one of those yellow envelopes put into his hand which, all the world over, contain a telegram, and immediately began to bustle and hurry the baggage on board, as if the Turks were entering at the other end of the town; but we had no idea then that the telegram regarded us.

He came on board with the interpreter and the Master of the Magazine, and we started up stream again.

By this time the Russians had turned their attention to card-playing. Small groups were clustered around sundry boxes and tubs, which were converted into extempore card-tables, and money was passing freely.

As the table was fully occupied, we made use of our portmanteau as one, where the doctor and ourselves dined, while Milano waited upon us. We had taken the precaution to order our dinner the night before, and to remind the cook when we came on board that morning, so we fared better than our incautious neighbours.

Our Serb friends were landed about three o'clock, at what appeared to be a wharf in the midst of a forest, but they were going to cross by a small boat to Drenkova, where the steamer, crowded as she was with troops, dare not stop, it being in Austria.

It was nearly 5 p.m. before we stopped again at a coaling place, and here the barges were drawn to the shore, and the men allowed to land; and then the sergeants, or whatever they were called, came on board the steamer and took the meat and bread; the meat was cut up on board, and each sergeant received a certain portion of that and bread for his men—the whole body being divided into messes of about twenty.

This and the coaling took a long time, and the evening shades were closing in before the men were re-embarked and we got off again.

We thought it would be very late before we reached Belgrade, or rather early, but we found that the steamer was to stop for the night.

We went down to see the cabin; it was crowded; some of the officers were sleeping, some playing cards, some smoking; it was impossible to remain there, we must camp out on deck, not a pleasant prospect amidst the night fogs on the Danube.

But here our good old friend, the engineer, stepped in, and most kindly offered to give up his cabin to us; we accepted it as gratefully as it was freely offered, and joyfully installed ourselves in it.

It was small, but comfortable, and we could sleep in peace there, while he slept in the engine-room.

The night came on, the fog thickened, and at last the steamer anchored for the night.

Even the untiring Russians were tired out at last, and silence sunk down on the vessel.

At daybreak we started again, and just after sunrise came to Semendria with its castellated wall, which we had not seen before, as it was pitch-dark when we passed it on our way down the river.

About eight we arrived off Belgrade. The Russians were all up and awake, and dressed in their best, and evidently expected a grand reception.

Poor fellows, we felt for their disappointment! They had come, some of them a thousand miles, to fight for Servia, and this was their welcome!

A few small boys cheered them in shrill voices as we steamed up to the wharf. An *attaché* of the Russian Consulate was in waiting to meet the steamer; that was all.

They trooped on shore with their pillows and blankets and *samovars*, the Cossack servants following with their baggage, and in a desultory manner wandered up to the town.

The men were marched off to some barracks prepared for them, and when all was clear we took leave of the captain and our kind engineer, and went on shore too.

We had sent a telegram to M. Dilbert to announce our coming, and asked him to get us quarters. It seemed afterwards that it never reached, and while I went to his house to ask where our quarters were, Dr, Leckie started off to find a corner for himself, and Louise sat on our trunk in the centre of the baggage like Marius amidst the ruins of Carthage.

My errand was unsuccessful. M. Dilbert had been up all night on

Red Cross duty and was sleeping. No one knew anything. If we could get into an hotel for an hour or two, they would send him to us.

Then back came Dr. Leckie; he had got one room in the best hotel, the Hirsch (German), Stanya (Serbish), Stag (English)—and this he would give up to us. If indeed it were true that there was no other vacant in the hotel.

By this time Louise, who had left Doïni very far from well, with the terrible malarious low fever, was utterly exhausted, and it was all we could do to drag her into the long coffee-room of the Hirsch, and get her some warm coffee.

I saw a kindly-looking woman behind the bar, and, going up to her, asked if there was no room, however small and humble, that we could have, as my friend was very ill.

"Then you are not Russians?" she said.

"No; English," I answered. "Why do you ask?"

"Because I will have no Russian *women* here." (The exact word she used had better be omitted.) "I have a nice room here. Andreas, Michael, take these ladies to No. 4, and send the chambermaid with hot water, and see that they have all they require."

Our troubles were ended; we were soon installed in a charming room, and while Louise rested, I went out to see what was going on, and to report our arrival at headquarters.

CHAPTER 27

The Turks in Belgrade

I had hardly turned into the Grande Place, before I met Herr Dilbert coming in search of us. I explained that we had found quarters, and he begged to remind me that for Red Cross workers there was a special tariff, and he should tell the people at the "Hirsch" that we were only to pay that. He added, "And I am very glad to see that you were able to catch the *Deligrad*; we hardly hoped it."

I was somewhat puzzled, and still more so when he added, "They are expecting you at the War Office. Your orders are waiting; you will have to start immediately."

For what place?" I inquired.

"For Paratjin," was the reply; "a great battle is expected on the Morava, and the wounded will all be sent there."

Now Paratjin was the very place where we had always felt that help was most needed; the wounded there had been more numerous, and suffered more than anywhere else; but the Russians had two hospitals in Paratjin, and in whatever town they took up their abode, they would at first have no one else, whether help was needed or not.

I started off at once for the War Office, and found both Dr. Beloni and Dr. Sava Petrovatz in their private bureau.

Both sprang up and greeted me with evident delight. "*Gut! Gut!*" said old Dr. Beloni "*Soyez la bien venue!*" said Dr. Sava Petrovatz. "So you did get the telegram?"

"No," I answered "What telegram? We only acted on your orders to come to Belgrade when we could."

"We sent you a telegram to start at once, and that the *Deligrad* was to wait, till you and your baggage were ready, to bring you back directly to Belgrade, that you may go on to Paratjin."

There was the explanation of the telegram in the captain's hand; the officials did not want us to leave—and this telegram would have been delayed in transmission to us. They had wilfully omitted to inform us when the *Deligrad* arrived, and they thought there would be no inquiry into the matter, so that, as we were on board, it was best not to give it to us.

Thus, we had accidentally done just what we were wanted to do, for though we were to leave Doïni, no special day or time was named.

I could not help suggesting that we had originally asked for Paratjin as our station.

"Yes," answered Dr. Beloni; "and I wish you had gone there; the Russians care for nothing but their own men. We have some rough hospitals there, and we sadly need your services and your stores."

Dr. Sava Petrovatz added, that we were to take charge of the Serb hospitals, under the head medical man; that no decent woman could work in a Russian ambulance, unless it were in that where the Princess Czartoriski superintended, and she would have no one in it but her own people.

He then gave me the official orders for transport, rations and quarters, and again holding out his hand, said as he held mine, "We are sending you to harder work than any you ever knew, and to win, I hope, higher honour, and we trust entirely to your charity and goodwill to us."

He begged us to send him a telegram about the state of the Serb hospitals, and what was wanted; and we parted with mutual words of kindness.

From all the Servian officials we always received the greatest kindness, and were treated with the highest respect; and we retain a grateful memory of their care of the strangers who came to their help.

On the way back to the hotel, I went to the transport-office, and found that it must be three days before we could get a waggon and post-horses.

I was not sorry. It would give us both time to get up our strength after the low intermittent fever of Doïni; but the reason was, that the Russians had taken possession of the transport-office, and claimed the right of taking everyone till they were all provided for, and Servians and volunteers, civil and military, had to wait their good pleasure.

These three days had to be passed in Belgrade, now, it might correctly be said, in Russian occupation. Even their letters were put aside in the post-office, and till they had all been served out, no one else could be attended to.

Had it not been for Mr. Spooner, the poor English epistles might have slumbered till now in dirt and oblivion. He got hold of them, and put them in his own little den, where he could always find them.

It was a decided case of "Save me from my friends!" The Serbs hated their Russian allies. Prince Milan and a few of his ministers might like them; but this was the national feeling—openly expressed by some, cherished silently by others.

It could not be otherwise. They treated the poor Serbs with a mixture of arrogance and contempt that was perfectly unbearable. They had occupied all the positions on the staff: nearly every officer in command, even down to lieutenants, was a Russian. The Serbs are by nature a kindly and courteous people. They address each other in the most polite way: "Favour me, my brother, by doing so and so," or, "Tell me such a thing;" and the militia now in the field were like our volunteer regiments; there were many landed proprietors, shopkeepers, and merchants in the ranks.

The fact of being an officer did not prove a man to be of superior rank to his privates.

These were the men—gentle, courteous fellows—who were kicked about by the Russians, with oaths and blasphemy: but, with the endurance and cunning of their character, they bore it uncomplainingly.

The day of vengeance came—we shall soon see how and when—and few of those tyrants returned to tell the tale.

I have heard it said to them, "You come here to help; why override the natives thus?"

"Help!" was the answer—"help a set of curs? No; we come to open our road to Constantinople, and you English cannot and shall not prevent it."

But to turn from this unpleasant subject. We had a spare day, and we went with Herr Dilbert to see the fortress and the Turkish prisoners, of whom there were about thirty.

There was nothing very wonderful in the fortress, but the view from the ramparts was most lovely.

We crossed a broad gravelled yard, and entered a long corridor, at the end of which was a large room, with a broad divan on either side, and on these divans lay some twenty Turks, enjoying a *siesta*,

They jumped up on our arrival, and, to our surprise, shook hands in a most friendly way with Herr Dilbert and several persons who had followed us in.

Some of them had visited Belgrade in days of peace, and all were on perfectly good terms with their captors.

They could not eat the usual rations, probably on account of some religious prejudice, and the government allowed each man a small sum a day; and Mahometan merchants, living in the Turkish quarter of the town, brought provisions for sale, principally bread and fruit. They drank neither spirits nor wine, but coffee and water. They were supplied with some tobacco, and bought more, for the money they had about them had not been taken from them.

They were tall, fine, clean-looking men. Their uniforms were well brushed, and they appeared in perfect health and cheerful spirits. They walked out every day about the fortress, and were permitted to go to the mosque with a single guard.

We then went upstairs, and the door of a small room was opened. A Turkish officer of rank was sitting at a table, reading, and rose to greet us.

Herr Dilbert and himself were old friends. The Turk had been in command of the fortress under the *pasha* in 1867, when Belgrade was finally evacuated by the Turks, and had visited many of the families in the town.

He spoke very good German, and said how strange it was that he should be a prisoner where he had commanded; but his old friends had not forgotten him, and, on the whole, he had no reason to complain. He thought he was better there than in the Morava Valley, where the Russians were.

He, too, walked out when he pleased, and was on parole.

These prisoners had been taken early in the war.

After the arrival of the Russians, *no quarter was given on either side,* except on the Drina, where the Russians were not in command, and where, however, there was little opportunity for the exercise of mercy to the enemy, so strictly enforced by General Ranko Alempits, because there was only desultory skirmishing going on.

This Turk, in fact, was quite a civilised gentleman.

There was a large establishment in the fortress for the making of bread for the army, and one for the clothes, which were all made on one pattern, and of one size. There were also some military prisoners, sent there for various misdemeanours, and who occupied themselves in carving wooden cups, tobacco-boxes and spoons, which they sold to visitors.

If all tales be true, there were sad scenes within those walls, when the cowards who fled from the front were sent down there and shot.

As we came out, we saw that the Grande Place was full of light waggons, waiting to take on the Russian volunteers, and we met the Russian adjutant fuming and fretting: "Quarters had been allotted to the prince in a dirty *café*; he must be changed. No great-coats had been served out; no orders issued. What *did* the officials mean by behaving in this way?"

We could give no explanation, and proceeded on our walk.

We went to see the English hospital. Dr, Laseron had gone to England to fetch two more sisters—rather an expensive way of getting help—and the sisters there hoped that they should be sent to the front.

I knew the hope was vain. Had they gone, Dr. Laseron would have insisted on going with them; and sundry persons in high places were resolved that he should stay in Belgrade.

It was rumoured afterwards that leave was applied for and refused. This might explain why so great a need as an ambulance, close to the seat of war, was not supplied by the National Aid Society. Otherwise, it is unaccountable.

Nothing could exceed the luxury of the hospital.

The stores of extra china, glass, and the quantity of wine and spirits was astounding; and we wondered who was to imbibe all this spirituous liquor, as the Serbs are not in the habit of drinking much.

There was a professed cook in a white cap and apron, and plenty of good food.

The breakfast-table of the "Director" (Dr. Laseron), his deaconesses, and the surgeons, was as elegant as an English breakfast-table; so was their afternoon tea. There was white bread, butter, and tea—delicacies not known upcountry.

Every bed was covered with a coloured blanket, and a Servian Testament and Prayer-book were placed on a shelf at the head of everyone.

This was very much objected to by the Serb officials and the archbishop, as an attempt at weaning the men from their national faith, and was certainly a breach of the principles of the Geneva Convention, which prohibit any interference in religious matters, and declare that "a wounded man has no nationality and no creed."

This shows the mischief of having an hospital nursed by a body of any one sect. The exclusiveness of many of these nursing sisterhoods is so great, that no lady can live with them and train with them, even by payment, unless professing the same creed.

In this case neither good nor harm was done; the men, many of them, could not read, and could not understand the pronunciation of

Serbish by the sisters; and the rest listened or read out of mere curiosity. Not one convert was made, not one man kept his books after he left hospital, and this money for printing the books specially in Vienna (it could have been done in Belgrade) was all wasted. It is to be hoped that the National Society did not pay for it.

The hospital altogether was very unpopular during Dr. Laseron's time, but was much better liked when he left and Mr. Attwood had the management.

At this time, as Dr. Laseron was away, there was a beautiful illustration going on of the old proverb, "When the cat is away the mice will play." The sisters were decidedly enjoying themselves, though they gave a propriety sigh now and then for "the dear doctor," and the conversation at the tea-table the day we were there was certainly very amusing. Several young men had strolled in and were having a little flirtation with the fair deaconesses, and we sat so late over the sociable meal, that the dinner bells of the hotels were ringing before we broke up.

Several of the correspondents were at our hotel, where also lodged "the Director," who preferred taking his ease in the inn to living in hospital, Mr. McKellar, who only paid flying visits to Belgrade, and several other English.

"To get to the front" was the one idea, and we were objects of great envy.

Next morning, I went down again to the transport-office; a waggon and pair of post-horses had been ordered for us at noon, but at 9 a.m. had been taken possession of by two Russian staff officers, who, although there were four places, refused to allow anyone to accompany them.

So another day passed on, and at dark when I went for the letters, the transport captain came up to me and said that he had had three angry messages from the War Office; that he had been obliged to detain the diligence going to Maidenpek and place it at our service, and that at eleven o'clock next morning it would be at the door of the Hirsch; also that we could do just as we pleased, but three Russian officers, who had to take a consecrated banner to the Army of the Ibar, begged we would permit them to accompany us. The message being a polite one, I was inclined to agree, and when I reflected on the fact that we should have to travel all night, I thought it might be better to have companions through a lonely country, and therefore sent word "Yes."

Our short preparations for travel were soon made, and at dinner we announced our approaching departure.

Our "good luck" was of course the subject of comment, and we congratulated ourselves that we should be in time, for no telegram had brought the news of a battle having been actually fought, though rumours of fighting past, present, and to come, filled the air.

We had one regret—that Dr. Walter Leckie was obliged to return to England; and as we had dismissed Milano, who in fact was at last compelled to return to the front, we had to go on alone; but we should meet our English friends, and we always had worked comfortably with foreign surgeons,—so except our natural sorrow at losing sight of our friend and companion of so many weeks of work and hardship, we did not feel in a state of despair.

CHAPTER 28

On the Road to Paratjin

Sunshine greeted our awaking next morning, and just as we were dressed a hasty rap came at the door, and hardly waiting for an answer, in dashed Mr. McKellar, a telegram in his hand.

All his men had been sent from Rashan to Lukovo; there had been fighting by Saitchar and now there was fighting near Deligrad. He should start as soon as he had been to the Consulate, and should pick us up "somewhere" in the front. He was off to try and get horses, and Mr. Cumberbatch, the English Consul's secretary, would see us off.

Away he flew, and we had hardly done our breakfast before the diligence came lumbering up to the door. Our portmanteau, in which were the instruments and the dry medicines, was packed in, and the invaluable box of medicines, chloroform, carbolic, and every other kind of medicine needed for the wounded, many of them given us by Mr. Bell, of Oxford Street, was also stored away behind.

We had repacked it, wrapping every bottle in cotton wool and lint, stuffing them into every corner, and filling them up level with a doubly folded sheet of lint, and *gutta-percha* tissue laid over all to keep things dry and snug; and we can cordially recommend this plan to all who are packing medicines to travel with an ambulance. Not a single bottle was broken, and the useful lint and cotton wool replaced the useless hay; much weight was thus saved, and a vast quantity of wool and lint can be taken in this way without forming a separate parcel or bale.

Under the uncertainty of our tenure at Paratjin, owing to the neighbourhood of the Turks, we went in "light marching order," and left a great many personal things behind, in the kind care of Madame Dilbert—all the space we could actually spare being filled with old linen, bandages, a pair of sheets and pillowcases for ourselves, two old tablecloths, and several towels.

The good hostess of the Hirsch, Marie, who had been cook at the

British Consulate, prepared us a basket of cold chicken, bread, wine, and of her own accord added two bottles of sweet aniseed liqueur. I objected, and said they were needless; but she and her husband, Ignace, shook their heads and said, "You will see! take our advice and the liqueur."

We yielded, and never was I so thankful that we had taken advice as I afterwards was that we had taken this, for those two bottles of liqueur saved, I verily believe, two lives.

Then we packed ourselves in, with our bundles of rugs and wrappers; Mr. Cumberbatch, who had been assisting us most energetically, bade us a kind farewell, and we jolted up the street to the post-office.

Here we found the three Russian officers and the banner, which was rolled round its staff and covered with canvas. As it was about fifteen feet long, it presented difficulties as to the packing, which were solved by the staff being tied to the diligence along it, forming a barrier that rendered one door useless.

Then the driver mounted; one young officer sat on the box, the other two, one of whom was a major, got inside, and off we started down the long *boulevard*, past the palace and "*Topschediry*," the summer palace of Prince Michael, never occupied since his assassination close by, and now used as a Russian ambulance.

This ambulance had been opened in the presence of the prince and princess by the archbishop, with a religious service, during which he solemnly blessed the house and all who should enter it.

The English hospital had been opened without any such ceremony, which is considered indispensable, even in beginning life in a new house, in Servia, and was therefore called by the people of Belgrade "The Unblessed Ambulance;" and its far higher death-rate was attributed to this cause by the people there.

When we came out on the open downs beyond Belgrade on this side, the wind blew bitterly cold over barren downs, and the poor Russian officers, who were very quiet, inoffensive men, shivered in the blast. Of the two inside, one could talk German, the other a little French, and we had spoken at intervals.

We offered them a large rug of mine, and a plaid shawl of Louise's, and they thankfully wrapped themselves up in them, and presented a most pacific appearance.

It was about four o'clock when we reached Semendria; we had already changed horses once, and we only halted here for five minutes. The country now began to be hilly, with fine woods. We wound up a road leading to a higher level, and just as it grew dark changed horses again at a large village.

We all now tried to sleep, and so the time passed till about midnight. We got to a large, rambling wayside inn in the village of Barzan, where the officers were to find the diligence to Kragojevatz and the Ibar.

But when the officer got off the box, we saw that he was a young, delicate-looking man, and that he could hardly stand. He was half-frozen, and had had nothing to eat since we left Belgrade.

He could speak no word of any language but Russian, but he could understand our signs as we broke off a large piece of bread, and the leg of a chicken, and handed him the cup of our flask with some liqueur in it. He leaned against the side of the diligence very faint from cold and hunger. We made him swallow the liqueur, and then eat the bread and chicken, and when he had done, he touched his cap, and with a pleading smile pointed to the cup. We gave it him filled once more, and he drew himself up quite revived. His comrades, who had been busy disengaging their banner, thanked us most heartily, and said he was not strong enough to come to this rough work, but he had insisted on it.

We parted, as people say, "with mutual regret," and went on our way to Paratjin.

It was just daybreak when we halted again at Jagodina, and there we got a little hot coffee.

At Tchupria we crossed the Morava, a broad, rushing river, now that the rains were beginning, and when we had just got a little further on, the driver turned round, and pointing down the road before him, said, "Paratjin."

As we rattled up to the post-office at Paratjin, we saw two or three officers standing there waiting.

One was a tall, elegant, handsome man, who announced himself as Captain Bogovitch, *commandant* of the town; another was a pleasant-looking, fair man, Herr Hadji Thoma, captain of the transport department, and with them were the quartermaster and the Captain of the Town.

We were warmly welcomed, and Captain Bogovitch said that a telegram had arrived during the night saying that we had started. Our cards were looked at as a mere matter of form, and the quartermaster was ordered to find us a room. This individual seemed much relieved to find that we were willing to go to the hotel till a room was found, as he was overpowered with business, and the whole party escorted us to the "hotel."

Shall we ever forget that place? We never knew its name, nor the name of the landlord. What it might have been in peace we cannot say—we have a curiosity to see; for what it was in war was a strange experience.

We entered a large, low room, opening on the street, with small tables about it, and a sort of bar in the background. A door led from this into a yard, surrounded by a covered corridor, from which the bedrooms were entered, their windows looking into the street at the side. In the centre of the yard were carriages, pigs, chickens, old harness, broken ploughs, and a dung-heap.

Into one of these rooms we were taken. It had been but lately vacated, and no one dreamed of putting clean sheets on the bed.

However, after a long struggle, we got some so-called clean sheets, some hot water, and a fire lighted.

Their stoves were curious affairs; inside the room was an iron pillar, with a pipe leading through the wall into a sort of oven outside. The fire was lighted in this oven, and the heat, when the door of it was shut, passed into the pillar in the room. The great objection was, that the room was always either too hot or too cold, and your neighbours stole your wood and lighted their fires from your hot brands.

By this time Louise was really ill. She had left Belgrade, before she had fairly recovered the effects of fever, and I was thankful to get her to lie down even on the unpromising bed, on which, however, we spread our own sheets.

We got some breakfast at the noonday meal, and when I went to order it, I saw two or three surgeons in uniform standing there, and Captain Bogovitch bringing an elderly man towards the door of the yard. He introduced him as the surgeon-in-chief, who would allot us our work; and the surgeon begged that we would, after the noonday rest, go to the central ambulance, where help was much wanted.

When he was gone, a tall, fine-looking man came forward, and introduced himself as Dr. Louis Barkan; he spoke good English and French, and was an Austrian. He said that he was most anxious to form another hospital, and begged for our services in it. Of course, we should, I knew, prefer serving under such a gentlemanly surgeon who could speak three languages, and we arranged it so. He was in the Servian service, and the elderly surgeon did just what Dr. Barkan told him. This senior was a Serb.

After dinner, as the noon-day meal was properly called, I went to the central ambulance with Dr. Barkan.

We crossed the road, leaving on our left hand the bridge, over a nearly dried-up stream, across which was the main part of the town, and the road to Deligrad and Alexinatz.

We then went on, down a road, which Dr. Barkan said led to Krushevatz, and formed a sort of suburb to the town, low one-storied buildings on either hand, till we came to a large building that had once been a *café*. In front was a village green, with scattered houses opposite.

The doctor opened the door of the ex-*café*, and I stopped short in horror.

"Come in," he said gently, "we want you so much; it is but the first sight."

I drew my breath and looked steadily in, and then followed Dr. Barkan into the ambulance.

CHAPTER 29

The Ambulance at Paratjin

A letter was published in the *Times* of November 3rd, 1876, signed in our joint names. This letter was read over, and fully approved of, by the English surgeons, and in it we said:

> We will not send a shudder of horror through the quiet homes of England, by describing the scene which, day by day, meets our view as we work there.

Nor will we now give details of that scene, yet a general description of it may afford an idea of what an ambulance at the seat of war really is, and we commend this chapter to the earnest consideration of all sentimental and romantic young ladies, who think it delightful to go and "bathe the fevered brow," or "fan the flushed cheek" of the "wounded hero."

War is a stern and dreadful reality, even in its pomp and glory. What is it when all the excitement of the battle is over, when only agonising groans and shrieks of pain can be heard, only varied forms of suffering seen all around? No romance, no sentimentality can stand the test of such an hour. It needs trained nerves and sobered thoughts to meet it.

The central ambulance consisted of a large room with fixed benches all round it; the door opposite the one by which we entered led, like that of our hotel, into a covered corridor with bedrooms. In this room was received every wounded man who came back from the battle in the front, about three hours away, at foot pace.

Here the dressings of their wounds were taken off, the chief surgeon inspected them, entered their names in a register kept for the purpose, gave them each a ticket, with the name of the hospital in the rear, to which they were to go, and then ordered the wounds to be re-dressed; whilst those too bad to be moved were placed in any vacant beds there might happen to be, in the Serb hospitals in the three houses close by, and in the bedrooms of the central ambulance.

Here it was that help was required to take off the dressings and then replace them, and this demanded some knowledge on the part of those so employed, which amateurs could not possess; yet this is what all who nurse in a war may be called upon to do.

The chief surgeon sat at a table in the centre by a desk, writing the tickets. Dr. Barkan walked about attending to the most serious wounds, and a young Serb surgeon and two Italian surgeons, who were in charge of the three small hospitals, occasionally came in to help. One of the Italians was a capital surgeon and a very good fellow; the other was a hopeless idiot, with long black curls behind his ears.

There were two or three *infirmiers*, whose work was to lift up crippled patients, take away dressings, and keep the cold water tubs plentifully supplied and the irrigators filled.

On this afternoon, the ambulance was crowded. Many wounded had come in from the battle on the Crevette heights, and so many more were expected that it was necessary to clear the ambulance as fast as possible.

The wounded men were sitting or lying all around the room, and were in turn inspected and dressed.

We worked hard, and as the autumn evening closed in, we had done all the cases, and Dr. Barkan gave orders, that all wounded brought in during the night should be "littered down" on clean fresh hay, and that all should be ready to begin work at 8 a.m. next morning.

We met Captain Bogovitch as we went back, and he took me into "our quarters." Even by the light of a dull lamp, they looked bright and clean, and they were, as he said, the best in Paratjin.

We shall never forget the kindly consideration of the captain and Dr. Louis Barkan, who had selected a room in a house, next door to the quarters occupied by himself and the other surgeons, so close that we could call over the wall of the yard if we needed anything—an arrangement which afterwards called out the warmest expressions of praise from our kind-hearted countrymen, the English surgeons, for, after all, we were two women alone in the heart of Servia, amidst utter strangers; but we always felt quite safe, and as comfortable as circumstances permitted, and we had the consoling conviction, that good work was to be done here, and that we were more wanted and more useful than ever we were in all our lives before; whilst everyone, high and low, treated us with respect and affection. We were really of service and heartily welcome.

I went home and found a rough supper going on. Louise was a little better, and much cheered by the good news of a clean, quiet home on the morrow, for I had arranged that during the midday rest we would migrate from the hotel.

I discovered some beer in a corner of the *café*, and we had some. The beer lasted till the English ambulance came that way, and then there was a beggarly account of empty bottles; but the "doctors" deserved it, and we could not complain.

The next morning was bright and fair; we went early to ambulance work, and at noon removed to our quarters.

It was a perfect specimen of a Servian house. A wooden gate opened from the road into an orchard, in which stood the house; one side of which, however, was flush with the road.

The door was in the garden end, and you entered a tile-paved hall. A door on the left led into the room we were to occupy—a large cheerful-looking one, two windows to the road, and two into the garden. All round the sides ran a narrow divan, covered with bright rugs and cushions against the walls; a red-tiled floor, a bed in one corner, and the usual iron stove in the other.

Two Serb women met us and kissed our hands; they were very glad, it seemed, to get rid of two Russian princes, and have two English women. Captain Bogovitch lectured them on the duty of the strictest kindness and politeness to us, and left us to arrange our goods and chattels.

There were difficulties about dinner: the rations were uneatable, and we could get nothing else.

We found that a kind of *table d'hôte* took place every day at 12.30 p.m., at the hotel. The charge was a *franc* a head, wine included; and we thought it best to avail ourselves of this, and give up our rations—two cups of weak coffee and two rolls of bread, small and made of Indian corn, were supplied to us from the doctor's table; for breakfast and at night a dish of some kind of meat, and a little soup; but all so bad that we only just managed to eat enough to keep ourselves alive.

The *table d'hôte* was a little better, but it was very scanty. There was soup, followed by the rags of meat they called *boullie*, stewed up with *capsicums* into the national dish, *paprikosh*, then some skinny fowls, and we had done.

Once there were apple-puffs, and I went into the kitchen and tried to buy up the rest of them, but they had been all bought up before.

Every day at dark—about seven o'clock—when ambulance work

was over, Louise laid the cloth—a clean towel—and put out the two glasses we had bought in Paratjin, and for each a pocket-knife and fork; one candle, in a brass candlestick, lighted up the festive board.

Meantime I, with an empty bottle reposing in a large basket, trotted off up the road, sometimes in pouring rain—for the weather had broken up—always ankle-deep in mud, for the transport waggons had cut up the road—and went to the hotel, where the room was at this time of the evening crowded with noisy Russians, and dim with smoke. And here I had the bottle filled with red wine from the cask in the bar. Half a *franc* was charged for this wine, but a little allowance made because I brought my own bottle; and this was for our supper. Later arrived from over the wall our plate of food, and half a loaf of black bread, and with this our supper was complete.

So much for our daily food. We had no newspapers, no books, and were always so very tired that, supper over, we crept thankfully into bed, and woke in the morning to a day exactly similar, the only early excitement being whether we should get our coffee or not, for it was a "movable feast," and it always came accompanied by a message that if the honoured *frauleins* would come immediately, the doctor would meet them and commence work.

The "honoured *frauleins*" were generally first in the field; and by the time the doctors arrived, for they had to look round the hospitals first, we had some men ready for them to see and register.

The men who had arrived in the night and the men who had come too late the evening before to send on, had slept in the room and in the corridors, and were waiting, while all up the road limped and crawled those who had found shelter in private houses.

Skirmishing was going on in front, there had been a battle by Saitchar, and these men found their way, one by one, to the central ambulance.

We had also to go to the hospitals to see to cases which had been sent there.

The Serb hospitals had no communication with the Russian ones. Each nursed their own men, but any Russians who had been in Serb regiments had to come and be registered, and were then sent back to the Russian hospital, to be transferred from thence to Russian hospitals in the rear.

Dr. Georgevitch was the Russian medical officer in command, and received the stores brought by the National Aid Society to the front. He naturally used them for his own hospitals. None ever found their way into the Servian ambulances. Later on, the English surgeons kept some of them for themselves, though they acted under the orders of M. Georgevitch, who had been made Director-General of the Medical Department in the field. He was always spoken of as a kind-hearted, clever, and active man.

Nothing could exceed the perfectly good understanding with which the old Serb chief, Dr. Barkan, and his Serb and Italian subs worked together with us, and wonderful was the jumble of languages—English, Russian, Serb, Roumanian, Wallach, French, German, and Italian; the English confined to Louise and myself, and Dr. Barkan always addressed us in that language, though he used German as a general rule.

He is about the only foreign surgeon we ever met who could ever understand English, and therefore those who go out to a war in a distant land, must know some language besides their own, unless they are serving in a body, and have amongst them two or three who are linguists.

Mr. McKellar is a perfect French and German scholar, and could arrange everything for the surgeons, several of whom spoke both languages.

One incident occurred that deserves notice. At the *table d'hôte* one day an elderly Russian lady came in late; her hair was nearly snow-white, and her face sad and anxious. Some slight civility on our part in making way for her, brought about an acquaintance, and she told us that her only boy, a student, had insisted on volunteering for the war in Servia.

The poor mother gave an unwilling consent, but on condition, that she accompanied the lad to the scene of action.

Being a woman of high position, she obtained leave; indeed, very many Russian officers brought their wives, nominally as nurses, though they never went into ambulance or hospital

This lady went with her son to Deligrad; beyond that she could not go. The troops advanced to the defence of the Crevette heights. All civilians, whatever their rank or employment, were ordered to leave Deligrad, and she, though she lingered to the last, lost sight of her son.

She was now seeking him. She could not hear that he was still with his regiment, and was certain that he was wounded, and in Paratjin.

We offered to assist in the search. The registry of the central ambulance did not give his name. Louise went with her to the Russian hospital. The Princess Czartoriska received them not too graciously, and had no information to give.

Madame then felt assured he was slightly wounded, and left in camp; unless, indeed, he were dead.

Two days went on, when a party of young Russian student volunteers, came down from the camp, and joined the *table d'hôte*. We all fell into conversation.

Louise mentioned the Russian lady, and her search for her son, and one of the students called out that he knew him. He was all right. He had slightly hurt his foot, or would have been down before this.

The lady came in, with her wild, sad look. She had been still searching for her lost boy, and we rushed to her with the good news, followed by the student, cap in hand. The poor woman burst into tears of joy. Dinner was impossible. She went to the transport captain to get horses to go to Deligrad and fetch him; but that day came rumours of coming battle, and strict orders that no one, "except on business," should go beyond Paratjin, and she was obliged to wait for coming events.

Day by day our work grew harder, and more wounded men came in, till that last sad week dawned in sunshine and ended in sorrow,— the week when the last battle was lost and won, and the Turk stood victorious on the so-called impregnable Djunis heights.

CHAPTER 30

Servia's Last Battle

On the morning of the 24th of October, 1876, an orderly came to summon us very early. A crowd of wounded had arrived, and must be sent on as soon as possible.

Off we went, and when we came to the ambulance, we saw that the little green in front was covered with men, some sitting round camp fires, some huddling together in huts of boughs, some lying on the ground, some still in waggons. The front door was blocked with men trying to get in and have their wounds dressed; and we had to go round through the yard. Here were as many more. We pushed our way through, and found the room crowded.

All that day we worked at the taking off the dressings and the re-dressing of the wounds, and as fast as one man was done, another took his place: and when we stood by the table where the dressings were, we were surrounded by a crowd of bleeding creatures, displaying their wounds, and calling on us in piteous tones to help them.

The dusk of an autumn evening closed in. Candles, stuck in bottles, threw a weird light over the scene. More carbolic dressing had to be made—old tablecloths cut up into bandages. The crowd and heat were intense, and the groans and shrieks all around most trying.

Just as things were at their worst, the door opened, and in came Mr. McKellar, his orders gleaming through the dusk. With him were Mr. Gimlet, a surgeon, and Mr. Cumberbatch, Mr. White's private secretary.

Mr. McKellar stopped for no idle greetings, only a shake of the hand, and telling Mr. Cumberbatch he, too, must help, and must go and fetch some bandages and *charpie*, he tucked up the sleeves of his Servian uniform, and went to work.

Dr. Barkan was in charge that day—the senior surgeon had gone to see his wife and children, who were at Tchupria, and send them off to Semendria—and was delighted at this unexpected aid.

We all worked till very late; and Mr. McKellar requested Dr. Barkan to find beds for two or three cases on whom he intended to perform operations, and asked us to take charge of them. He also telegraphed to Mr. White, to say what a fearful state of things was going on in Paratjin, and that we were working hard, and must have help; also, that tents must be sent up to form a front ambulance.

We strolled together to our quarters, and parted. Mr. McKellar and his party were on the road to Lukovo, to see what was going on there, and to bring back his three surgeons to the front by Deligrad; and next morning they left.

Affairs were just as bad next day. All night long waggons brought in wounded; and again, as the evening closed in, the scene was more dreadful than words can express. Again, the door opened, and in came three Englishmen. One of them we recognised as Mr. Barnington Kennett. His exclamation, as he looked around him, showed how horrified he was. The others were Mr. Sandwith—not Humphrey, but a young cousin, one of Sir Edmund Lechmere's surgeons—and his companion, Mr. Brock.

Mr. Kennett suggested taking eight of the worst cases to Belgrade. Dr. Barkan gladly accepted the offer, but this shows how sadly an ambulance was wanted in the front.

Mr. McKellar had left three cases. Mr. Sandwith and Mr. Brock left several more. Eight were to go to Belgrade, a journey of forty-eight hours, in the heavy ambulance waggons. Every one of these should have been safely housed in a good clean ambulance, for to nurse them properly in the Serb hospitals was impossible, more especially as one—the only one where there were unluckily two or three vacant beds—was superintended by the little Italian doctor, who was so stupid and not qualified, and would persist in changing the English dressings as soon as put on, till we gently hinted that no interference could be permitted with the cases belonging to the English doctors.

Mr. Kennett kindly gave us a good store of lint bandages and *charpie*, and next morning departed with his eight wounded to Belgrade. He did his best, as he always did; but if the expense of the waggons, drivers, attendants, and horses were taken into account, as compared with the number of wounded brought to Belgrade, it will be found to have been a very expensive process. I have an impression, but I may be mistaken, that the waggons only made four journeys to the front. If so, they only took thirty-two men, but the accounts of the National

Aid Society, if they are ever given, are so given in the rough, that it is impossible to arrive at a correct idea of details.

Mr. Sandwith and Mr. Brock found a conveyance, and went on to Deligrad.

We were not to be left unaided, for at noon next day back came Mr. McKellar from Lukovo, and with him Mr. Hume and Mr. Boyd, bringing with them the wounded from Lukovo.

Beds had to be found for the worst cases, and they worked hard all day. The gallant young fellows themselves lifted the wounded out of the waggons, placed them on stretchers, and carried them into the room.

More and more wounded arrived, and more severely wounded. We had on the preceding day a sad proportion of men who had wantonly shot off the forefinger of the right hand, so as to incapacitate themselves from further military service; but now we had men with the most hideous wounds, such as might haunt a nightmare dream—some brought in on stretchers who died before we could touch them, some who must die ere morning dawn.

Operations went on all the next day, the men were left in our charge with instructions as to extra diets, which indeed had been given to all the "English" cases: soup, eggs, wine, and *raki*.

Every man had a ticket pinned to him, "English Hospital, Belgrade," and we wrote the same in German over every bed. It was pleasant to see how proud and pleased the men were; how, when we came to them, they pointed to the ticket and smiled, whilst others made signs that they, too, wished to be labelled "English".

It was fully arranged that night between Dr. Barkan and Mr. McKellar, that the weather had broken up too much for tents, and that Dr. Barkan would take up a nice house next door to the ambulance, which we would prepare, and take charge of; that one English surgeon should be left at Paratjin, who could mess with the doctors, and that all the wounded they sent back from the front should be placed there under his care and ours.

This was the exact position of affairs:—

The surgeon-in-chief, Dr. Barkan, finds a house and furniture, and has us, as nurses for it, in whom the English surgeons said they had every confidence.

Extra diets, medicines, and clothes, are to be found by us, the superintendents of this hospital, as the English surgeons needed all their medicines in front, and had no clothes for hospital use of patients; and the beds in this house are to be at the disposal of the English surgeons, who are to send back men from the front, ticketed "English Ambulance, Paratjin," and these cases are to be taken care of till they can return to operate upon them, or, after operation, till they are well enough to be sent to the rear. It would appear a most suitable arrangement.

The National Aid Society had no ambulance in front, had refused to form one, and there was no time to receive fresh orders from England, or to send up stores from Belgrade, so Dr. Barkan stepped in to the rescue, backed up by ourselves and our stores. And yet this well-intentioned proceeding was met by a most discourteous and ungracious letter on Colonel Lloyd-Lindsay's part, who never wishes any work done unless he has the arrangement of it himself; not that he ever does a hand-stroke of ambulance work, or knows anything personally about it. More of this later on.

Early next morning we heard heavy firing, and word came that there was heavy fighting in front.

I went to the hotel to tell Mr. McKellar, and he and his comrades were off as fast as horses could carry them to Deligrad.

Dr. Barkan had got the house, and as the wounded came in but slowly today, we worked at getting it ready, and arranged about stoves, but Captain Bogovitch, who came by that way, suggested that we had better wait till next day to buy them, which looked suspicious.

In the course of the evening I went to send an official telegram to Dr. Sava Petrovitch, and found Captain Bogovitch watching at the office to inspect all telegrams. He was a cousin of Prince Milan's. I asked him how the battle went. "Very badly as yet," he said, frankly.

When we went for our dinner, we found that the front police-post had been removed from Deligrad to Paratjin, and half the room was parted off, and used as a police-office. Every cart or carriage that came was stopped, and not allowed to pass over the bridge, beyond which was the long, main street of Paratjin, with houses—some one-storied, some two-storied—on either hand, and which led on to the Deligrad road.

All that day we heard the boom of the heavy guns and the firing of musketry. It ceased at sunset, and we expected crowds of wounded—none came; but towards night hundreds of unwounded men passed through the streets to the rear.

But we were very tired; too tired even to speculate on what was the probable result of defeat.

When I went to the post-office to look for a stray newspaper and letter which arrived now and then (the *Guardian*, by the way, sent by kind though unknown friends in England, came very regularly), I was handed a telegram from Mr. Boyd to Sir Edmund Lechmere, warning him not to come to Deligrad, as there was heavy fighting in front.

Most English telegrams were brought to us, as the only resident English, to keep till their owners came.

We had heard of Sir Edmund's probable arrival in Servia, but did not know he had come.

We had thought this probable all day, for every wounded man, however bad, had been sent to the rear, and waggons had been going continually down to Jagodina full of wounded; also, many had been told not to stop there, but to go straight on with their load of sufferers, and on going round the hospitals with the extra diets, we had missed several of our English cases. Very few men were left.

That evening on going for our wine, I saw a crowd in the street and a carriage dashing past. It was Prince Milan; he drove amidst dead silence to the palace, just up a street behind the hotel. Whilst watching his progress I saw a body of Cossack cavalry coming over the bridge, with their lances upright, and in the midst an officer and his staff. It was General Tchernaieff, coming in from the front to meet the prince. He, too, went to the palace, and was lost to sight; what passed in that meeting no one knows, but events proved that the prince was convinced further resistance was useless.

Our first sleep was broken by a loud tapping at the glass of the window. We started up. "That's the order to be off," we said, but called out, "Who is there?" in sundry languages.

An English voice answered, "It is I, Spooner, from Belgrade; you have got a telegram for Sir Edmund Lechmere; please give it me."

"All right," we grumbled; "we thought you were the Turks."

We dressed hastily, and let Mr. Spooner in. He had arrived that evening with Sir Edmund and Lady Lechmere, with the intention of going on to Deligrad.

We gave him the telegram. He told us a few pieces of Belgrade news, and then he left, and we slept soundly till early dawn.

The sad story of that day's battle has been most picturesquely told by Archibald Forbes in the *Daily News*. We met him at Jagodina a few days later, and he said that the heights of Djunis ought to have been impregnable.

Another English gentleman told us, that he believed five thousand Englishmen would have held them for six months against the whole

Turkish Army.

The Russians who defended them had been primed with *raki*, as old histories tell us they were, on the night before Inkermann, and the priming had been a little overdone. It might have answered possibly for a wild charge, but it did not answer when men had to stand steady and repulse an attack.

The Turks began to climb the heights. It was said they came up in a splendid style—as the Germans at Spicheren. They were cool, and steady, and sober, and Abdul Kerim Pasha was one of their best generals. The Serbs saw this; it was hopeless to defend the heights against such odds; why should they stay to be slaughtered? They owed the Russians many a heavy grudge; they would not be killed to help them, so they tucked their muskets under their arms, and quietly walked away to Paratjin, and to home in the villages and towns beyond.

It was said, and on good authority, that 4,000 Russians fell that day. The same number was given me afterwards by the Russian adjutant, whom we had met on board the *Deligrad,* and who burst into tears as he told the tale.

Is it therefore surprising, that there is, even at the present moment, between the people of Servia and the Russians, an honest, hearty hatred?

If Russia gains her ends, she cares little what becomes of Servia, and this the Serbs know well. It is only the Russian party in the government who profess any respect or affection for Russia. The people know well what all the cant of "holy cause" means, and nothing will force them into active measures to aid the Russians.

The militia may be called; you may "call spirits from the vasty deep," but will they come when you do call them? The militia may not flock to the standards in the numbers they did in 1876—certainly cannot, for so great was the number of wounded, enfeebled, or crippled for life—so great also the number of men rendered unfit for military service, by their own act, that there must be a serious diminution on the rolls, and if they do respond, it will be as an apathetic, unwilling body of men, from whom hope and enthusiasm have been crushed out together, not by the cruelties of the Turk, but by the iron hand of the Russian.

Those who live at a distance cannot judge of their feelings; those who only rushed up to the front and down again, do not know the Serbs.

We do not profess that these, our opinions, are infallible. We relate faithfully what we saw and heard, and the impressions we deduced from all that went on around us, and we leave it to our readers to decide if these impressions are correct or not.

Chapter 31

The Retreat

The sun was shining but faintly when we woke next morning, and when we went to the ambulance there was a strange stillness and emptiness about the place.

We had seen the Russian ambulance waggons with all the stores pass down the street as we left the house, and when we entered the ambulance, Dr. Barkan sat there, idly scribbling on a bit of paper.

A few men were scattered about, and we prepared to begin work. "The orderlies have dressed them as best they could," he said. "The order has come to evacuate the town; the wounded are nearly all gone. I shall see that you go when we do; you had better go and get all ready."

We went back, and while Louise finished our small preparations, I went to the hotel to hear the latest news.

I met in the street the Circassian prince and the adjutant. I recognised many a Russian we had known on the *Deligrad*, even our friend of the grey fur dress, but our singer of comic songs was nowhere; he had fallen at Djunis.

The street was crowded, huge cannon were being dragged to the rear; waggons of wounded were going slowly along. I recognised some of our men in them, and, strange to say, amidst all that fearful confusion, one of the men ticketed "English ambulance" made his way down to the hospital at Belgrade.

The hotel was more crowded than ever, officers were shouting, half-drunken men lying about, waggons packing in the yard, horsemen dashing past. Captain Bogovitch and Herr Hadji Thoma seizing every pair of horses they could, to take somebody or something to the rear.

The telegraph was receiving and sending a perfect storm of messages. The prince was in his palace. General Tchernaieff with him; nobody could find anybody else, and still down the broad street went the great guns, slowly dragged along by teams of oxen, and men sullenly tramping over the stones inch deep in mud; while amongst the mob, carts made their way, laden with all the household goods of the flying villagers—frightened women, tugging the tired horses along, and large-eyed children sitting amidst the cocks and hens on the top, the cow and calf tied behind, all the stock, except the pigs, who as a refugee told me, were as obstinate as the pigs of other lands, and would not go forwards, but backwards, and so were left for the Turks.

After the manner of the Serbs in general, I thought. Oddly enough, when some of these refugees went back, they found their pigs still grubbing about. Was this owing to the fact that the pig is regarded as an unclean animal by Mussulmen?

When I entered the hotel, I found Mr. Spooner and Lady Lechmere. Of course, the *Deligrad* expedition was given up, and they were about to return to Belgrade. Had there been time to send a telegram there they probably would not have started, as all the horses had more to do than they could get through, and every additional person or carriage added to the work; whilst the wounded, whom they came to look after, had all been sent to the rear. Sir Edmund Lechmere was in the yard unpacking some quinine for distribution. If they had arrived a few days before, it would have been of great use, and it was most kind of him to bring it.

I asked them to take our little chest of valuable medicines. They had no room for us, as two wounded Russians were going with them to Jagodina.

I met the captain of transport in the passage. "You are going with Herr Lechmere?" he said.

"No," I answered; "they have no room."

His brow clouded over. "I know not where to find more horses," he said.

Captain Bogovitch came up hastily. "I will arrange," he said. "Come with me, Herr Thoma; some of the prince's horses are standing in the stable. We will send the English ladies with a pair to Semendria."

No, thank you," I said. "We are ordered to follow the wounded to Jagodina. Why Jagodina; can you tell me, Herr Hadji Thoma?"

"Because," he answered, "the Turks may come up and cut off the road by Tchupria; beyond Tchupria is the second line of defence, and if we fight again, it is there that the struggle will take place."

"And why are we off in such a hurry?"

"Do not say a word," he replied, "to create more panic. There is not a man or a gun between us and the Turks."

"Pleasant news!" I remarked. "And why are they not here already?"

"Just because they never follow up a victory. They might easily have been here last night. They will probably arrive tomorrow. When will you be ready to go?"

"After dinner; about two o'clock. We *must* see the ambulances cleared first."

"The Russians went off at daybreak," remarked Captain Bogovitch, "and left some of their wounded to be sent on after them."

"So, it appears," I said. "Then you think we must go today?"

"Yes, certainly. Besides, there is no work here now, and all the civilians will have to evacuate tomorrow."

I went home, and found all ready. The day had changed to dull, gloomy, depressing weather; and the circumstances were depressing—fear, and flight, and terror all around; a broken army retreating piecemeal to the rear; a cruel foe in front.

The Turks had not stirred as yet. So said the people coming in from the outlying villages. We had breathing time, and we went round the hospitals. Not one man remained in them. We went into the central ambulance. In one corner was a stretcher, on which lay a poor fellow, whom they had taken from his bed to put into a waggon. He was dressed once more in his blue coat (he was a regular); but he was going a longer journey than to Jagodina—he was dying—his breast heaving heavily, and his eyes closing. The orderlies sat around in silence; and one, bringing a lighted taper, crossed his hands, and put it into them.

We stood silently by, and in a few minutes all was over. We closed his eyes, and bade the orderlies bury him before they left, and mark the place.

He was the last of the patients left. Our work was over; and we went to fetch our baggage, and start for Jagodina.

Herr Hadji was at the hotel, rejoicing: the prince had most gladly lent us a pair of horses, and capital ones they were. Our medicine chest had gone in the carriage to Belgrade, and for us they had found a waggon with plenty of clean hay, in which we nestled, with our few goods and chattels around us. The captain and the *herr* bade us, not farewell, but "*au revoir*" and we rattled down the road to Tchupria, a warning cry from the driver, one of the prince's servants, making everyone pull aside to let us pass. How we bumped along! The good man could not have driven faster if the *Bashi Bazouks* had been behind. But the horses had to be back in Paratjin that evening for the prince's use next day.

It was not dusk when we reached Tchupria, and crossed the Morava, and beyond it saw the lines, with men working to strengthen and complete them; but we did not stay our progress to inspect them.

We passed many waggons of wounded, and many wounded men who could walk, all on their way to Jagodina.

It was said in one English paper at the time, that as the prince passed through the streets of Paratjin the wounded were lying about.

This was simply not the case. Every wounded man came to the ambulance, and was sent on from thence. They could not pass the sentinels on the bridge, or the police-post at the hotel, without giving their name and number, and were not permitted to pass out of the town without the ticket, of which I have spoken, to say to which rear hospital they were to go. The later ones, who could travel far, were all ordered to Semendria. No nearer place was considered safe: and even the wounded from Tchupria, in care of a capital Roumanian ambulance, had been sent to the rear.

All that department was in most perfect order, as far as Tchupria: beyond, as we shall see, there was confusion and misery, easily accounted for. While order was still preserved in front, where the headquarters' staff was stationed, it naturally fell off in the rear. The farther from the scene of action, the wilder were the rumours. It was believed at Jagodina, when we arrived, that the Turks were in Paratjin, and Krushevatz; but, as I have said, amidst all the confusion, there was perfect order at Paratjin.

I was in the street when the prince arrived, and therefore can speak certainly. There was no single wounded man there, except in waggons. It would have been our duty, had we seen such a scene, to report it at once, and have the men taken to ambulance, to be fed, have their wounds dressed, and be registered.

A few were sent on without their wounds being touched, but only as far as Jagodina, and because the waggons could not be delayed; but every man was registered, and the orderlies from every Serb hospital went with their wounded.

The order of evacuation ran,—first, the wounded; then their attendants, doctors, and nurses; then the authorities of the town, with their archives and business papers; next, the general public (who might get away meantime as best they could, and must not stay beyond their turn); and, lastly, the military.

Dusk was just closing in at evening time when we reached Jagodina, a town of one long street, like Paratjin; but the roofs of the one-storied houses extended over the side pavement of red tiles, and so formed covered walks.

We drove up to the best hotel, and were thankful to get a bedroom. But that hotel was worse than Paratjin.

There was a *café*, off which opened a room for dinners beyond; instead of the usual yard was a passage with bedrooms on either side, and at the end of the passage was the stable, full of horses.

Our room was very small, and half full of plants put by for the winter. No single comfort or even convenience of life was there—a dirty bed, a table stained with wine and ink, and on which lay tobacco ashes and relics of the last tenant; no chair, no *toilette* apparatus, but a wooden stool in the corner, with a small cracked basin and an empty jug.

The smell of the stable penetrated into the room; and the trampling of the horses, and the jingling of the chains that held them to the crib, went on by day and night.

We looked around in dismay, but it was of no use, so we made the bed, with our waterproof-sheet over the dirty mattress and our own sheets over that, a railroad-rug and a shawl for blanket and counterpane, and our pillow-slips over the heavy cushions that represented pillows; and then we went to supper with what appetite we might, and finding the dining-room full of Serb officers—who had never been to the front, and were accordingly in most valiant mood and very bright uniforms—we withdrew to a corner, and the host, who was most kind and courteous, brought us some roast turkey, well cooked and nicely served.

The cuisine of that hotel was the best in Servia—except at Belgrade—and for the information of future travellers, I may state that the cook (an Austrian by birth) is gone to the hotel at Kragojevatch, which can therefore be well recommended.

We sent off telegrams to Drs. Barkan and Sava Petrovatz at Belgrade, telling the one where we were, and asking the other for orders. The Paratjin one did not get an answer, which we attributed, and rightly as it seemed, to the crowded state of the wires, for it did not reach for two days afterwards. The Belgrade one brought an answer, but it left us to judge for ourselves, as evidently nothing was settled; and we decided to await the arrival of Dr. Barkan, who was expected next day.

We were not of course aware that an armistice was being arranged, nor did we know it till we reached Semendria. We fully expected to have to work at Jagodina, and resolved to adopt the Paratjin plan—get a room as quarters in the town, and dine at the hotel.

The fugitives had not of course come on as fast as we had. Many halted for the night at Tchupria, in spite of the fear of the Turks cutting off the road. Their tired horses could get no farther, and the bullock waggons made a whole day's journey of the distance, and of course had halted for the night.

The officers soon dropped off, a few Russian soldiers disposed themselves to sleep on the benches in the *café* and dining-room. Jagodina subsided, and we tried to sleep amidst the smell of india-rubber, stables, and plants, and the noises of the said stables. Sleep under such circumstances can never be very refreshing, and we woke in the morning feeling very much as if we had been sitting up all night.

CHAPTER 32

From Jagodina to Semendria

We vainly expected news next day; it poured with rain, and everything looked cheerless. Where were our friends? and where were the Turks? We felt sad and dull all day. Next morning, suddenly, while sitting with our room-door open, we heard English voices—how pleasantly they sounded!—and directly afterwards out of the room opposite, came two gentlemen, one of whom was the very Dr. Costello whom we had left in Belgrade, and the other an American surgeon from Vienna, Dr. Bodemann, and we met as old friends and agreed to dine together.

In the course of the morning our heavy baggage came down from Paratjin, but the drivers only said that Herr Hadji Thoma had said "Go to Jagodina with the baggage." The Paratjin people were some of them coming away, and some of them staying there, and no one knew anything of the Turks.

This was incomprehensible. Dr. Costello and Dr. Bodemann had come away in all haste from Krushevatz, but still this was nearer to Djunis than Paratjin, and this was the second time that everyone had been ordered to leave the town. Certainly, the Turks had not advanced. What were they about?

In the evening came another Englishman, who was working with Dr. Ziemann, and at noon next day Dr. Ziemann himself.

He was on his way to Djunis, in spite of the Turks, to see what had become of the wooden barracks he had built there for the refugees, and more especially of the blankets, with which he had provided them. He was sure that the Turks had got the blankets, and he should go and claim them back.

How we all laughed, and wished he might get them; but such a brave, energetic, cheerful man was never seen. Our spirits rose as we chatted together, though we all were puzzled what to do and where to go.

Reports were more bewildering than ever; all that we could find out by inquiring at the hospitals was that they were full from Tchupria—the waggons from which of course had got before us to Jagodina; and that the Paratjin waggons had gone through in the night to Semendria. Posharevatz was now spoken of as the centre of work, but this looked unlikely.

There was nothing for it but to wait, and amuse ourselves as best we could, and employment suddenly sprung up. Dr. Costello and Dr. Bodemann had gone out in search of under garments; they could procure none, and they came back, and in most hesitating tones suggested that if we would renew the kind offer we had made of furnishing them with a few articles, they would gratefully accept it.

We on our part said that one of our boxes had come nearly to pieces, and if they would open it and mend it, and take out what they wanted, they would be more than welcome. We had sent for a Serb carpenter, who positively refused to come, on the ground that he himself was packing up.

No sooner said than done; the two gentlemen went to work with a will. We entirely unpacked one chest, and Dr. Bodemann mended it in most workmanlike style. This occupied all the afternoon; all we wanted was news. We had a cheerful supper together.

On the 3rd of November, which was next day, it poured in torrents, but I went to see for telegrams from Paratjin. While I was in the office came the official news of peace, or at least of a prolonged armistice. This was indeed good news, and we all rejoiced. We resolved to go to Belgrade as soon as possible, and I went to get horses and a waggon. The transport captain, on my giving the name of Herr Hadji Thoma, promised us a conveyance at 8 a.m. next day, and Dr. Ziemann did get one to Paratjin.

We were up bright and early on the morning of the 4th, but the Russians walked off with our waggon, and in despair I went to try and hire a conveyance. Dr. Bodemann had asked us as a favour to take to Semendria his late landlord, Herr Johann, a merry, humpbacked little tailor, who had been obliged to fly from Krushevatz, to which place he had returned after the first exodus, having left his wife and children in Austria. He was an Austrian, and spoke capital German. We had consented, and never was a common act of kindness so well repaid.

Little Herr Johann ran about with me; he was very anxious to get to Semendria to catch the boat to Basiach, and at last he found a waggon and horses, which we hired, at a reasonable price for war, though an exorbitant one for peace time—about two sovereigns of English money.

Our baggage was packed, and we were ready, when to our horror the horses were taken out to be shod, a process, including the driver's dinner, of two hours.

We got off at 1 p.m., leaving our heavy baggage to follow. Dr. Bodemann and Dr. Costello most kindly taking charge of it, and we crawled out of the town and along the road beyond.

Herr Johann then discovered that the driver did not intend to go farther than Barzan that night, intending to reach Semendria the night after, and though we begged him to go one post beyond, he persisted that Barzan was the best place to stop at.

When we drove up to this posting hotel, we found it full of Russians, and no beds to be had, and were advised not to go to the next post, as they knew that was full too; but to turn off the road to the left, and go a couple of miles to Baterschin, a large village, where we should find accommodation.

Evening was closing in, the sudden evening of lands that have no twilight, and before we had gone a mile to the left it was dark.

We drove along a narrow road where the boughs of the trees met over our heads, and not a sound was to be heard. How glad we were to have Herr Johann, who spoke Serb perfectly.

Suddenly we saw the red glare of fire through the trees. It was the watch-fire of some Serb soldiers who were sleeping around it, and camped about were the heavy waggons going to the rear, which had halted for the night.

No one interfered with us, and we groped along. At last we emerged into the open and came into a town; but this place was full of the officers and soldiers of the 3rd Reserve, called up to defend the last lines. They were drinking and singing, and did not believe in the peace.

Every hotel and *café* were crowded, and Herr Johann at last went to the house of the Captain of the Town and demanded quarters for us.

We waited quietly in the waggon, and presently found ourselves surrounded by several officials. We sat up in the hay, in as dignified a way as circumstances permitted, wondering what was the matter, and found that they were in the most polite way requesting us to accept the hospitality of someone nearby. We bowed our thanks and retreated from the pouring rain into the hay.

The waggon went slowly on, Herr Johann splashing by the side through the mud. It stopped, and a servant-girl with a lantern came to the side; we got out and found ourselves at the end of a long passage, between two houses, covered in, but open at each end; going on through this, we came to the yard with its covered corridors and rooms off it.

A bright-eyed, pleasant-looking woman welcomed us, and showed us into a charming room with a bed, actually a clean bed with a coverlet of lace lined with blue silk!

If we had been old friends instead of stray strangers, we could not have been more kindly treated. We produced our own supper from our basket, gave Herr Johann some, and, refusing to trouble the kind hostess for coffee, showed her our bottle of Négotin wine; we made each other perfectly understand that we came from Paratjin on account of the "*Turken*," and were going to Semendria, and that we had been nursing the wounded.

She soon left us, and we enjoyed a good night's rest in the clean, sweet bed. Herr Johann promised to call us at 3 a.m., as he said we should have a long day of it to Semendria, and ought to be there before dark.

It did not seem that we had slept an hour, before his tap came at the window, and we started up and struck a light. It poured with rain, and was pitch dark.

The good woman got up and insisted on making some hot coffee. I was too anxious about the waggon and the baggage, and the coming day, to take any. We thanked her as best we could, and, as she had brought her children to see us, we put a silver *gulden* in the baby-boy's hand.

We never knew who she was, or what she was—that she played the part of a good Samaritan to houseless strangers we do know; and we shall always hold her in grateful remembrance. The maid and the lantern lighted us to our waggon, and we started.

At first all went well, except that the rain would penetrate through the tent that covered our vehicle, and that it was so dark we could not see the horses' heads. At last we turned into the main road as day was breaking, and here began our troubles.

With daybreak the heavy rain of the night changed into cold sleet, and bitter wind; we tried to shelter ourselves, in vain, it seemed to penetrate the very bones, and we vainly hoped that as day grew on it would get better, but instead of that, it got very much worse.

We were now on the main road; the mud was ankle deep; the horses splashed into it at every step, and our progress was naturally very slow.

It was broad daylight, when we stopped at the first post-house to rest the horses and let the driver breakfast.

By this time, we were perfectly benumbed, and the bitter wind seemed to blow even more keenly as we stood still.

Herr Johann came out and said there was nothing to be had but *paprikosh* and "*raki*," and implored us to take a little of the latter. It was so nasty and fiery, that we turned from it in disgust, and tried to warm each other by keeping close and covering ourselves quite up. Our feet ached with cold, in spite of the hay; and the driver was so long over his miserable breakfast that we sent in a dozen messages, and at last he came and we started off again.

We never wish to think of the sufferings of that day and the scenes around us.

We were now on the main road, along which tramped the fugitives of the defeated army—some so worn and weary that they laid down by the roadside and died where they lay; some struggling on to the last; all around mud, and sleet, and cruel wind. Half a dozen held on to our waggon, which was going at foot pace; it afforded them a little shelter, for the wind was straight ahead. We passed waggons with wounded in them, and wounded men tramping along; we could not help them, all were involved in one common trouble. How we could live through the day was our thought.

We covered up our faces with shawls and blankets; we could not look out, the sleet so cut our faces.

Slowly the morning hours rolled on, and at last, in spite of the wind and sleet, we got at our basket and the liqueur.

We were faint with cold and getting sleepy, and I verily believe it saved our lives. We gave some to poor Herr Johann, who was sitting in front, and so arranged the waterproof-sheet as to give him some of it; the snow lay upon it, here and there melted into pools, and we also gave him a small blanket.

It was past noon when we stopped at Orissa, and pulled up at an hotel. With difficulty we got out and entered it, taking with us our wet shawls and rugs.

There was a fire in an iron stove in the middle of the room, and the master offered to light us one in a private room. This we accepted, as we could dry our things.

We ordered some dinner, and while waiting for it about a dozen of the wretched fugitives came slowly in and crept to the fire. A long consultation ensued amongst them, and they produced a couple of *piastres*—all they had—and asked for some *raki*.

This would entitle them to stay for a few minutes by the fire.

We asked Herr Johann to inquire of them where they were going.

It appears that they had walked from Deligrad here, and were going to Belgrade. They had spent every farthing they had till they got to Semendria, where they would report themselves to the Captain of the Town. Some of their comrades were weak and sickly, they had fallen behind, and then all was over.

We suggested to Herr Johann that we would pay for *paprikosh* and *raki*, with a large loaf of bread each. The hot *capsicums* in the hash would be good for them.

Herr Johann explained, and they rose as well as their stiffened limbs permitted and touched their caps with some Serb expressions of thankfulness.

After dinner we started again, dried and refreshed; but the rain and sleet were as bad as ever, and we got very tired and worn. At last, at sunset, the clouds broke, and we rose up to breathe the air. We were coming into a town, and we hoped it was Semendria; but no, the horses tramped on through the mud, and now the driver quickened their pace, and we drove through a large village looking cheerful in the sunlight.

We always regretted that we did not halt there for the night. We should have avoided much trouble; but we pushed on, and darkness fell on the way.

We seemed an age going up a steep road between high trees, and then down again; we were so weary now, and Louise feeling very faint from the effects of the cold. It was just here that, two nights afterwards, wolves attacked the horses of the English ambulance. A little farther on and the lights of Semendria came in view, and soon we were rattling over those dreadful stones once more, having been twenty-two hours on a ten hours' journey.

We drove up to the hotel; not a bed to be had! I invaded the dining-room and found Baron Mundy, the Inspector of Hospitals. He sent out a surgeon with me to a private house. Everywhere every bed was taken up for Tchernaieff and his staff, and had been so for two days.

Now, as Tchernaieff's staff amounted—when he did come—to about ten gentlemen, none of whom objected to sleeping half a dozen in a room, this was perfectly absurd, but was only one instance of his profound arrogance and selfishness.

We tried every hotel in vain, and Louise was now so ill that she implored us to get the waggon into some covered stable or yard, and let her lie there, but this I could not think of, the hay was so damp.

One more wretched *cafané* remained, and here Herr Johann tried, and this time with success. One dirty room was vacant, and while I saw to our wraps, Herr Johann nearly carried her in and laid her on the rude bed.

The room smelt of dirt, but I made up such a bed as I could and gave her what food we had left. She was too ill to eat, and I could only trust to sleep to restore her.

The morning revealed the filthiness of the place. Herr Johann brought some coffee, and I told him that we could not remain there. I found that the steamer for Belgrade was not to start till next day, and said I should go to the hotel, find the Captain of the Town, and demand quarters.

I set off and missed my way back. The intelligence was that there was no bedroom in the only practicable hotel, and that I could not see the captain till eleven o'clock, but that we could go and get our breakfasts there; so ordering our waggon, we got ourselves and our traps together, and set off for the hotel.

Herr Johann's traps consisted of one bundle, containing a shirt and a pair of boots, all that remained, as he said, of his house and thirty years' work; but never mind, land could not run away, he should go back some day, and he should be sure at least to find his pigs.

Many months later we heard that he did go back, and, as the Turks had never entered Krushevatz, found his home and furniture as he had left it.

I propped up Louise in a chair by a sunny window; and she looked so ill that even the waiter who brought our coffee pitied us both, and told me to go into the dining-room and find another waiter, whom he described.

I followed his advice, and told my new friend that I would give him a silver *gulden* to find us a room. He looked cunning, and in ten minutes came to fetch us, and took us upstairs to a room just vacated by some officer gone on temporary duty to Belgrade, whose muddy saddle, sword, and belt were piled on a table in the corner.

Two good-natured Austrian girls were remaking the bed, and hastened to get it ready. I never felt more thankful than when I laid

Louise down to rest at last, in comfort and clean sheets. She was still shivering with cold, but a large fire was lighted in the room and threw its heat into the iron stove, as well as looking cheerful, when the door of the stove was opened.

About 7 p.m. she was so much better that I persuaded her to come down and have some dinner, and directly afterwards we went upstairs and locked the door, in case Tchernaieff and his staff should arrive.

This long-expected event took place about eleven at night, and the noise and clatter were something appalling. Our room-door was violently shaken, but resisted all attempts, and when the "staff" had retired we slept soundly.

There was bright sunlight next morning; the steamer was to arrive about 11 a.m., and when I went to the wharf, I saw the large barge of the English ambulance, which was to be towed with us to Belgrade.

It was splendidly arranged, but it only made two or three voyages; it was too late, and the expense must have been very great.

Noon passed, and no signs of the steamer; about two o'clock she was reported in sight, but a long way off; and we ordered our baggage down to the wharf and I went to see our order carried out.

The river being low, a broad expanse of slippery mud lay between the actual bank and the water, and over this I had to make my way. Baron Mundy kindly helped me over some very slippery parts, and I began to wonder how I could pilot Louise, weak as she was, over such a difficult path.

I turned to go back when all was done, and then I saw an astounding sight!

Louise was coming slowly but safely along on the arm of a huge Cossack, dressed in the usual fur-lined coat. He had to stoop on one side, as he supported her with one strong arm, and under the other were tucked her shawl and a little blue-striped pillow, our companion in many wanderings.

Not a word was exchanged. Slowly and solemnly they came over the slippery ground, till they arrived on the wooden wharf; here he deposited her on our portmanteau, her shawl and pillow beside her, and with a low bow withdrew.

"How on earth did you know that man?" I asked.

"I did not know him," Louise said. "I wanted to follow you, and I began to slide about; he came up, took my shawl and pillow from me, and put my arm through his. He never spoke a word."

"And a perfect gentleman he is," I said, "whoever he may be; he saw you in trouble, and helped you out of it!"

This day was a strange exception to the bitter cold of the preceding ones, and the snow that fell next morning. It was as lovely as a June day in England, and we enjoyed sitting on the wharf and looking around us.

The ambulance barge was anchored close by. Two of the English surgeons were there, and we watched with interest the stretchers coming along over the rough broken ground, bearing the wounded to the barge. They were principally Russians, from hospitals in Semendria, going to the hospital at Topschedery, near Belgrade.

But how gently and tenderly did Mr. Hume and Mr. Boyd see that those stretchers were carried carefully on board, and themselves help when some rougher place than usual had to be traversed.

They looked so bright and cheerful too, models of brave-hearted, merry English gentlemen, not afraid of hard work, not ashamed of showing that they could be as gentle as a woman.

At last the steamer came, and we got on board. When all was ready, and the barge had "fallen in" behind, we still waited till General Tchernaieff made his appearance with the staff, and walked grandly on board.

But this gentleman deserves a more detailed description than befits the end of a chapter, for we have seen many generals, victorious ones too, but never one half so high and mighty as General Tchernaieff.

Chapter 33

Belgrade Under the Russians

General Tchernaieff was a short man, by no means of imposing appearance; his eyes were small, with heavy lids; his nose, large; his complexion, a muddy red; and his hair and moustache of no particular colour.

His manners were as reserved and haughty as if he had been a successful and celebrated man—indeed, rather more so.

Though not a large man, he required a great deal of room. There was a deck cabin, which was taken up by his staff, for his smoking-room. On going down below, I was entering one of the ladies' cabins, when a young *aide-de-camp* greeted me with, "Get out; dis de General dining-room." I retreated, and tried the ladies' cabin the other side, with no better success: this was "de General sleep-room."

Luckily, a steward came by, and to him I appealed, and he turned furiously on the Russian.

"What do you mean," he said, "by taking up all the cabins? You may have that one for all of you," pointing to the first cabin. "There are not many ladies on board, and we shall be at Belgrade before night; but this one you cannot have."

"General Tchernaieff requires it," was the surly answer.

"Does he?" said the Austrian steward. "Let me tell you, these ladies pay for their passage as well as your master, and English gold is better than Russian any day."

The *aide-de-camp* retreated, and the cabin remained free.

These said *aides-de-camp* were very young men, with wasp-like waists, and shakos with plumes of white feathers.

Their clothes were so clean and new, their gold aiguillettes and sword-belts so bright, that we came to the conclusion that they had left them in Semendria before they went on the campaign, and picked them up as they came back.

The general and his *aides* grouped together on the deck, and looked contempt at the outer barbarians. We were infinitely amused at this, but still more so with the Austrians.

The boat was, of course, an Austrian one, and on board were three or four Austrian officers, who, like all their nation, were most courteous and polished, speaking German with so soft an accent as to take away all its harshness.

They smiled good-humouredly at the airs and graces of "the Cossacks," as they called them; but they kept their own place, and were not to be put out of temper, or out of the way, by the fussiness of the *aides-de-camp*.

When dinner came on, we all placed ourselves at the long tables; but a great delay took place in serving.

The *aides* hovered in the passage, and seizing the dishes carried them off into the general's dining-room.

At last, an Austrian officer, with half a dozen orders on his breast rose up, marched into the passage, seized the two waiters, and made them deposit the dishes they bore on the table in the saloon; after which we helped ourselves.

So, the day passed on. In the evening some men of the crew sang songs on the quarter-deck; and the general condescended to listen, and even to smile, on which all the staff smiled too.

It was dusk when we reached Semlin, and the Austrian officers landed, and quite dark as we steamed up to the wharf at Belgrade.

We noticed an unusual number of lights on the wharf. The general and his staff hurried to the side of the ship, to be ready to leave it first; and then we saw a group of officers, with crimson shakos and white plumes, and soldiers bearing lighted torches attending them.

It was Prince Milan and his staff. He had come back from Paratjin by road, and passed through Jagodina by night, therefore we had not seen him; and he had come to meet General Tchernaieff.

But none of the people were there. No popular greeting met the unsuccessful Russian general. In silence he landed, and was conveyed away in the prince's carriage.

For ourselves, we were thankful to be greeted by M. Dilbert's apprentice, who had been sent to meet us by his master, to whom we had telegraphed from Semendria, and who was at the hospital on duty.

He led us up the steep steps into a brightly-lighted hotel, called the "National," where we were tolerably comfortable.

The snow lay deep on the ground next day, when we went to the

War Office. Herr Sava Petrovatz welcomed us warmly, and was very anxious that we should work at the military hospital in Belgrade if many wounded came down; but, as it turned out, not many did, and most of those were Russians, and taken into their three hospitals.

These Russian hospitals were the despair of good Baron von Mundy. It is impossible to enter into any details as regards the lady medical students who acted in them as nurses. Sufficient to say, that no Englishwoman with any notion of self-respect could work in them, even if she were allowed to do so; and that a high official and an experienced judge told us, that "the Russian ambulances and hospitals were models of everything that they should not be."

The Russian Red Cross Society is enormously wealthy; they took stores back from Servia unused that would supply fifty ambulances. It cannot be too often repeated, that they will accept no personal help, and need no other.

Various societies are now appealing for help for the Eastern sick and wounded; but let the English people before they respond to these appeals ask one solemn question, and demand a decided reply:—*Do the Russians or Turks give quarter?* Do they not slaughter every man that falls into their hands?

The Servians did give quarter till the Russians came; after that *none was given on either side.* The proof of this is, that in all Servia there was but one wounded Turk, and we have every reason to believe there were no wounded Serbs or Russians in the Turkish ambulances.

Is it right to send assistance to such savages?

It is a premium on murder. A man whose hands are red with the blood of some helpless and wounded enemy—is he to come back, possibly wounded himself, and be treated with every care and kindness? Humanity itself revolts against it.

It matters not what the theory is; it matters not what nominal orders are given from headquarters; we know what the practice is—*no quarter is given.*

But, to return to Belgrade, we had to tramp through snow and mud. Every carriage was taken up by the Russians. Every hotel was full of them except two—the National and the Hirsch, which refused to receive them.

At the National a Russian officer had kicked a poor woman with his spurred boot, because he thought she had cheated him of a *piastre*; and the Hirsch was kept by an Austrian, between whom and the Russians there seems to exist an hereditary hatred.

Then we called on Herr Philip Christich, He was depressed, but not despairing. He had great hopes that a European Conference would do much for the Slav provinces, and blamed the late war as rash and useless. He kept much aloof now from the court, which was overrun by Russians.

Our days in Belgrade passed slowly along, but we waited there for two things—first, to see if we were required for any work, and next by request till the statutes of the Order of the Takova were altered, so that it could be given to women, and that our crosses might be presented to us.

We found our old friends, Ignace and Marie of the Hirsch, had taken an hotel, which they proposed calling "The Crown Prince of Servia," and were to get into it in a few days; and they begged us to go with them into their new abode. We had no particular affection for the "National," though the people were perfectly civil. It was so much out of the way; and therefore, we did migrate, much to our regret afterwards, owing solely to the Russians.

A specimen of our life at the "Crown Prince" will be a fair specimen of what the Servians suffered from the Russians.

It appeared that this hotel had been for some time so far shut up that it did no business, and therefore it had been taken up as quarters by the Russians.

When Ignace took it, and occupied it, he gave them notice to quit, and they refused to go. They paid about two *francs* a room a night, and a dozen or so slept in one room. They were not profitable tenants, and the habit they had of sitting up all night gambling and drinking was an uncomfortable one for other guests.

The principal offender was the "*Herr Major*," a brute of a Russian, belonging to the Presbajinsky Guards, whose one aim in life was to insult everybody who was not a Ruski, and who hated the English with a bitter hatred.

One of them on hearing that we were English spat at my feet, and on my asking if he did that on purpose to insult my country, he did it again.

Louise was so far from well that she had to remain much in her room, and when I went out on business I was obliged to leave her locked up and take the key, for, if not, the Russian officers would open the door and annoy her by rough and insulting remarks in German.

We should have gladly left but that, besides the reasons I have given, Louise was not fit to travel. Dr. Humphrey Sandwith and Baron

Mundy both ordered change of air, but we could not venture to start.

One day there was a great dinner in the place. I went down and had a struggle to get something for us to eat. Poor Marie bewailed her fate, and "excommunicated" the Russians, and I got leave to walk off with what I liked, and carried it upstairs.

The band of the headquarters staff was crammed into the *café*, and nearly blew the roof off with their brass instruments, and the noise went on till daybreak.

About midnight a quarrel broke out: Ignace refused to supply more champagne, till some of what had been drunk had been paid for, and a Russian officer drew his sword and tried to cut Ignace down. Some Serbs present in the *café* interfered, and a "free fight" ensued.

The police came in and the quarrel subsided; but a *fracas* was always occurring, and there was no redress; all wrongs committed by Russians, all complaints against them, were to be laid before the general—Russians were not amenable to Servian laws. They paid what they liked, and did what they liked, and there was no redress.

The poor people of Belgrade groaned and said "they should prefer Abdul Kerim Pasha," who was at Alexinatz; and really we thought he could not have been so cruel, and his soldiers would have been more sober.

Just about this time I had a message from the English Consul that I was to go and see him when convenient; so, wondering what he wanted, I betook myself there and met the usual kindly reception. He apologised for troubling me—"he knew all about it, but Lloyd-Lindsay had written, or rather his secretary, to ask by 'what failure of duty on the part of the officials of the National Aid Society in Servia, it had been left to Miss Pearson and Miss McLaughlin to do their work'"—or some such phrase.

They had seen our letter in the *Times*, and I will quote the paragraph that offended their lordships.

Extract from letter in *Times* of November 3rd, 1876:—

Paratjin, October, 26th, 1876.

The great want here is some place in which to receive the severely wounded sent back from the front. They have only open waggons to travel in, and the weather is bitterly cold. It is here that the National Aid Society should have had their hospital, not in Belgrade, where it is not wanted; but if a small one could be opened, it need not be so luxurious, or with such wastefully costly fittings as the Katherine Hospital in Belgrade. Something much more rough, ready, and inexpensive would do, and could be carried on at a trifling cost. We have, however, through the kindness of Dr. Barkan, one of the chief surgeons here, procured a ward in the ambulance for five beds, which will be at the disposal of the English surgeons (now all in the front), and under our special care, and we may be able to find another somewhere else. We are thus working hard and happily together, though personally we have nothing to do with the National Aid Society, nor have we received one farthing from it, and we shall furnish the extra diets required out of the funds intrusted to us by our kind friends. We are glad thus to be able to help the National Aid Society in the style of the little mouse that gnawed the rope that bound the lion

We cannot conclude without paying a just tribute of admiration and esteem to the surgeons sent out by Sir E. Lechmere and the Order of St. John—brave, active, kind-hearted, skilful, never sparing themselves when work is to be done. Messrs. McKellar, Sandwith, Hume, Boyd, and Attwood, at Belgrade, are all that surgeons should be. They deserve the thanks of England for having so nobly vindicated her courage and her charity.

"Well," I said, "those surgeons were taken over by Lloyd-Lindsay; they were the officials in the front; no one could find any failure in duty on their part; moreover, some of them read the letter before it was published, and liked it."

"To be sure they did," said the consul; "but what am I to answer? I know all about it; but I must give your explanation."

"I do not see that I am bound to give one; but rather than those gallant fellows should be blamed, I say that the National Aid Society do not understand their work, or they would have had an ambulance in front; that the chief medical officer agreed with the English surgeons on that subject There was no time to telegraph to England and call a committee meeting together, 'that day week to consider and report on the application'. There was no one there with funds to start an ambulance, ourselves excepted, and we gladly took up any work that lay to our hand; and knowing the antipathy of two of the officials of the National Aid Society we did not wish to ask for any grant from them, but we could not see men die because of their red-tape stupidity. Their workers are splendid. It is their chiefs who are failures."

The consul smiled. "Am I to deliver that literally?"

"Of course, and as much more as you like to add."

"I shall add that you have been working superbly."

"Thank you; we only tried to do what we could."

After which we shook hands—the English method of showing our appreciation of each other—and chatted on indifferent subjects and passing events.

But it was not a gracious proceeding on the part of the National Aid Society. If their officials in the front had failed, that was no fault of ours; we were only trying to repair that failure in the cause of humanity.

But they did not fail. Every man of that gallant little band, including also Mr. Gimlet and Mr. Bennington Kennett, was worth a hecatomb of committee men in England. They knew what was wanted, and they did it, and we tried to help them; that was a plain duty.

The committee in England knew nothing but what Lloyd-Lindsay chose to tell them, and could be no judges of passing events.

Necessities vary in war every day, and the committee were sitting over their comfortable fires in their quiet homes, speculating on news from the front, a week old, while their officials were braving snow and wind, and sleeping on straw, half-frozen and half-famished; and we were *roughing* it, to say the least of it, in the work far away in a half-civilised land, all forgetting everything but how to carry on the work best, and to help each other—and after all this to have this ungenerous questioning going on!

The sooner that Society is broken up the better.

All England knows it pretty well now, with its crass ignorance and its obstinacy; and soon, let us hope, better chiefs, and more liberal principles, will supersede bad management and ingratitude to honest workers.

The weather grew worse and worse, and there were rumours that the Danube would soon be frozen and navigation cease.

The prospect of a winter in Belgrade with no work to do was not enlivening, and the doctors strongly advised our going southwards for the winter. This we resolved to do when practicable.

Everybody who had been to the front seemed congregating in Belgrade. All the Russian volunteers came down and were in great distress.

They had spent nearly all the money given them by the Slavonic Committee on starting, and what they had not spent was gambled away in Belgrade.

Every night high play went on in the *café* of our hotel, and gold passed freely; and when Ignace insisted on shutting up, the gamblers adjourned to their own rooms, and play went on till morning.

Quarrels were of constant occurrence, and there was no peace day or night.

All over the city were complaints of Tchernaieff and his officers, and his soldiers. Sometimes the general interfered, sometimes he did not.

It was said that there were men on his staff with whom the ex-editor of a Russian paper could not interfere, and so many a wrong went unpunished.

Therefore, the feelings of the citizens may be imagined, when one morning drums and trumpets sounded, Russian soldiers were paraded in every street and vacant place; a grand celebration was announced to take place at the cathedral. Every officer was in full dress—and all this was because it was General Tchernaieff's birthday.

The Serbs looked on in sullen silence. They had no part in all this rejoicing; their one aim and object was now to get the Russians out of Servia; and under what difficulties and delays it was accomplished, the journals of the spring and early summer of 1877 have told.

We paid an evening visit to General Likovitch and his wife. He had lost a leg in the Crimean War, fighting against us, but we were not the worse friends for that. He can still ride on horseback, and is regarded as one of the most gallant officers of the Servian Army.

He prided himself on only speaking Serbi Russian, but his wife, a Russian, spoke German and French; and with her he had travelled to France, Germany, and Italy; still the general knew the words "good wife" in every European language, and made us laugh by his odd pronunciation of them.

He had been in command on the left wing of the army of the Drina, and had received the Order of the Takova for his services; but when the Russians came, he, like many others, felt aggrieved at the prominent place they took, and, finding no fighting going on, changed to the Army of the Ibar, where he hoped to find active service.

He so far succeeded that he was present at some skirmish, in which he was slightly wounded and taken to Jagodina, where his wife went to nurse him.

He was one of those who at first welcomed the Russians; but, when they felt the iron yoke of their would-be friends, turned from it in sadness and disappointment, and he may be regarded as the best type of a native Servian officer.

On the 1st December the "Katherine Hospital" was given over by the National Aid Society, and Dr. Laseron and his deaconesses departed for Berlin *en route* to England.

Dr. Attwood, one of the English surgeons sent out by Sir Edmund Lechmere, and who had had charge of the hospital, most nobly took it upon himself to keep it open, as there were ninety-six badly wounded there, and it was not finally closed for two or three months more.

The Russian ambulances began to depart, and to re-embark their stores in such quantities, that we remarked at the time there was enough for another war.

One interesting thing we saw—the best-managed, charity in Belgrade.

The Countess Joannini, wife of the Consul-General of Italy, is one of our "American cousins," and therefore we have a right to be proud of her energy and good judgment. She is herself the daughter of a diplomat, and has lived some years in Servia.

She got up a soup kitchen—or rather a dinner kitchen—every day at eleven o'clock, and was always there herself. Soup with good meat and vegetables in it, and loaves of bread, were given to bearers of tickets—a plentiful portion, sufficient for dinner and supper, and, if care was taken, a little for breakfast also. Such a boon was this considered that refugees quartered in the country applied to change to Belgrade to benefit by the good daily meal; and it relieved a class who were not touched by the money and clothing distributions.

This class consisted of what we may call small farmers and their families, who had fled before the advance of the Turks. They had saved all their clothes and furniture, and were too proud to accept money gifts or ask for relief, while their appearance was so respectable that some of the distributors of funds did not suspect their true position, and passed on to the ragged, noisy claimants, who moved from place to place, and thus received relief four or five times over.

These poor people could live on this daily food till spring-time came, and they could return to their homes and sow their crops, and exist on the produce of their farms.

And this relief cost so little—about 6*d.* of English money a-head a day. Had this "kitchen" been better known, I think very many charitable persons would have seen that it was, after all, the most effectual and best way of giving help.

Our stay in Servia was drawing to a close. A few days of faint sunshine melted the snow, and the Danube ran blue and free again.

We arranged to depart, and to go by way of Austria to Italy, a new and hardly known way, but a most interesting one.

We took leave of our friends at the War Office; the Order of the Takova was conferred upon us, but the crosses themselves were not ready and were to be sent through Count Joannini. We said goodbye to Herr Philip Christich and his son-in-law, Herr Hadji Thoma, and to Dr. Humphrey Sandwith and the good Dilberts, and all our friends; and one bright day in December we embarked on board the Austrian steamer for Semlin, and left Servia possibly for ever, for though Herr Hadji Thoma came to Rome, and begged us, on the part of the War Office, to return and take charge of the nursing department of all the Servian ambulances, in case Servia went to war, we refused, on two grounds: first, we did not believe that Servia would go to war again; and next, that for a year at least we did not feel we should be in a state of health to undergo again such hardships and fatigue. We must rest.

And so we departed—the first English women to land there on Red Cross work, the last to leave. The war was over; the wounded all cared for, our task there was done, and we went to seek new strength for any work or duty that the future might have in store for us.

CHAPTER 34

From Belgrade to Venice

The little steamer took us in ten minutes to Semlin, and here Austrian sentinels prevented the passing of any passengers on shore without showing their passports.

Warned by the trouble we had with our baggage at Drenkova, we had been to see Prince von Wrede, the Austro-Hungarian *chargé-d'affaires*, and had procured from him a letter charging all whom it might concern, to let us and our baggage pass, and to afford us all help and assistance.

The prince is a talented and gentlemanly man, most kind in his intercourse with the people of Belgrade, and yet, because he is the representative of Austria, he is regarded with distrust and dislike.

We had very little baggage now. Before we left Belgrade, we had given to the impoverished medical department all our spare medicines and instruments, lint, and wool, for which the prince thanked us most gracefully in the *Belgrade Gazette*. Dr. Ziemann and Dr. Humphrey Sandwith had the spare clothing for the refugees, so chest and bale were all disposed of.

We were very glad we had that letter, for directly I showed it we were allowed to pass, our passports returned to us, and the baggage sent on untouched, while other people had a good deal of trouble.

Moreover, no one was permitted to go on the Vienna boat—ourselves excepted—as it was not to start for a couple of hours, so we had choice of places in saloon and sleeping cabin, and arranged ourselves comfortably.

It was impossible to walk into the town of Semlin; the sun had melted the snow, and the mud was ankle deep; nor indeed was there anything to see worth the trouble of a walk, the one object of interest there being the ruined castle of John Hunyady, who delivered Belgrade from the Turks, which stood on the top of a high hill close by.

Semlin overlooks the junction of the Save and the Danube; it stands on flat ground, and the fortress of Belgrade on the opposite shore looks down upon it.

We were off at last; Belgrade was lost to sight, and we felt that we had left Servia.

The captain came and talked to us, and spoke of the impalement supposed to have been seen on the banks of the Save, and the wigging which had been given to the steward of the Save boat for his mendacious statements; "and even if it were so," he added, "which, however, we can disprove; there is no proof that the Turks did it."

"Was not that part of the Servian shore," I asked, "close to the advanced guard of General Alempits' army in Bosnia?"

"Yes," he answered; "too close for any such thing to have happened; they must have known of it if it had been so; and I think we have heard of impalements practised in Bosnia by others than the Turks. I mean the so-called vampires, dead bodies supposed to be animated by the evil spirit of someone, and who suck the blood of the living; these bodies are taken from the grave and impaled."

"Yes," said an Austrian colonel, who had joined us. "I have heard of that; the old superstition prevails, even in parts of Hungary."

"And there is another explanation," the captain went on; "men often mount those tall poles to look out for fish, and they twist their arms round the crossbars to support themselves, and they remain perfectly quiet and still. The cross-bars are originally intended to extend the nets, which are hung up to dry, and when these nets are cast in the river the fishermen watch them from the top of the poles."

In short, it appeared that there were half a dozen explanations of what had been asserted to have been seen, besides the improbable one of an impalement by the Turks close to the army of the Drina.

We leave these accounts to the consideration of the reader; no one in Servia believed in this story, though they were ready and anxious to accept all probable tales of Bosnian and Bulgarian atrocities; no one attempted to deny that there have been impalements, but this particular one is a most doubtful matter.

It may be observed, that seaweed drying, and other explanations given elsewhere, were not alluded to. The argument was based on the fact, that a body presenting the appearance of impalement, or actually impaled, might have been seen, and yet have had nothing to do with the Turks.

Let it not be imagined that we have any sympathy with that nation;

acts of cruelty and ferocity have justly been ascribed to it; but are the Russians clear of such a charge? and when we know that in this war in Servia no quarter was given, can we excuse the brutality of such doings?—are they not even worse, because carried on by Christians professing to come as saviours of the oppressed?

It was dark when we reached Neusatz, a large modern town; we had passed Karlovitz before.

On the other side of the river was Peterwardein, a rock-built fortress, and here a bridge of boats 840 feet long crosses the river. The citadel is an important one. The town which clusters round it is very small.

The scenery on this part of the river is pretty, but not bold; but as it was night and very cold on deck, we retreated to the sleeping cabin.

There was a singular arrangement here. If a passenger chose to pay a florin, the mattress bed was covered with a sheet; a pillow and a counterpane were added, and it was possible to undress and have a good night's rest; but if the florin was not forthcoming, there was nothing but the mattress.

The steamers had always been so full that we had slept in the saloon, but this was not allowed when there was room below; the saloon was kept empty all night, and in consequence was much more agreeable next day.

Another morning of sunshine, the river dancing along as if delighting in the last few days of liberty before it was captive in chains of ice.

We enjoyed the bright, fresh air, and the comfort, cleanliness, and quiet of our steamer.

There were a few Russian officers on board, who had lunched in the saloon when first we left Semlin; but when the steward came round at night, to take payment for the provisions consumed during the day by each passenger, and examined their tickets, he found that they were second-class passengers.

They insisted upon it that officers with second-class tickets travelled first-class. The captain was called in and said, not foreign officers on an Austrian boat; they must pay the difference, or leave the saloon, and they elected to leave the saloon.

We saw them in the morning sitting on the bow of the vessel much crestfallen; they were going home, *via* Vienna.

It was just dusk when we reached Mohacs, the railway station on the Danube for Southern Austria.

It is now but a small town; here was fought that terrible battle between Solyman the Magnificent and his enormous army of Turks, and Lewis II., King of Hungary.

The battle took place in May, 1526. It was a fatal day for Hungary and Christianity: 22,000 Christians fell on the field out of 30,000—amongst them two archbishops, six bishops, twenty-eight magnates, and the flower of the Hungarian chivalry. The king, in attempting to escape, got into a marsh, where he was smothered in the mud, near a village called Czeczi.

Another battle was fought here in 1688, when the Duke of Lorraine defeated the Turk. This was the last invasion of Hungary by them, and it may be hoped (1877) that never more may Turk or Russain set foot on the fair land of Austria; for it has been truly remarked that, if where the Turk plants his horse's feet no grass can grow, where the Russian comes no man may raise his head.

We landed at Mohacs, and the good-natured steward and his boy ran on shore with our baggage and put it in the railway station. We felt delighted at being once more in a civilised land, and all we had seen of Austria and the Austrians had led us to form a most favourable opinion of them.

They are a pleasant people to travel with, most kind and courteous, and this gracious manner pervades all classes; it is delightful to hear them talk German, all the harshness is gone, the language flows on softly and sweetly.

We were greeted at Mohacs with the intelligence that the express through train had gone, and we could only get as far as Funfkirchen that night. We had been told of a very good inn here, "The Wild Man," and preferred going on there to stopping at Mohacs.

The distance was a short one, but we went at a foot-pace. All around Mohacs are mines of brown, dusty coal, used for fuel on the steamers; and at Villany we halted a long time, while coal trucks were being shunted backward and forward. We reached Funfkirchen at last, and, to our surprise, found an omnibus waiting to take us to the hotel.

It seemed to be a large town, but as it was dark, we could see nothing of it.

The hotel was large and good, for so out-of-the-way a place.

We left it at 5 a.m., to catch the through train to Pragerhof, and our bill, which was printed in two languages, is a curiosity.

One language is Magyar, the other of course German. Here is a specimen of it.

HOTEL ZUM WILDENMANN.

Note:—

	f. w.	
Lakas / Logis von	1 60	Lodging.
Stearin qyertyn / Stearin-kerzen	0 40	Candles.
Etkek es italok / Speisen und getranken	1 80	Eating and Drinking.
Vaspályai szallitas / Bahnfur	1 0	Omnibus to and from railway.

Another item, "*Istello jämlek*," I believe to be "porter for baggage," but we never could find out. At the end of the bill is printed in German, "Thanking you for your kind coming, requesting you to return.—Ignace Wybyad."

Let all who wish to travel in Southern Austria take warning by this—nothing was spoken or could be understood but this Magyar, and a German *patois*.

The country we ran through that morning was very pretty, wild, and thickly wooded. We came to a station called Kanitza, where we had to change carriages, or rather had to wait for the train from Agram to Pragerhof.

At Kanitza we met an English gentleman, Mr. Franklin, who turned out to be an old Norfolk friend, and gave us some interesting details of the surrounding country. He was the agent of a London firm of timber merchants, who had bought all the forest round for many miles. The trees were to be cut down, sawn into planks, and sent to Trieste, to be shipped for England. Mr. Franklin said that he had, before February or March, very many thousand trees to mark for cutting.

The forests abound in game, and there are many wolves; in the winter time, when the frost is very severe, they have been known to come almost into the streets of Kanitza. Shooting parties are formed, with the peasants as beaters; they go out for several days together, and bring back enormous quantities of game. There are also wild boars and deer.

Kanitza, though small, is a pretty, cheerful-looking town, and would be capital headquarters for a shooting expedition. When the woods are cut down, the land will be put into cultivation. At present they are as untouched as the backwood forests of America.

Near Kanitza are rich mines of ore, of several kinds.

It was quite dark when we got to Pragerhof, a large and important town, and had to wait two hours for the train to Laibach and Nabresina. Fortunately, it was a moonlight night, for the scenery was most superb. The mighty Oestrica Spitz lifted up its head crowned with eternal snow. It is 7,700 feet high, and the loftiest of all the mountains in the surrounding provinces of Styria, Carniola, and Carinthia.

The railroad follows the course of the river, winding amidst mountains, at first clothed in wood. We stopped at a little station close under the huge cliffs, where there was just room for the road and the station between them, and the river. We looked and saw the mountains closing in behind and barring our way in front.

A powerful engine was put on, and we gradually worked our way upwards, till on the top we found ourselves passing though the most picturesque and wild scenery imaginable. Not a tree, not a shrub, not a blade of grass, was visible all around us; only the weird hills of white stone, ghostly in the pale moonlight—the far-famed Julian Alps.

It was daybreak before we left them and ran into Steinbruck, from whence to Laibach the way led through a lovely country, with wood and water, and fertile plains and valleys.

Laibach is a large town of Roman origin, once destroyed by Attila and his hordes.

We had only taken our tickets as far as that place, having been assured at Funfkirchen that we should reach it at 7 p.m., and intending to sleep there; but on explaining to the guard that we now wished to go on to Nabresina and Venice, he most kindly advised me to go straight into the ticket-office and get tickets for Venice. He would not let the registered portmanteau be taken off the platform; and if I showed the ticket for it at the baggage bureau, they would change it for one to Venice, and he would have the portmanteau re-labelled while I was absent, as we had but five minutes to stop there.

Everybody was so quick and civil that all was done before five minutes were over, and we were fairly on our way to Italy.

Near Laibach are the celebrated caves of Adelsburg, but we were too weary and worn to care for sightseeing.

Everyone who has travelled to Trieste from Vienna knows how lovely is the view from Nabresina: the road is on the height, and far below are the blue waters of the Adriatic, with the shores of Dalmatia on one side and Italy on the other. The view is perhaps even more lovely beyond Nabresina, where we changed carriages for Mestre and Venice. All along that road view after view opens up like a panorama, till at last Mestre is reached. The passengers for North and Central Italy left our train, and we ran over the viaduct way, and into the station of Venice.

A few more minutes and we were out on the little wharf, and stepping into our *gondola*, floated through the still, calm watery streets, through narrow byways, round sharp corners, where the peculiar warning cry of the *gondolier* announced our coming, till we emerged into the glorious sunshine that turns the waters of the Grand Canal into a golden stream, and saw the palaces on either side, with their quaint, rich architecture telling of the civilisation of ages, and the glories of bygone days; and the hardships and rough life of Servia faded in the distance, and we felt at last we had come to a land where we might rest.

Belgrade, le 1 Janvier, 1877.

Chere Mademoiselle Pearson—

J'ai eu le plus grand plaisir en apprenant de la bouche même de son Altesse la Princesse Nathalie que S. A. le Prince Milan a daigné vous accorder à, vous et à, Mademoiselle MacLaughlin la Croix de Takova. Je les ai reçues l'autre jour, et je me suis empressé suivant votre désir de les remettre à M. le Comte Joannini, Consul-Général d'Italie, pour vous les faire parvenir.

En vous offrant mes sincères félicitations j'ai l'honneur de vous presenter mes meilleur compliments l'occasion de nouvel an, et suis,

Votre devoue serviteur,

Philip Christich.

Mes respects à Mademoiselle MacLaughlin.

Adventures in Servia

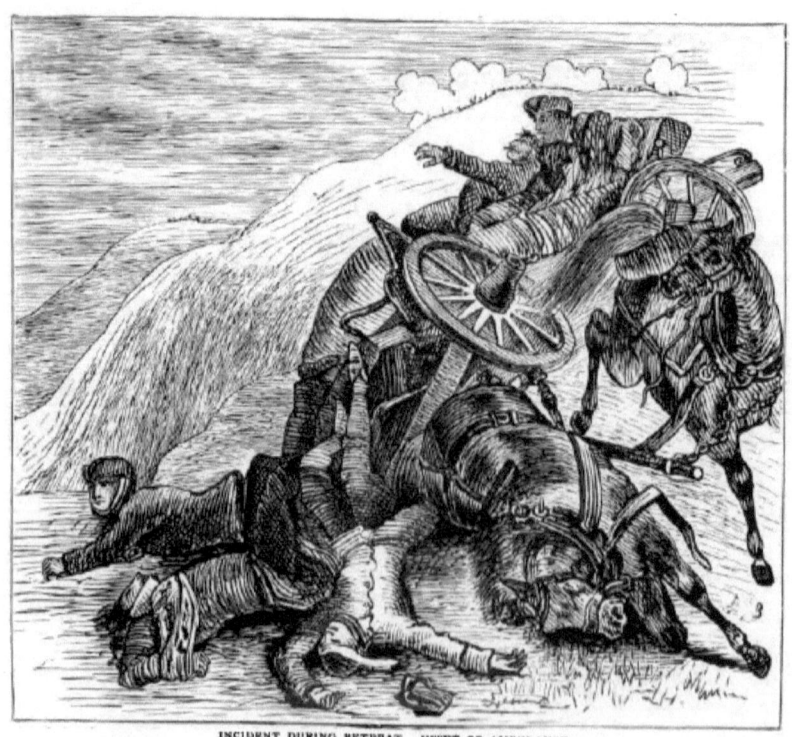
INCIDENT DURING RETREAT. UPSET OF AMBULANCE.

Contents

Preface	195
Depart for Belgrade	197
We Meet Colonel Bragg	205
The Contract Signed	208
A Dirty Hospital	211
Radicalism	217
Rough Travelling	220
A Narrow Escape	229
Baron von Tummy	233
Von Tummy Blows Me Up	248
An Unpleasant Ride	251
Prince Obolenski	258
A Mysterious Resemblance	264
A Trip to Jubovac	270
A Lovely Evening	281
Strange Conduct of Savrimovitch	291
Good News	299
We dispose of a Pig	303
The Attack	310

Astounding Horsemanship 327
Letters from Home 347

Preface

When my esteemed friend Dr. Wright asked me to edit this work and also to write its preface, I agreed to do so, but not without a considerable amount of hesitation and diffidence, for I was loth to run the risk of marring what appeared to be a very excellent book by my own necessarily imperfect workmanship.

The good doctor, however, placed the matter before me in such a light, that I felt constrained to comply with his wishes.

I cannot lay claim to the "pen of a ready writer," therefore I trust the public will excuse what may appear to them to be a halting style. And now to the real business of my preface.

I have the author's word for it that at least three out of every four of the incidents herein narrated really took place, and that to the fourth only such proportion of romantic dressing and spicery has been added as would enable it to harmonise with the rest.

Moreover, I am desired to state that every character depicted in these pages had its living prototype.

Thus Marie, Colonel Bragg, Savrimovitch, Colonel Philipovitch, the ruffian Pauloff, Dr. Ibaum, etc., represent real personages, whose names even, in some cases, have been preserved. The quarrel with Von Tummy, the upsetting of the waggon, the fight for the bed, the pig incident, the occupation of the cottage, the description of the battle, are all fairly accurately described; and the conversations with Russian officers about India and with the Nihilists are reported almost verbatim.

Facts are stubborn and eloquent things, and I can say nothing stronger in behalf of these pages than that they treat, for the most part, of absolute facts.

My duty to Dr. Wright prohibits me from drawing this preface to a close without making some reference to the painful circumstance that my distinguished friend has as yet received no considerable token of the public favour. As he pathetically puts it:

"Monarchs don't seek his medical advice, kings consult him not, and sovereigns neither summon him to their sick-bed sides, nor find their way, in another sense, into his coffers."

The doctor says he occasionally sees a person clad in prints, but never any one "*en prince*," and he reminds me, moreover, that though Pope lays it down as an axiom, that "whatever is, is *Wrights*," yet he gets hardly any of it at all.

Now this, I maintain, emphatically and without fear of contradiction, ought not to be, and I would respectfully intimate to the potentates of Europe, that unless they patronise the illustrious doctor more largely than they have hitherto done, there is some fear of his throwing physic to the dogs, and becoming, if not a Nihilist, at least a desperate Radical.

I state this entirely on my own responsibility. May those whom it directly concerns take it seriously to heart.

A. G. Farquhar-Bernard, M.R.C.S.
(Late surgeon of the Servian Army)

CHAPTER 1

Depart for Belgrade

Late in July 1876, whilst the war between Turkey and Servia was at its height, I, at that time a medical student, resolved to pay a visit to the latter country with the double view of making myself useful, and of gaining experience in the profession I was striving to enter. I mentioned my project to my particular friend and chum, Henry Winter, of whom I shall speak for the future by the sobriquet he had received from the students at our classical hospital—*viz.*, Hiems. Hiems fell in with the idea at once, and agreed to accompany me.

As a preliminary step we wrote letters to several newspapers announcing our intention and our readiness to take charge of stores for the sick and wounded at the seat of the war.

We were soon overwhelmed with packages of pills, jars of extract of beef, bales of cotton-wool, parcels of lint and bandages, and bottles of quinine, etc., etc. These, with a case of surgical instruments, a cutlass and revolver apiece, and a somewhat scanty supply of clothing, which included, nevertheless, our volunteer uniforms, each adorned with a Geneva cross on the arm, and our preparations were complete.

The day of our departure arrived. We proudly donned our uniforms, which, though rather the worse for wear, still had the advantage of looking as if they had seen service, and took our places in the train. We intended to travel to Vienna by rail, and from thence to Belgrade by the Danube steamer. Our journey was uneventful, except that our uniforms attracted more attention than was altogether pleasant.

The French mistook us for Germans, and scowled angrily at us, and the Germans took us for Frenchmen, and regarded us with cold hostility. In fact, wherever we went, people seemed to wonder who on earth we were, and what the dickens we wanted.

At Salzburg we were accosted by a stately and elegantly-attired lady of middle age, who informed us that she was the Princess Woronzoff, and saying that she was delighted to see Englishmen espousing the Servian cause, requested us to convey the sum of five *napoleons* from her to the Servian sufferers by the war.

This we promised to do, and she bade us farewell. We arrived at Vienna late on a Friday evening, and stayed there until Sunday morning, putting up for the time at the Goldenes Lamm Hotel; and Hiems utilised the time by coaching me up in the broad-sword exercise, at which he was a proficient. He was particularly careful to teach me the hanging guard position, and I flatter myself that I learnt it thoroughly. It certainly is a very striking attitude, and when my cap was cocked properly on one side, and I had my big boots on, I must have looked very killing.

The next morning, we repaired to the steamboat quay, full of eager anticipations of what we considered would be the most interesting and picturesque part of our journey, for Strauss's favourite waltz had led us to believe that the Danube was both beautiful and blue.

We were, however, grievously sold. From Vienna to Belgrade, there is simply no scenery at all. The banks of the river are flat and dreary-looking, and the water itself is brown and dirty, so we soon turned our attention to our *compagnons de voyage*.

In the boat with us were a dozen handsome lads, all clothed alike in dark-grey tourist suits, and who seemed to be under the charge of a tall, military-looking man.

We ascertained that they were some of the King of Bavaria's pages.

These lads appeared to be greatly impressed by our romantic uniforms and martial appearance, and presently one or two of them, who spoke English fairly well, entered into conversation with us. They were particularly curious to see our cutlasses. We showed them the weapons; and I believe that I made a profound impression upon them, and convinced them of the invincibility of English seamen by frowning fiercely and trying to show, cutlass in hand, the hanging guard I had so recently acquired.

The jealous Hiems endeavoured to dissuade me from flourishing my sword, by the remark that the young Germans would only laugh at me. I did not believe him, and am happy to say that my efforts extorted from one of my audience the acknowledgment that he thought Englishmen were very brave and hardy, and that he attributed their love of adventure to the rough nature of their sports, such as "*the* football and *the* cricket," and so forth. A corpulent little Hungarian doctor, too, watched our proceedings with great interest, and very politely proffered us each a cigar.

"Gentlemen," said he, when we had all three lit up, "is it true that you are going on the Servian side?"

"Quite true," responded Hiems, puffing vigorously at his cigar and nodding.

"And you are Englishmen, born in England?" interrogated our new friend.

"We are Englishmen, but not born in England," responded Hiems. "I was born in Ireland."

"And I in India," said I.

"An Englishman, born in India!" replied the Hungarian lifting up his eyes and hands with astonishment; "and yet you are going on the Servian side! It is amazing! It is incredible! Don't you know that the Russians are the enemies of your country, and that they want to get Constantinople?"

"I know that we fought them and beat them in the Crimea," replied I.

"Yes, and England did very well; she did right then. And what are you going on the Servian side now for? Don't you know they are the same as the Russians, and that the Russians have got up this war? Why are you not on the Turkish side?"

Hiems replied that we went as medical men, and not as combatants.

"That's worse," answered our little friend; "for as fast as the Turks knock a man over, you set him on his legs again!"

"Then again," said I, "the Servians are short of medical men."

"So much the better," said this bloodthirsty little Magyar, "the war will be over all the sooner then. No, no; you take my advice, and go over to the Turks!" His Russo-phobism did not prevent him from chatting very pleasantly with us afterwards, and he proved a most agreeable and interesting companion.

Dinner was served in the saloon at seven o'clock. Our Hungarian friend and a large party, however, did not dine then, but stationed themselves at the other end of the saloon, where I heard him telling the others that we were Englishmen.

"They are Englishmen, Englishmen!" said he, with a graceful wave of his handkerchief towards us; "and one of them was born in India. They eat a good dinner, you see. They have each had a plate of soup and a beefsteak with eggs, and some sweets, and now they will both have coffee. Ah, no! One of them, you see, has tea———" (here he

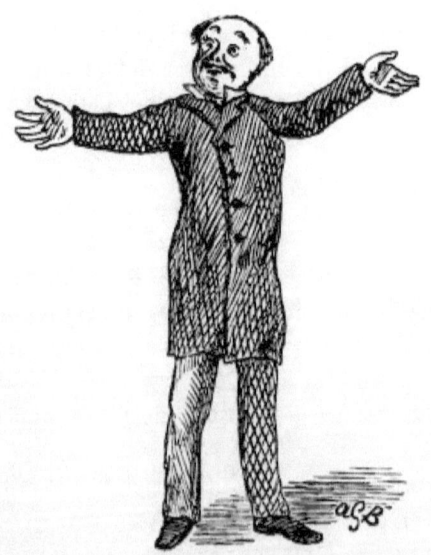

THE HUNGARIAN GENTLEMAN TELLS HIS FRIENDS THAT WE ARE MAKING AN UNCOMMONLY GOOD DINNER.

stepped quietly up and looked over our shoulders), "and the other has coffee. Englishmen," he repeated, as he retired on tiptoe to his seat again; "Englishmen—one of them born in India—and they have eaten a most excellent dinner!"

When the boat stopped at Pesth our eccentric little acquaintance went on shore; we remained some time longer to see our luggage transferred to the Belgrade boat, which lay alongside our own, and met him no more.

"Five o'clock! Belgrade in half an hour!" such were the sounds which, roared in a stentorian voice by the steward, roused me from a pleasant sleep, the sixth morning after we left Charing Cross. I was wide awake in an instant, and dressing quickly hastened on deck; but a thick mist hung on the river, and Belgrade was still invisible. The sun's rays soon, however, dissipated the haze, and there, within a few hundred yards of us, lay Belgrade, an imposing array of white-walled, green-roofed buildings and churches with glittering spires, rising terrace on terrace to a considerable height above the water's edge.

It looked so bright and beautiful that Hiems and I were in ecstasies of delight, and congratulated each other again and again on having selected so charming a spot for the basis of our operations. The boat presently drew up alongside the jetty, and a tall Servian official in a smart blue uniform with very broad scarlet stripes down the sides of his pantaloons stepped on board and collected all the passengers' passports.

Then came a number of drowsy-looking porters, who began to overhaul the luggage and solicit patronage for the different hotels. We selected one who seemed more active and was tidier than his fellows, and instructed him to convey our things to his hotel, the "*Königin von Griechenland.*" The man instantly summoned four or five assistants, each of whom, in an indolent and casual manner, commenced dragging one or two of our packages after him. We followed their chief up a steep flight of steps, cut in the hill or cliff on which Belgrade stands, and they followed us, droning a dismal and most unmelodious ditty in chorus.

These steps were converted by a number of beggars into a kind of rag and deformity bazaar. On one of the lower steps sat a miserable creature, who, from some freak of nature, had been born without any arms; at the other end of the same step sat a blind, toothless old man, who mumbled forth a request for a *piastre*, and who was clad in such unsavoury garments that we felt almost plague-stricken as we passed;

a little above was a frightful dwarf, a victim apparently of goitre; above him again was a man whom accident or war had deprived of both legs; then came a deaf and dumb woman; and so on right away up to the top of the steps.

The "*Königin von Griechenland*" was not an imposing-looking edifice; however, it seemed as good as any of the other hotels, and was fairly comfortable. We were shown into a bright, clean-looking room with two beds in it. Here we had a glorious wash and changed our linen, and then went down into the coffee-room, where some dozen persons were smoking cigarettes, drinking coffee, and playing billiards. For breakfast they brought us excellent coffee, fresh eggs, and white bread-and-butter.

Seated at the next table was a portly old priest with flowing locks and a rosy—a suspiciously rosy—face. For some time, this reverend gentleman surveyed us minutely, carefully, and critically. Nothing from the top of our caps to the soles of our boots, and from our black cross-belts to the little red Geneva crosses embroidered on our arms, escaped his scrutiny. At length he rose with slow and dignified gravity, and bowed, and saying some words in a language which neither of us understood, seated himself opposite to us at our table. As he was a priest, we rose and returned his salute, and then shook our heads to betoken our ignorance of his language.

Nodding to us again, the new-comer beckoned solemnly to one of the waiters, and gave him some instructions in an undertone. Then turning to us with a smile and another nod, he said, interrogatively, "*Ingleski?*" (English.) Hiems said "*Ja*" and I said "*Oui*" in our best German and French. The priestly face beamed with smiles, and then the waiter brought in three large glass flagons of foaming ale. The priest pushed one of these to Hiems, another to me, and taking the third himself, he motioned to us to drink. As we raised the glasses from the table, he clinked his against ours with much cordiality and another series of smiles and nods. Then leaning back on his seat and folding his hands on his lap, he surveyed us again. At last it occurred to Hiems to try him with German; so pulling himself together and pronouncing his words as carefully as possible, he said:—

"*Sprechen Sie Deutsch, mein Herr?*"

"*Ne—nein*," replied the priest, shaking his head once more.

"I'm afraid it's no go," said Hiems, with a sigh; "and it's a pity, too, for he seems an uncommonly nice old fellow. I wish we could have expressed our appreciation of his kindness better than by grinning and nodding at him."

"So do I," said I; "but I don't see how we're to do it, except by getting him to drink with us."

Hiems reflected for a moment, then suddenly brightening up, said to me, "You know you used to be a swell at Latin at school, old chap. Try if you can't polish up some of it now. I have heard that all foreign priests talk Latin."

"That's not at all a bad idea of yours, Hiems," said I, not without a little pride. "What shall I say to him?"

"Say—why say, 'How do you do?' to him, and ask him to have another drink."

"Confound it, Hiems, ask me to say something sensible. How the dickens do you expect me to translate sentences like that?"

"What! can't you translate them?" asked Hiems.

"No, of course not," replied I. "The Romans never said things of that sort to one another."

"What dummies they must have been, then," replied my friend in disgust.

For a few seconds we were silent. All at once Hiems brightened up again.

"What is the Latin for 'This'?" said he.

"What?" said I, not knowing what he was alluding to.

"*This*" said he again with considerable emphasis.

"Which?" said I, quite puzzled.

"What a fellow you are! Why *This*, the article, noun, adjective, pronoun, or whatever you like to call it—*This*."

"Oh ah! Now I see," said I, perceiving that he meant the word *this*. The Latin for this is *Hic*."

"Why could not you have said so before then?" replied he, tartly; "and what is the Latin for *is?*"

"*Est*," rejoined I, without a moment's hesitation.

"And for 'beautiful'?"

"*Pulcher*."

"Now we are getting on," said Hiems; "and for 'beer'?"

"I don't know. Call it wine, *vinum*."

"All right; that will do, I suppose." Then to the priest, "*Hic est pulcher vinum*."

For a moment our companion was puzzled. Then his face beamed with a smile of intelligence. He nodded, grasped Hiems by the hand, and said,—

"*Bibamus alterum poculum.*"

Then he began to speak Latin so fast and fluently that I could not catch a single word. But before the waiter could be called, I was relieved from my embarrassment by the sound of martial music in the street. Every one—priest, billiard players, and ourselves—hastened to the window and looked out. A long and solemn procession was approaching—the funeral *cortége* of an officer who had been mortally wounded in the recent fighting. At the head of the column marched a military band playing the Servian Dead March, then twelve priests with banners and flags, a regiment with arms reversed, and last of all the coffin borne on the shoulders of eight men. The lid of the coffin, as is the custom in Servia, was removed, so that the pale face of the dead man was visible. His breast was covered with flowers; two soldiers marched behind, one bearing his sword and the other his cap. The procession slowly filed past, and when we looked round—lo! our jolly friend the priest had disappeared.

Chapter 2

We Meet Colonel Bragg

Left to ourselves, we held a consultation as to what our next step should be. We both fancied that Servia was a very small country, and imagined that we were but a moderate distance from the front.

This illusion was quickly dispelled by the *maître d'hôtel*. From him we learned that the scene of action was at least one hundred miles away, also that an English officer, Colonel Bragg, who commanded a newly-raised squadron of cavalry, was then in Belgrade.

This was indeed acceptable news. His camp, we were told, was only about two miles away, at a place called Topchidere, on the other side of the town, and we determined to offer our services at once.

It was now about half-past ten o'clock, and intensely hot. There was not a cloud in the bright blue sky, and the sun's rays beat down with fierce and dazzling power on the white and dusty streets. We, therefore, fortified our muffin-shaped forage caps with *puggarees*, after the Indian fashion. Amongst other things I had brought out with me were a pair of india-rubber half-Wellington boots, very loose about the uppers, and shiny like goloshes. I was rather proud of these, and being anxious to make a favourable impression on my distinguished fellow-countryman, I determined, in spite of Hiems' protest that they were "ridiculous," to wear them.

After a dusty walk we arrived at Topchidere. The cavalry camp, which contained only a score or two of tents, was in a large field. We had no difficulty in finding Colonel Bragg's quarters, being directed thither by a good-natured little doctor, who introduced himself to us as Dr. Ibaum, and offered us each a pinch of snuff. Our reception by the colonel was not encouraging. He was talking to a tall, good-looking young fellow, who turned out to be the special artist of an English illustrated paper, and as he approached we heard him say:—

"Who the —— are these beggars, and what the —— do they want

here, I wonder?"

The artist looked towards us, and burst out laughing. Nothing daunted, however, we walked up to the tent, and Hiems, saluting politely," said:—

"Colonel Bragg, I believe?"

"Hulloh!" said the colonel to his friend, "they're English!" (*Then to us.*) "Yes, Bragg's my name. What can I do for you?"

"We are medical students, just arrived from England, and hearing that you were organising a body of cavalry, we have come to offer you our services," said Hiems.

"D——d good of you," said the colonel, "but I don't think we want any surgeons. What stores have you got with you?"

We replied that we had a good supply of quinine, *Ipecacuanha*, Condy's fluid, opium, strapping, bandages, cotton-wool, prepared oakum, lint, etc.

"Hum—well, you can send them over here, if you like, and I'll just think the matter over; but—you were never going to the front in those idiotical boots, were you, sir?" said he to me.

"Indeed, I was, sir," said I, rather angrily, for his contemptuous tone and manner of speaking nettled me.

"More fool you, then," said the colonel.

I was so incensed at his rudeness that I turned on my heel and would have left him there and then, had he not sung out in a kinder tone:—

"Come, come, my lad, don't be riled. I'm a blunt soldier, and always speak my mind. Shake hands; there!" and he held out his hand with a rough good-nature that almost made amends.

"By the way, though, my lad," said he, "if you can't take a joke in good part, you'll hardly do for a campaigner; blows are harder to bear than jokes."

"Not when you can return them, sir," replied I, haughtily.

"Well spoken," said the colonel. "So, you are really anxious to go to the front?"

"Yes," we both replied in a breath, "and we don't mind if we get a little fighting as well as doctoring," added Hiems.

"Well," said the colonel, with a fierce twirl of his moustache, "I guess you'll get a good chance of both if you come with me. I shall not forget you, only bear in mind that it will probably be two or three weeks before we shall leave for the front, for my men beat creation for stupidity at drill, and will want a lot of licking into shape before they'll be fit to face the Turks. What's your hotel?"

We told him.

"Very well, then; you'll hear from me before we leave. Good morning;" and lighting another cigarette, the colonel turned away from us and resumed his conversation with the artist.

We left the camp, not over well pleased with our reception, and were walking moodily homewards, when we were hailed by a loud "*Yai! Gospodina!*" and, looking back, we beheld a soldier running after us, with a piece of paper in his hand. On taking the paper we found the following words written on it, "Dr. Ibaum make to the English gentlemen his esteem, and will say to them a few words." The soldier pointed to our right, and there was the doctor, snuff-box in one hand and hat in the other, beaming on us with the kindliest of smiles.

"Eh!" said he, "my dear friend, you have seen the Inglis camp, eh? And how love you Kol-o-nel Bragg, eh?"

We replied that we thought Colonel Bragg a first-rate soldier, but that we were disappointed to learn that he was not going to the front for two or three weeks, as we were anxious to get to work immediately.

"You will to work now, aha! Then I will say what I will do," said the little doctor, puckering up his face into a look of the most unfathomable profundity. "The Minister of the Health here, Dr. Savar Petrovitch, is great friend to me." Here he drew himself up and looked very important. "I will speak to him for you, and he shall make you some work very soon—quick—aha—eh?"

We made an effort to thank him, but he stopped us at once.

"For what," said he, "will you thank me? All Inglismen my friend; I love him. But you, you will to work for my country; why will you then to thank me? No, no, I thank you! I will now," continued he, "to walk with you some way. Will you let—eh, my Inglis friend?"

We were only too glad of his company, and the kind-hearted little man was good enough to walk back with us as far as our hotel, and when he left us, it was with a promise to call for us the next morning, and accompany us to the offices of Dr. Savar Petrovitch, the Minister of Health.

Chapter 3

The Contract Signed

True to his promise, Dr. Ibaum called for us at ten o'clock the next morning, and accompanied us to the War Office, where we were introduced to Dr. Petrovitch.

Dr. Petrovitch received us kindly. He was a small, slightly made, but good-looking man, with dark eyes, whiskers, and moustache, and spoke French very fluently.

We informed him that we were anxious to go to the front, but he replied with a smile that they had plenty of medical men there, but were greatly in want of them at Semendria and Belgrade.

"You can choose between the two places," he said. "Belgrade is the more agreeable; there is more society there, and you won't be so dull. On the other hand. Dr. Ibaum works at Semendria, and will look after you if you go there. I have promised Baron von Tummey, our inspector of hospitals, not to send any more surgeons to Deligrad, but to keep them for our hospitals at Semendria and Belgrade."

This was terribly disappointing, and we should probably have declined the offer, in the hope of getting to Deligrad with Colonel Bragg, but for Dr. Ibaum.

"Come you with me," he said, coaxingly. "You shall be glad all the tay long. You shall eat— ah! very much and good—and you shall drink—oh! you shall drink wine and beer and *café*; you shall have horse and you shall have dog; you shall have money—oh! much money,—and you shall not work."

"That won't do for us," said I. "We want to work. We have come here for the sake of working."

"Aha!" said the little man, his eyes gleaming with satisfaction; "you will to work, you shall work then—plenty work—as much as you will to do, and you shall have money. How much money will you to have?"

We replied that we would be content with £2 per week and board and lodging.

"Yes, yes; you will to have two pound Inglis per the week—yes, that is *vier ducaten*" (four *ducats*). "Yes, I will speak with Dr. Petrovitch. Will you so good to wait one minute? Aha! I come quick back." And, taking Dr. Petrovitch by the arm, he left the room with him for a moment

When they returned, Ibaum bore in his hand a couple of papers.

"Gentlemen," said Dr. Petrovitch, in French, "we are quite willing to engage you as assistant surgeons at a salary of four *ducats* a week; we will provide you, moreover, with board and lodging. I cannot promise that you shall go to the front, but you shall not be forgotten should an opportunity offer. Will you allow me to see your passports and certificates?"

We complied with his wish, and finding the documents satisfactory, the papers before mentioned were handed to us to sign, and we were informed that our engagement was completed.

No one perhaps was better able to revive drooping spirits than cheerful, chatty, little Dr. Ibaum. After the arrangements were made, out came the inevitable snuffbox. He insisted on our taking a pinch, then linked his arms in ours, and led us out of the room.

"Now, my dear friends," said he, looking from one to the other of us, and giving us both a gentle pat on the back, "we shall be no more grievous. If you will be sad, I will, too, to be sad, but we will not be grievous. After our work we have done, we will sing Inglis song and Servian song, and we will dance;" and suiting his actions to his words, he adopted a dancing step and broke out into a merry *tra-la-la!*

That evening we dined with the doctor at his hotel. He was an excellent host, and gave us a first-rate dinner *à la serbe*. We began with *papricash*, a kind of tomato soup. Then came caviar, fried schill, and cray-fish, then pork cutlets and beefsteaks served with potatoes and poached eggs. Portions of roast goose and roast turkey figured most conspicuously in the meat course. Then we had sweet omelettes and pancakes called *palachinkas*, and wound up with dessert and coffee. For drinks we had a native wine called *Vaslauer*, which resembled Burgundy in colour and flavour; champagne, and a spirit made from plums, called *sligievitch*, which had an agreeable odour, but, to my mind, a most horrible taste.

After dinner the doctor waxed very jovial and communicative, "I lof," he said, "ze Englis charactaire. Ze Englismans lof horses and togs; all Englismans lof horses and togs, and will hunt much. When I have knowed ze excellent good Englis charactaire, then have I self taught mine self ze Englis tongue, and speaks him not fine, but so also too not wicked."

Shortly afterwards our papers arrived from the War Office, and Dr. Ibaum informed us that we were to start for Semendria at six in the morning.

CHAPTER 4

A Dirty Hospital

Next morning the doctor made his appearance with military punctuality. We breakfasted together and paid our reckoning, and left the hotel, much to the disappointment of the landlord, who doubtless had hoped that we should stay a week or two with him. Nevertheless, the good man was overwhelmingly polite, and accompanied us to the top of the steps leading to the landing-place, where he remained bowing and rubbing his hands as long as we could see him.

Before embarking we had to run the gauntlet of the beggars, who displayed their deformities and mumbled for *piastres* with redoubled vigour as we approached. Dr. Ibaum looked at them kindly with a complacent satisfaction. He evidently regarded them as pathological curiosities, and appeared to be as proud of them as a cockney of the most famous lions of London. He stopped and spoke to a great many of them, and gave a copper or two to all.

A dirty little steamer was waiting at the quay. We went straight on board with our baggage, and as soon as we had stowed it away made ourselves comfortable in the fore part of the boat. The scenery became rather more picturesque as we left Belgrade. On the Servian side of the Danube the ground undulates, and forms a succession of slight eminences, upon one of which Belgrade is built.

Just opposite to us, on the flat Hungarian shore, was an Austrian block house, in front of which paced a sentinel, whose bayonet glittered brightly in the sun. At some distance off we saw a large town, which Dr. Ibaum told us was Semlin. The water here was anything but clear, still it was not so muddy as we had seen it higher up.

The Danube is so shallow in the greater part of its course that vessels drawing more than three or four feet of water have to proceed with the greatest caution. We were going with the stream, which was very strong, yet I don't think the boat throughout the journey ever went at a greater rate than seven or eight knots an hour, so that we were afloat nearly three hours, although the distance between Belgrade and Semendria is barely twenty miles.

However, the weather was lovely, and the air fresh and pleasant, the sun not having as yet attained its full strength. The arrival of a steamboat was evidently a remarkable event at Semendria, for the landing-place was crowded with people. The majority of them were dressed *à la Turque*, in baggy knickerbockers, jackets, and *fezzes*; only a few wore European costume. Our uniforms at once made us objects of such interest, that we were followed about by a crowd, much to the delight of Dr. Ibaum, who astonished the multitude by speaking in English.

The hospital at which we were to work was a tumble-down wooden building of two storeys. It stood some twenty yards back from the roadway, and the ground in front was fenced with a rough, irregular wooden paling. In one corner of this enclosure stood a disused pigsty, which gave forth a very disagreeable and piggish odour. The hospital was built on a most irregular plan. It jutted out here and went in there in the oddest fashion. The upper storey was reached from the outside by a rickety wooden flight of steps, which sloped into the yard.

We were met as we entered the latter by Dr. Ibaum's colleague. Dr. Lazar Stephanovitch, a short, thick-set, coarse-looking man, who conducted us into one of the wards on the ground floor. This was a room some thirty feet long by fifteen wide, paved with tiles, and lighted by eight small windows, four on each side. The windows did not open, and there being no other means of ventilation than the door, the stench was terrible. The floor, too, was in a very dirty condition.

In this delightful place some twenty wounded men were lying on as many beds. Every now and then one of them would utter an exclamation of pain, but the majority of them bore their sufferings patiently, and some were even chatting cheerily. There were no female nurses in the establishment, their places being taken by soldiers chosen for the duty by lot. These men did not strike me at first sight as being suited to the work. Like most of the Servian peasantry, they were clumsy, good-natured simpletons. I saw directly that there would be plenty for us to do, and wished to set to work at once; but Dr. Stephanovitch informed me that their patients' wounds had all been dressed for the day. I pointed to the windows, and expressed my dissatisfaction at the ventilation. He replied that the building was a makeshift for a hospital, and that they were compelled to make the best they could of it. Then, after addressing a kind word or two to each patient, the doctors invited us to accompany them through the other wards, of which there were three.

Throughout the hospital I found the condition of things much the same. The men had fairly comfortable beds, and were well fed, but there was an utter want of ventilation, of cleanliness, and, as I have already stated, of properly qualified nurses. Dr. Ibaum also told me that they were very short of splints, bandages, and disinfectants, and that our supplies would be most acceptable, so we arranged to send them into the hospital that evening. Neither he nor Dr. Stephanovitch would accept the money we had collected in London, so we enclosed it in a letter, and sent it off to Dr. Petrovitch at the War Office.

The two doctors informed us that they began work at the hospital at six in the morning—and usually completed their rounds by ten o'clock, after which they took it in turns to remain on duty for the rest of the day. We were requested to be there at six also, and they expected to receive in a day or two a large batch of wounded men from the front, so that we must be prepared for hard work. We had some little difficulty in finding any lodgings within a convenient distance of the hospital, and were compelled to be content with a large room in a pretty one-storied house, the front of which was overgrown with flowering creepers.

The room looked clean, and had a large window which opened on to a little piece of front garden. The bed linen, we were glad to observe, was snow-white. We asked Dr. Ibaum to settle the terms, and after a little chaffering with the landlord, he arranged that we were to pay one *ducat* a week for board and lodging—terms which we considered astoundingly moderate, although Dr. Ibaum informed us they were very high, and explained that he had not been able to manage better for us, because the war had forced up the price of everything.

When we had secured the room, the kind little doctor invited us to accompany him to the house of a relative who was overseer of the extensive vineyard belonging to Prince Milan in the neighbourhood of Semendria, from which he acquires a considerable portion of his revenue.

After a delightful walk through an undulating and beautifully wooded country we reached the vineyard. The house of the overseer, M. Ristovitch, stood on a little eminence in the centre of the vineyard, commanding a view over a great part of the estate. Our approach, therefore, was soon perceived, and with true Servian hospitality M. Ristovitch came forth to meet us, and invited us to join his family. The party consisted of M. Ristovitch and his wife—a comely middle-aged lady—Mademoiselle Ristovitch—a pretty brunette with beautiful dark eyes and luxuriant black hair—and a Bulgarian girl, Mademoiselle Miloikovitch, taller and slighter than her companion. There was a restlessness and self-possession in the manner of this fair Bulgarian which reminded me considerably of Miss ——, the popular English burlesque actress, whose voice, too, hers much resembled.

We were soon on the most friendly terms, and odd as it may seem, our quickly-formed intimacy was in some measure attributable to the mosquitoes with which the house and vineyard swarmed. The Servian name for mosquitoes is *Kamaratz*, and we excited not a little amusement by calling them *Karamatz*, which, I believe, means elephant, or some other huge animal. From the attacks of these pests our entertainers, both ladies and gentlemen, defended us in a manner at once original and simple.

While I was speaking, a mosquito settled upon my face. M. Ristovitch perceived it, and promptly succoured me by crushing the insect between his finger and my skin; and this proceeding, which was frequently repeated, was as amusing to us as our mis-pronunciation of *Kamaratz* was to them—nay, more, the younger ladies especially came to our assistance so frequently, and with such bewitching grace, that they made a very deep impression upon our too susceptible hearts.

Hiems was captivated by the beautiful Servian, and I was led in chains by the lovely Bulgarian. After dinner tobacco and cigarette papers were produced, and we all—ladies as well as gentlemen—fell to smoking and drinking coffee. Before leaving England, I entertained a narrow-minded and bigoted objection to ladies smoking, but the charming grace with which these fair Sclav damsels put a cigarette to their pretty lips, took a little whiff, and then with an elegant turn of the wrist and play of the hand, removed it, breathing forth small puffs and wreaths of fragrant smoke, caused my prejudices to melt away.

Presently the young ladies sat down to the piano and discoursed excellent music, and Mademoiselle Miloikovitch sang a Bulgarian love song, of which I did not understand a single word—more's the pity—to a quaint and plaintive melody. Then, to our dismay, we were called upon to contribute to the entertainment. Hiems, who could play a little, strummed forth his stock waltz, "The Beautiful Blue Danube."

This our entertainers seemed to regard as a special compliment to them and their muddy river, and they applauded enthusiastically. Then came my turn. My treacherous friend declared that I had a superb voice, and sang exquisitely. This absolutely false statement filled me with confusion and despair. In vain did I cough and use my handkerchief, and protest that I had a frightful cold. My villainous comrade told them not to believe me, so the two ladies, particularly Mademoiselle Miloikovitch, led me firmly but gently to the piano, and fixing their lovely eyes upon me, alternately coaxed and commanded me to sing an English song. My *rèpertoire* at that time was very limited, consisting only of "God save the Queen," and the "Perfect Cure!" I selected the former, and sang it as well as I could to a one-finger accompaniment, played by myself. They recognised the air immediately, and joined us in the chorus most harmoniously, and after it was over, were pleased to greet my humble and discordant effort with prolonged applause.

Emboldened by this success I was tempted to sing the "Cure," much to their delight and amusement Dr. Ibaum seemed more pleased than anyone else, for he clapped his hands and shouted "Bravo! Bravissimo!" until he was hoarse, and then went about informing everyone that these were real English songs. When he had somewhat recovered from his excitement, he sat down to the piano himself, and shouting out, "Dance, dance!" he commenced playing in admirable style the "*Soldaten Lieder*" waltz. At this the girls signalled to us to help them, and we wheeled the furniture from the centre of the room, and then ...

Alas! the pleasantest meeting comes to an end. When we had had a few most delicious waltzes, Dr. Ibaum informed us that it was time to set our faces homeward again, so we thanked our new acquaintances for their hospitality, and prepared to bid them *adieu*. All insisted, however, on accompanying us to the vineyard boundary. Presently our revolvers became objects of interest. Ristovitch and Ibaum expressed a desire to see their effect upon the stump of an old tree. We readily complied with their request, but our revolvers being "Bulldogs," weapons that make a tremendous report, and with which it is almost impossible to hit anything, the shooting was very indifferent.

Mademoiselle Ristovitch put her fingers in her ears, and gave a pretty little scream every time we fired, but Mademoiselle Miloikovitch seemed greatly interested, and presently, to my surprise, asked me to load the weapon for her, and to allow her to have a shot. I did so after some remonstrance. As I handed the pistol to her, a singular change came over her face; the fresh colour died away from her cheeks, the amiable light in her eyes was replaced by a fierce sparkle, and her lips were sternly compressed together. Taking a steady aim, she fired three successive shots at the tree, and the third time succeeded in hitting it.

Dr. Ibaum subsequently informed me that several of her relations had been massacred by the Turks in 1875, and that she herself had shot two *bashi-bazouks* in making her escape.

Chapter 5

Radicalism

Besides the Servian hospital to which we were attached, there was another in Semendria, supported by the Russian Red Cross Society, and of which all the staff were Russians. On our return we found awaiting us an invitation to spend the evening with the Russian doctors, and as Ibaum was going, too, we accompanied him. We were received with hearty courtesy, and as we expressed a wish to see their hospital, they very kindly took us over it. The arrangements there were as excellent as those at our place were faulty. The ventilation was first-rate, the wards were beautifully clean, and the air in them smelt fresh and pure. Venetian blinds to the windows tempered the heat of the sun.

There were four wards, each of which contained about twenty wounded men, and to each ward was a trained nurse. These nurses, indeed, were lady medical students. When we entered, one of these ladies was applying a bandage to a man's arm with a skill that I have never seen surpassed. Adjoining the hospital was the house in which Dr. Cutemoff and the rest of the staff resided—a long one storeyed building, with rooms of considerable size. The evening being cool and pleasant, a table had been taken in the garden and spread with a substantial meal. Tea, coffee, beer, wine, spirits, sardines, preserves, caviar, soda-water in syphons, jars of tobacco, books of cigarette-papers, grapes, and jugs of milk were displayed in tempting profusion.

After we had all partaken of this good cheer, the tobacco and cigarette papers were handed round, and a general and cosmopolitan conversation began. Only three of the lady medicals were present, the other one remaining on duty at the hospital; but the three who honoured us with their presence were really shining lights in their way. None of them could be called beautiful, but they all had clever and intelligent faces. The plainest of the trio, indeed, a Mademoiselle

Dinah Mitykoff, struck me as being the cleverest. The conversation was carried on by different members of the company in French, German, Russian, and English, amid the clattering of glasses and clouds of tobacco smoke. This Mademoiselle Dinah Mitykoff, next to whom I was sitting, began by abruptly asking me if I was a radical.

"No," replied I, "I am a liberal conservative." She fixed her eyes upon me (they were blue eyes, not very large, but uncommonly sharp and bright) with a somewhat contemptuous expression, and then after a short pause blew forth from her lips a cloud of cigarette smoke, which completely concealed her face for a moment, and asked me "why I was not a radical."

"Because I appreciate law and order, and dislike extreme views and measures," replied I, somewhat nettled at her contemptuous manner; "and radicalism means the subversion of order, and consists of nothing but extreme views and measures."

Again, she looked at me with the same aggravating expression; then she said, "When you are older and wiser, sir, you will know that radicalism means progress."

Considering that she did not seem more than a year or two older than myself, her rebuke amused me greatly. I replied, however, that I did not admit that radicalism was synonymous with progress; on the contrary, I thought it tended to disorder and chaos, and consequently retrogression, and I added that most eminent radicals were either furious fanatics or unpractical dreamers.

"You are wrong, *monsieur*," said she. "We radicals are the most practical people in the world, and, for my part, unless I believed in the progress of mankind in this real and tangible world towards greater liberty, happiness, and knowledge, I should discard all faith in religion. Mark my words, the time is not far distant—nay, it is almost at hand—when kings and emperors will be swept aside, and even distinctions of nationality will cease to exist. The whole human race will live together in harmony and brotherly love, and though my country seems one of the most backward now, she will be foremost in leading to the change."

"Amen," said Dr. Knifem, one of the surgeons, in a deep voice, moving his chair closer to us. "The changes Mademoiselle Dinah Mitykoff foresees will assuredly come soon, but they will be preceded by a universal and terrible revolution—a tornado which will blow away the tyrannies and abuses that now infest and poison the world. Then, woe betide the enemies of human progress!"

"What will you do to them? Will you cut their throats?" said I, with a smile.

"Yes, like rats," said he, a fierce gleam shooting across his face.

"You are a radical, I presume?" said I.

"I am an enemy to tyrants and a friend of liberty. Call me what you like—radical, socialist, or nihilist—anything you please," replied he.

"But, my good sir," said I, "there are great numbers of persons who, like myself, believe themselves to be really greater friends of progress than you radicals, but who are strongly opposed to extreme measures and revolution. Are we, too, to be knocked on the head?"

"You must decide for yourself, sir, which side you take when the critical time comes, and if you choose the wrong side, you will have only yourself to thank if you suffer for it."

"And you are so convinced that your views are right, that you would make war on other nations to promulgate them."

"Yes, we would make war on tyrants," replied he.

"What!" said I, "and kill thousands of your fellow-creatures, bombard towns, and bring ruin and desolation on hundreds of happy homes?"

"I have told you already, sir, that we would even make war in support of our views. I know as well as you that war is a horrible and atrocious thing, but at the very worst, it can only affect a fractional part of one generation, whereas untold generations would reap permanent advantage by the triumph of our glorious cause."

"Come, come, ladies and gentlemen," said Dr. Cutemoff, "that is enough of politics for the evening. You'll never make converts of each other by argument. I never yet came across anyone who was argued out of his convictions. Let us have a game of cards."

Chapter 6

Rough Travelling

The next morning, we were up betimes. The Servians are early risers, and the landlord and servants of the hotel were up and about before five o'clock.

Dr. Ibaum called for us—gay and festive as ever—and brought his English dog, Bee-lee, with him, a pretty little black-and-tan terrier.

"Aha! my friends, my friends," said he, "how you to do this early morning? Have you slip well, eh? Are you slippy steel? (Sleepy still.) No! good-good! Will you to snuff? No? So, so. Here, Bee-lee, my Inglis tog! Bee-lee I Inglis name! Ah! he come to see my Inglis friend. Inglis tog will to see Inglis man. Eh—ha! ha! ha! Beelee, say you how do now—good tog!"

Bee-lee sat up on his hind legs and held out a paw.

"Bee-lee good beggar, jolly good beggar—eh?" said the doctor complacently to us.

We were amused by the doctor's droll language and loquacity, and Hiems replied that the dog was a first-rate beggar.

"Yes," said the doctor, "I have teached him all myself, when he was small pup-dog. But come, my dear friends, now must we to the hospital go. Bee-lee shall to carry my stick, and I will take your arm." So, saying, he threw his cane into the garden, when Billy rushed after it with a shrill yelp, seized it, shook it, after the manner of dogs, and finally trotted off with it—wagging his tail rejoicingly, and looking round every now and then to see if we were following him.

A few minutes' walking brought us to the hospital, where we found Dr. Stephanovitch already at work. We lost no time in following his example. I was requested to attend to the out-patients. These consisted, for the most part, of men who had received slight wounds about the face or arms, also a good many malingerers, who to avoid going to the front had mutilated themselves by placing a finger over the muzzle of a rifle and pulling the trigger with the other hand.

Some of these fellows had punished themselves much more severely than they had intended, and in one or two instances their hands were completely shattered, and, as might have been expected, they displayed very little fortitude whilst having their wounds dressed. As there was no special out-patients' department, I attended my cases in one of the wards, in which, at the same time, Dr. Ibaum was engaged with the in-patients, some of whose wounds were of a very painful nature. To my surprise, those who were waiting their turn laughed at the contortions of their suffering comrades as a capital joke, whilst a few minutes after, these, in their turn, would be laughing at the grimaces of the other unfortunates.

The Servians are naturally a kind-hearted race, and this apparent heartlessness was due, evidently, to a keen sense of the ludicrous. I have seen Servians roll over one another in fits of laughter at a very feeble joke. The Servian doctors prized our Condy's fluid very highly. After its introduction, the mortality, so they said, was distinctly diminished, and wounds to which it was applied certainly healed up with great rapidity. The rest of our supplies also were of considerable service, particularly a large case of Liebig's *Extractum Carnis*. The Servians make excellent soup, but do not understand beef-tea, and many of the patients who could not take the soup on account of its greasiness, were able both to take and enjoy the former.

With the consent of Drs. Ibaum and Stephanovitch, one of the uppermost panes in each of the windows was knocked out and replaced by a small Venetian blind; and to impress our soldier nurses with the importance of cleanliness and set them an example, Hiems and I sprinkled the floor over with diluted Condy's fluid, and swept the ward out ourselves. The soldiers looked on with approving smiles, and we thought we had made a great hit. We were, however, mistaken. The next morning, I found the floor of my ward untouched. Putting on a stern expression, I beckoned one of the soldiers up, handed him the broom, and motioned him to set to work with it. The man, however, impudently, amid the laughter of his comrades, returned the broom to me, and motioned to me to sweep.

I was so indignant that I seized him by the collar and turned him out of the ward, bestowing a kick upon him as soon as I had got him outside the door. The fellow did not mind being turned out of the ward, but objected to the kick, and aimed a blow at me in return, whereupon I was compelled, in self-defence, to knock him down.

I then handed him the broom once more, but he sulkily refused to take it. I was puzzled what to do for the moment. Suddenly a happy thought struck me. I took the commission I had received from the War Office out of my pocket and showed it to him. On it was the State seal. This seemed to make a great impression upon him.

I then mentioned in succession the names of Prince Milan, M. Ristic, and Dr. Sava Petrovitch, looked very grave and determined, and once more handed him the broom. The soldier took it without a word, and set to work immediately. I then showed the commission to the other men, and repeated the talismanic names to them, with—I am happy to say—the same success. After this they always behaved with the greatest civility, and I never had occasion to complain again of the untidiness of the ward. Hiems had some trouble also, but Dr. Stephanovitch interfered, and compelled the soldiers to obey him.

We were very short of splints at this hospital, and had to improvise them out of old boxes or anything that came to hand. We showed some of the most intelligent of the men how to dress wounds, and in a short time they became really zealous and useful assistants.

Stephanovitch and Ibaum worked hard and unremittingly, and we also did our best, but in spite of our utmost efforts, mortality amongst the severely wounded was very high. The Servians have an invincible repugnance to amputation, and many lives which might have been saved were lost through obstinate refusal of the men to submit to the operation. At the front the soldier's consent was not asked, but in our hospitals no operation was permitted without it.

The Servian transport system—for the wounded—at that time also was extremely defective. Semendria was more than eighty miles from the scene of action, the roads were, in many parts, extremely rough, and yet scarcely any of the waggons in which the wounded were conveyed had springs. Travelling, even for those in sound health, was far from pleasant, whilst the sufferings of wounded men—with, in many instances, unset, fractured limbs, and exposed to the fierce heat of the Servian sun—must have been something almost too shocking to contemplate.

The journey from Deligrad to Semendria in these waggons occupied from two to three days. It is not surprising, then, that many of the severe cases were moribund when they reached us, whilst not a few actually died *en route*.

The work of the day at the hospital over, we used to spend our evenings in various ways. The most agreeable, perhaps, were passed with the Ristovitch family, whom we occasionally entertained at our quarters. Our landlord, a genial old Serv, on these occasions placed his whole house at our disposal, and his wife—a kind-hearted, buxom, but withal active dame—would bustle about the house making the necessary preparations. After tea the young ladies gave us lessons in Servian, whilst M. Ristovitch smoked his cigarette and looked on, and his wife knitted, and every now and then offered a suggestion.

How we enjoyed ourselves!

We generally had two lessons every week—one at M. Ristovitch's house, and one at our own, and at one of the latter we had quite a little adventure. Hiems and I had been out for a walk. We had gone as far as the old fort at Semendria—a ruined castle built by the Turks about the middle of the fifteenth century, and a very favourite resort of ours, for we used to wander amongst the ruins and hunt for snakes. A species of adder abounds there which attains a considerable size, and which the Servians hold in great dread. I have killed them quite four feet in length. The Servians say that the bite is fatal.

On the day in question, we turned over a huge stone in our search, and in so doing disclosed a very fine snake. The creature gave a fierce hiss, and endeavoured to escape, but we belaboured it with our sticks until it appeared to be dead, and then we took it back with us in triumph. At home it was placed in a basin of water to cleanse it from the blood and dust, and left in one of the rooms whilst we prepared to receive our visitors. They did not arrive quite punctually, and we went a little way to meet them, and brought them back with us. As usual, tea was served in the garden, and our lesson begun there as well; but during the course of the latter the sky became darkened with storm clouds, and ere long a flash of lightning, followed by a terrific peal of thunder and a shower of hail, drove us indoors. We repaired to a room adjoining that in which we had left our snake.

The storm was so fierce whilst it lasted, the lightning so vivid, the crashes of thunder so deafening, and the downpour of hail and rain so heavy, that for a few minutes all remained silent. Gradually, however, as the storm abated, we resumed our conversation, and were very soon busy at our lessons. For some reason or other I was rather more backward than usual on this occasion, and my teacher was on the point of administering a lecture to me, when a loud hiss, followed by a scream from Mademoiselle Ristovitch, startled us all. There, in the twilight, for it was now getting dark, we discerned our captive gliding across the floor. For one second Hiems and I stared at one another in blank

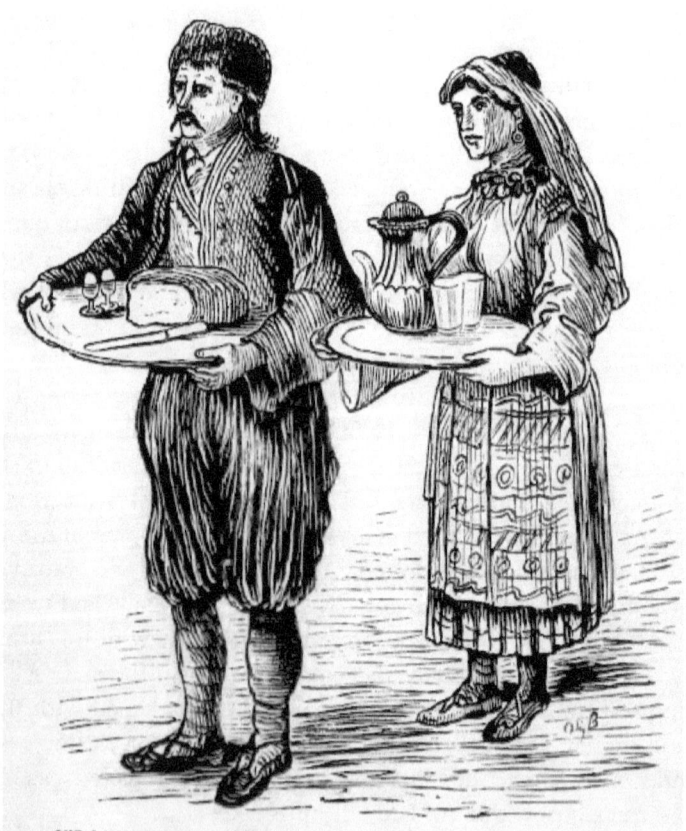

OUR LANDLORD AND LANDLADY AT SEMENDRIA BRINGING OUR BREAKFAST.

dismay; all was commotion and panic. The three ladies, tucking up their dresses after the manner of the sex when crossing a muddy road, perched themselves on chairs.

M. Ristovitch armed himself with the hearth brush, Hiems seized a stick, and I a wooden stool, and we advanced to attack the reptile, which retreated into a corner, and with erect head and fierce hisses stood at bay. The contest was short and sharp. The snake made a sudden dart at me, which, luckily, I succeeded in receiving on my stool, and the next minute my friends had struck it down, and I had crushed its head. This affair made Madame Ristovitch so nervous and uncomfortable that her husband decided on returning home at once. The storm had now completely passed away. The western sky was still bright and flushed with gold and crimson by the setting sun, the moon had risen, and the stars were beginning to twinkle. Altogether it was a beautiful evening. M. Ristovitch took the lead on their homeward journey with his wife, Hiems followed with Mademoiselle Ristovitch, and I brought up the rear with Mademoiselle Miloikovitch.

Now whether it was due to the storm or to the fine weather which followed, or to the influence of the planet Venus, which certainly was twinkling very brightly just then, or to the pale moonbeams, or to the lively manner in which Mademoiselle Miloikovitch had mounted a chair and maintained herself there during our combat with the snake, I cannot say, but I felt at that moment desperately in love with her.

For several minutes we walked on in silence, but although I did not actually speak, I was several times on the verge of doing so. What I wanted to ask her was, "What is the Servian name for love?"

At last, I did venture to speak, but the sound of my voice frightened me. I could get no further than "what." Three desperate efforts I made to get out the phrase, but each time my voice and courage failed me.

Fortune, however, favours the brave, and at last she had compassion, and helped me. The part of the road we were now traversing was rather rough, and in the silvery moonlight I saw that Mademoiselle Ristovitch had taken Hiems' arm. I therefore ventured to offer my arm to my partner, and, to my great joy, she at once took it. What a thrill of delight I experienced when I felt her fingers resting on it! The contact, light as it was, inspired me with fresh courage, and clearing my throat I dashed at the sentence once more, and this time succeeded in getting it all out.

"If you please, *mademoiselle*, what is the Servian word for love?"

Mademoiselle Miloikovitch fixed her large dark eyes on me for a moment with an expression in which surprise and amusement were equally blended, and then, to my great disappointment and discomfiture, replied, "I have given one lesson today already, M. Alfred, and I certainly am not going to give you another now. Besides, there are lots of things I want to talk about. For instance, I want to know if you have ever been a soldier?"

"I have been a volunteer," replied I, proudly.

"Can you shoot well?" said she, looking at me approvingly.

"Not well for an English rifleman, who are the best shots in the world, still I could hit a man at two hundred yards," I replied.

"I wish I were a man instead of a woman," said she, with sudden energy, "I would enlist in our army immediately."

"What a singular wish," said I, considerably surprised.

"A singular wish, M. Alfred! Do you not know that my relatives have been murdered and my dear country overrun and rendered desolate by those hateful wretches—the Turks? What would you think if your own land were invaded by hordes of cruel barbarians, smiling villages and happy homes turned into blackened heaps of ruins, and innocent, defenceless men, women, and children shot down and hacked to pieces? It has been my cruel lot to see all this take place before my very eyes, and I care not what anyone thinks, and I repeat it—I long for vengeance, and I often think of going—woman as I am—to the front and firing a shot at our accursed enemies."

Mademoiselle Miloikovitch spoke with such fierce emphasis and excitement, that for a moment I was thunderstruck. At last, I said, "*Mademoiselle*, I sympathise most deeply with you, and I am very certain that were I in your place, I should feel precisely as you do now."

"What," said she, eagerly, "would you recommend me to go to the front?"

"Heaven forbid, *mademoiselle!*" said I, "unless you went as a nurse; and even then, I don't think it would be a wise step on your part, as you have had no training."

"What aggravating things you men are! You are all alike; you all say the same thing; and there's not a bit of sense in a single word you utter!" said she petulantly; then with a laugh she added, "I expect you think me very strange. All the same, soldiering apart, I wish I were a man! Your greedy sex monopolised all the sensible occupations, and left us poor women nothing but nursing and needlework."

"Pardon me, *mademoiselle*, but I do not think you quite do justice to our unfortunate sex. In my humble opinion, the ladies— who in the long run always have their own way—have allotted all the really disagreeable work to us men. Who works harder and gets worse paid than the doctor? Who gets more abuse than the lawyer, or more sneered at than the parson, or more hard blows than the soldier, or is more hated than the politician? On the other hand, what can be more delightful than looking after a number of merry, innocent children, or more profitable than needlework, which provides you with new dresses, etc.?"

"M. Wright," said Mademoiselle Miloikovitch sternly, at the same time withdrawing her hand from my arm, "you are talking nonsense, and you know it. I shall not walk with you if you continue to do so!"

"My dear *mademoiselle*," said I, in considerable alarm, "pray forgive me; I most humbly apologise. Ah, *mademoiselle!* can you think I would presume intentionally to offend you?" and I contritely tendered her my arm again.

"I cannot say whether I will forgive you or not," replied the young lady, still walking apart from me, "that will depend entirely upon your behaviour for the rest of the evening. Now I want you to tell me, if you can, why the professions should not be as open to women as they are to men?"

"At the present time, *mademoiselle*," replied I, "there is, in my humble opinion, no good objection, speaking theoretically, to women, who are fitted by taste and inclination, and have been suitably educated, entering the professions. Practically, I scarcely think the world sufficiently advanced for such a step. Women are, speaking generally, purer and more refined than men, and they exercise an immense influence over our sex for good, which may be termed a home influence. Take women away from home, and send them into the world as it now stands, what would happen? They might gain in intellect, but I believe they would suffer morally by the change, and their influence for good be converted into an influence for evil. With the spread, however, of real thoughtful religion and knowledge, and the mental elevation that will accompany them, men and women will be able to work indiscriminately together, and then their so doing will have a good effect rather than otherwise."

"And how long, oh! most profound philosopher," said Mademoiselle Miloikovitch, "do you think it will be before this will happen?"

"I cannot say," replied I. "I don't believe the world is ripe for it just yet. It rests very much with you ladies when it will take place. You have an instrument at your disposal more powerful for moving the world than Archimedes' lever."

"What is that, *M. le Philosophe?*" said she.

"The force of your example, *mademoiselle*. When the ladies make up their minds to do a thing, it is said they always do it. Now there are 500,000,000 ladies, young and old, in the world. Let these 500,000,000 irresistible beings resolve that the world shall take a decided step in the direction of goodness, progress, and enlightenment; and let them, with that end in view, one and all, give us poor men the benefit of their powerful example, and heigh-presto! the change would be effected at once."

"Do you mean to insinuate then, sir," said Mademoiselle Miloikovitch, with an air of mock gravity, "that we ladies are not setting you a good example now?"

"Far be it from me, *mademoiselle*, to insinuate anything so utterly false," replied I; "but I thought it might be possible for your sex, as a whole, to undertake the measure more vigorously."

"Hum, M. Alfred, you are a provoking prevaricator. I will wait for six months to see if the world profits by my good example, and takes a step in the right direction; but if it shows no signs of improvement then, I will become a professional woman at once. But here we are at home, will you come in? No? Then *adieu!* and many thanks for your instructive and philosophical discourse."

"*Adieu, mademoiselle,*" replied I, attempting to give her hand a tender little squeeze; "will you tell me next time the Servian for that little word?"

"You must wait until next time, M. le Philosophe," said she, withdrawing her hand, "and see. *Adieu* again."

CHAPTER 7

A Narrow Escape

Close to the old fort was a secluded spot by the river side. Here, morning and evening, Hiems and I were wont to bathe. The Servians tried to dissuade us, declaring that the river abounded in poisonous water-snakes. The weather was so intensely hot, and we were so fond of the water, that in spite of the alarm occasioned by this information, we bathed regularly, at least once a day. Neither of us ever saw a water-snake nor anything like one, but it is not impossible that some of the adders, of which there are great numbers close to the water's edge, may, for divers reasons known only to themselves, occasionally indulge in a swim in the river, and that this was the origin of the Semendrian belief in water-snakes.

The night after my stroll with Mademoiselle Miloikovitch, I was singularly sleepless. I lay thinking a long time of our conversation. I felt vexed at having been so timorous, and kept conjuring up in my mind's eye some bolder suitor stepping in before me and winning her affections. "Surely," I thought, "so beautiful and interesting a young lady must have shoals of admirers;" and tossing about on my bed, I resolved that next time I would make a formal proposal, and secure her for myself at once. This notable resolution calmed me a little, and I presently dozed off, but my sleep was fitful and broken by all kinds of senseless dreams. At five o'clock I rose, determined to refresh myself for my day's work by a swim in the river. I tried hard to persuade Hiems to accompany me, but the only response elicited from him by my eloquent appeal was an inarticulate mumbling, followed by a loud snore, so I set off by myself.

Arrived at the bathing place I quickly undressed and plunged into the river, which here was very deep, and about one-fourth of a mile in width. I was a very indifferent swimmer, but the water was so pleasant that I struck out boldly, and was soon far out in the stream. The strong current carried me along for some distance, so that when I turned to swim back, I discovered, to my consternation, that I was a long way from the place where I had left my clothes, and was drifting towards a small row of huts which lies a little beyond the old fort. I did not wish to land in front of these huts, as people were already moving about on the shore, and I foolishly endeavoured to swim against the stream to the point from which I had started.

By exerting myself violently I succeeded in making a little progress at first, but I was quite two hundred yards from the shore, and beginning to feel dreadfully tired. Still, I struggled on, and succeeded in diminishing this distance by another fifty yards. By this time, however, I was nearly exhausted. A kind of numbness began to creep over my limbs, and I could scarcely strike out at all. Recognising my danger, I endeavoured to make straight for the shore, but the numbness continued to increase, and I soon saw that unless someone came to my assistance, I would be quite unable to get to land at all.

Cursing the folly which induced me to venture out so far alone, I shouted again and again for help. No one seemed to hear me, and I despairingly renewed my struggles. I thought of Mademoiselle Miloikovitch and of Hiems, of dear old England, and the friends and relatives whom I might never see again. Then drowsiness came over me—with the dim, vague idea of how comfortable the cottages on the shore looked, and how bright and green were the trees behind them, then I lost all consciousness. Luckily for me, a fisherman on the other side of the river had seen me turn in the water, and noticing the little progress I made, started to my assistance just as my strength was beginning to fail me. I had a very narrow escape, for he saw me sink twice before he could reach me, and just caught me by the hair as I was going down for the third time.

It was a long time before I recovered my consciousness. My first sensations were those of extreme misery and discomfort. There was a choking sensation at my throat, and I felt most horribly sick and faint. Then I was made to swallow some strong spirits, and on opening my eyes I saw, as it were, in a mist, Ibaum, Stephanovitch, Cutemoff, and my dear friend Hiems, the latter—God bless him!—sobbing as if his heart would break, and swearing at himself for not having gone with me to bathe, and praying for my recovery, in one and the same breath. Dr. Ibaum seemed scarcely less agitated, and when I opened my eyes, he flung away the glass of cordial he held in his hand, and rushed into my friend's arms, and the two hugged and jerked each other about—I can't say danced—in such a comical manner, that, ill as I was, I could not help laughing.

"Hurrah! hurrah! hurrah!" shouted Hiems; "he's coming round fast! Look there; he's laughing; hip, hip, hurrah!"

"Yes, yes; he have smile wit his mouth. I have seen so mine self, eep! eep! oorah!" and the two danced round again. Meanwhile Stephanovitch and Cutemoff had been working indefatigably (and, indeed, so had the others, until I opened my eyes and their feelings overcame them), trying different methods of artificial respiration upon me, chafing my limbs, and putting hot applications to my chest, etc.; and at last, they had succeeded in completely restoring my temporarily suspended animation.

"By Jove, doctor!" said Hiems, extricating himself from Ibaum's embrace, "he's coming round grandly. Let us make his bed comfortable for him, and he will have a good sleep."

By this time, I was able to breathe very well, and with a heart overflowing with gratitude I tried hard to thank my kind friends for their goodness, but they refused to let me speak, and tucking me up in dry and warm blankets, bade me go to sleep. As I felt very heavy and sleepy and weary, I was not long in following their advice. My last recollection of that memorable morning was seeing my dear old Hiems seated by my bedside, looking anxiously into my face, and good Dr. Ibaum stealing noiselessly about the room, now darkening the windows, and now chasing a noisy little mosquito from my bed.

But my troubles were not over yet. On waking from my sleep, I had a violent shivering fit, followed by a sharp pain in my side, great difficulty in breathing, and high fever.' The water I had drawn into my lungs caused a severe attack of pneumonia. For some days I was in furious delirium, and whilst in this condition the wildest and most extravagant fancies filled my brain. Now I thought I was on the battlefield, surrounded by *bashi-bazouks*, who, in spite of my furious resistance, bore me to the ground, and thrust their weapons into my chest and side. Then again, I would fancy I was walking about in a beautiful meadow with Mademoiselle Miloikovitch, plucking gorgeous flowers and offering them to her.

Suddenly a hollow moaning sound filled my ears, and a vague and indefinable feeling of dread came over me. Then, instead of Mademoiselle Miloikovitch, appeared a terrible and menacing figure, and the hollow moaning sound changed to a loud roar of advancing water, from which I would try to escape; but the figure by my side held me fast, and the waters overtook and overwhelmed me. This form of delirium was followed by a complete unconsciousness, during which time I believe I must have been asleep, for I awoke one morning to find the pain in my chest and difficulty of breathing nearly gone, and feeling comparatively comfortable. Hiems and Dr. Cutemoff were in the room, standing near the window, and talking in whispers. I had a vague idea that something had happened, but I could not recollect what, so I called out in a voice so weak and strange that it surprised me:—

"Hulloh! Hiems, where am I, and what is the matter?"

In a moment the two were at my bedside. "Thank God, my dear boy," said Hiems fervently, "for your recovery. You have been desperately ill. Once or twice we actually gave you up. At one time you were fighting, raging, and raving like a demon, so that it took three or four of us to hold you down, and you called me an infernal *bashi-bazouk*, Dr. Cutemoff a vile Circassian, and told Ibaum and Stephanovitch they were a couple of Turkish devils, and that if we would let you get up and try your hanging guard, you would take us all singlehanded. You told us fifty times over you were a British subject, and dared us to touch you, on pain of incurring the wrath of the British Empire."

"What a trouble and nuisance I must have been to you all!" said I, pressing Hiems' hand. "I am sure I can never, never repay you for all your kindness."

"Shut up, old chap," said Hiems; "you've nothing whatever to thank me for. The little I have been able to do I would have done for anybody who was as ill as you have been, much more then for an old friend. I'm sure, under similar circumstances, you would do the same for me."

"That I would, a thousand times over," replied I, gratefully.

"Very well then, you see we are quits. But now hold your tongue, old boy; you have done quite enough talking for the present. Hulloh! where's Cutemoff? Ah! here he comes with some beef-tea and jelly. What a regular trump he is, isn't he? Don't answer. So are they all."

And indeed, nothing could have exceeded the kindness I received from all quarters, and I owe the kind friends who attended me during my illness a debt of gratitude I can never repay.

CHAPTER 8

Baron von Tummy

Thanks to a sound constitution, I was soon up and about again, so that three weeks afterwards I was able to set to work at the hospital, and this, moreover, in spite of a severe disappointment which befell me in the temporary annihilation of any amatory designs upon Mademoiselle Miloikovitch. M. Ristovitch received a summons from the *Skuptchine*, or Servian Parliament, to proceed at once on business of importance to Paratchin, a town some sixty miles from Semendria, and not very far from Deligrad, which was at that time the headquarters of General Tchernaieff's army. As Mademoiselle Miloikovitch had relatives there, he decided upon taking her with him. Consequently, when I recovered, I found that my fair lady had gone, and that for the present I could hope for no opportunity of informing her of the state of my feelings.

A personage made his appearance at Semendria a day or two after I resumed work, who drove all thoughts of love-making out of my head. This was Baron von Tummy, the celebrated Austrian surgeon, who was acting at the time as Inspector-General of all the Servian hospitals. His advent was preceded by the arrival of a large batch of wounded and invalided soldiers from the front. They were so numerous that every available corner in both hospitals was occupied. Most of the invalids were suffering from dysentery, and were as ill as they could be, and many of them emaciated to skeletons. Many of the wounded soldiers, too, were dangerously hurt, so that, as might be imagined, we all had our hands pretty full.

Baron Von Tummy was a very remarkable man, both for intellect and personal appearance. He was very short, very stout, and very clever; in fact, weighty both in mind and body. In height he was perhaps five feet two inches, but he must have been nearly two yards in circumference. He might have been fifty years of age, and he had iron-grey hair, beard, moustache, and whiskers, and a stern and resolute expression. The day he arrived all the doctors mustered at the hospital to receive him. Everything was as neat and shipshape as possible, but though the wards were clean, two things were painfully evident—the defective ventilation and the overcrowding.

Our first impression of Baron Von Tummy was decidedly agreeable. Considering his great size, he was remarkably active, and waddled along at an astonishing rate. He was dressed in the uniform of a colonel in the Servian army—*viz.*, a brown tunic with red facings, a row of gilt buttons down the centre, and three gold stars on either side of the collar, blue pantaloons, with a very broad red stripe down the sides, and a naval officer's peaked cap. He carried no sabre, but bore in his right hand a huge white cotton umbrella, lined with blue, with which he shaded himself from the sun. The first thing the baron did on entering the hospital was to shut up his umbrella, pull a very wry face, stop his nose with his fingers, and charge at the windows with the point of his gingham. *Smash, crash*, and *crinnel!* and a shower of glass descended on to the floor. Then, turning to me with startling abruptness, he said, in excellent English:—

"Phew, that's a d———d sight better, Mr. Englishman, isn't it?"

"A great improvement, sir," said I.

The baron's grimace and whimsical energy excited the risibility of the servants and soldiers present, and they all began to chuckle and grin. Von Tummy stopped short and glared around him with a fierce growl, and the alarmed bystanders checked their hilarity directly, all except one unhappy man, who did his best to restrain his mirth, but ineffectually, and broke every now and then into a smothered guffaw.

In an instant the redoubtable umbrella descended on his head with a sounding thwack, and as the man turned to flee, his departure was expedited by the forcible application of the baron's foot to his back.

As soon as order was restored again, the baron completed his inspection of the wards, formally presented Dr. Stephanovitch with a copy of a book he had published on hospital management, shook hands very affably with Hiems and myself, and took his leave.

On my expressing surprise to one of the doctors at the baron's familiarity with the English language, he told me that he (the baron) could converse fluently in twelve European languages, and that curiously enough he paid especial attention to oaths and expletives, so that when annoyed he would sometimes swear in half a score of different tongues.

Some days after I received a despatch signed "Ludwig Von Tummy." It informed me that I was selected to take charge of a batch of forty wounded men who were to be sent from Semendria to Belgrade; that I should have two Servian medical students as assistants, and that I must be in readiness to start by steamboat the next morning. Poor Hiems looked round to see if there was a despatch for him, and was sorely disappointed not to find one. However, he consoled himself with the reflection, that, had he been sent, he would have been deprived of the society of the charming Mademoiselle Ristovitch.

Presently Ibaum and Stephanovitch looked in. They also had received orders from Von Tummy to get the wounded men in readiness. They congratulated me heartily on my good fortune in being selected for the service, but there was, at the same time, something mysterious in their manner. They nodded and winked and whispered to one another in a way that puzzled both Hiems and myself. It was evident that both wished to say something to me, but that neither liked to begin. At length Stephanovitch asked me in German whether I preferred the charge of sick men or wounded. I replied that it was immaterial to me, but that other things being equal, sick men required less looking after. "Ha," said little Ibaum, with an air of great satisfaction, "you will like bester to take ill people?"

"No, I don't say that," I replied. "I merely say that sick men will probably require less looking after."

"So—so—good—most good," said Ibaum, nodding his head. Then they smiled and winked at one another, and shook hands with me over and over again, and departed, leaving the mystery unsolved.

The next morning, we were up at six o'clock, and at the hospital by half-past. There all was noise and masterly inactivity. Several of the soldier servants were lounging about, chattering away at the top of their voices. A few were engaged in the removal of the wounded, but were doing it in the most casual manner—joining in the general conversation and exchanging repartees with the loungers with the most perfect indifference to the groans of their unhappy burdens. These unfortunate creatures were deposited by twos in little carts littered with straw and hay, and driven slowly to the landing-place, there to await embarkation. Early as it was, Drs. Ibaum and Stephanovitch were already there, superintending operations. As soon as the former saw me, he came forward, and greeting me cordially pressed me to have some breakfast with him in the hospital. Believing there was a lot of work to be done, I declined.

"My so good friend," said Ibaum, "there is not more wounded men to go. They have all early this morning gone; there is the laster two!"

"Goodness me!" said I; "you must have been up very early this morning."

"My dear friend," replied he, "I was very early to rise this morning. The Baron Von Tummy is a very punctual man—oh, most punctuallest! So come in, you, and the dear Hiems, and have a few breakfast here!" It was quite true—all the invalids who were to be removed had gone, so we yielded to Dr. Ibaum's hospitable importunity, and had a "few breakfast" with him. During the progress of the meal, I noticed our host once or twice exchanging signals with Stephanovitch, and wondered thereat, but reflecting that their idiosyncrasies were no concern of mine, I went on with my breakfast, and said nothing.

As soon as the meal was concluded, we went to the river side, where the wounded men were awaiting the arrival of the steamboat, which was to convey them away. The latter was now within half a mile of us, and rapidly approaching. As soon as Ibaum saw the boat, he produced a field-glass, and adjusting its focus somewhat pompously, scanned the steamer with a haughty and commanding air. Suddenly he turned very white, dropped the glass out of his hands, and uttering a hollow groan, literally staggered against Stephanovitch. The countenance of the latter, too, underwent a sudden and ghastly change, like that of a man who is seized with an attack of cramp in the stomach, and both of them uttered simultaneously the name Von Tummy!

Following the direction of their glances, I saw on board the vessel, and looking over its side, the fierce, resolute countenance of the illustrious Von Tummy! But though the great man's expression was ferocious, yet, as he was not looking at either of the terror-stricken Servian doctors, I was quite at a loss to account for their panic.

Meanwhile the steamer glided up to the landing-place, and the object of their dread waddled ashore, and, strange to say, saluted us all with gracious cordiality, and then gave orders that a stack of hay, which stood in a field close by, should be demolished, and the hay spread over the deck for the wounded men to lie on. Now it so happened that the hay belonged to a farmer who intended consigning it to Belgrade for sale to the military authorities, and who hoped to reap a large profit by the transaction.

The consternation of this individual, who happened to be standing by when the hospital servants began to carry out the baron's injunctions, was piteous. With anguish depicted on every feature, he hastened to Von Tummy's side and energetically remonstrated against this summary proceeding. The baron's reply was a terrific scowl and a savage ejaculation, which evidently meant "Shut up!" The foolhardy farmer, however, persisted in pleading for his goods. The baron gave him another black look, and then, as lightning flashes fall from a storm-cloud, leaped upon him, and inflicted, first a heavy blow upon his nose, then a second on his stomach, which doubled him up, and finally put him to flight by a volley of kicks.

Meanwhile the soldiers, with the usual Servian indolence, were very slowly pulling down the stack and trailing small bundles of hay towards the ship. The lazy spectacle exasperated the irascible and energetic Von Tummy beyond measure. Seizing a long carter's whip from a bystander, he rushed amongst them and lashed into them furiously, shouting with every stroke "*Heite!*" (make haste!), followed by a string of untranslatable and unsavoury Servian and German oaths. The effect of this well-timed onslaught was excellent. The demolition of the haystack was greatly accelerated, and the hay was promptly conveyed on board and arranged on the deck. Hiems, with his hateful love of punning, remarked, with a grin, "That it was but natural that a whipping should make the Servians smart," a joke which, in spite of my respect for the baron, nearly made me ill.

Apparently satisfied and restored to good humour by the results of his severity, the baron linked his arm in mine, and leaning on me, said that he would now inspect the wounded men.

As we approached the convoy of invalids Ibaum and Stephanovitch were once more seized with the same unaccountable panic—especially Ibaum, who hurriedly muttering something about an operation which must be immediately performed, fairly turned tail and bolted. Stephanovitch, though pale as death, stood his ground.

Arrived beside one of the patients. Von Tummy, apparently not noticing the singular conduct of the two Servian doctors, asked the man what was the matter with him.

"Dysentery, sir."

"What!" roared the baron, "aren't you wounded, then?"

"Oh, wretched fool!" interposed Stephanovitch, "what are you talking about? Your Excellency," turning to Von Tummy, "the man has a severe wound in the head, and does not know what he is saying."

"I see no wound in his head, sir," replied the baron, giving Stephanovitch a keen glance. "Why——" (here Von Tummy thundered forth a string of expletives in half-a-dozen different languages), "the man isn't wounded at all! Get out of that" (tearing off the sick man's coverlet); "be off!" (giving him a kick, and then to next soldier), "What's the matter with you?"

"Dysentery."

"Oh, indeed———" (oaths), "take that, and that!" and with a kick and a thump he sent him about his business as well, and so on, right through the convoy, until he had weeded out all the sick, leaving only the wounded there. The spectacle, in spite of its cruelty, was ludicrous enough. There was the corpulent Von Tummy, rushing furiously hither and thither amongst the half-clad, emaciated Servians, whilst they stalked away in all directions, holding their garments about them, as fast as their wasted legs would carry them.

It seems that both Ibaum and Stephanovitch greatly preferred surgery to medicine, and when they received instructions to send away forty of their wounded, conceived the idea of getting rid of several of their sick at the same time. They were under the impression that Von Tummy was on his way to the front, where he would probably stay some time, and hence their terror when they recognised him on board the steamboat. Stephanovitch received a terrible lecture from the baron, but as for Dr. Ibaum, I believe he got off scot-free. Nothing happened after this to hinder the embarkation of the remaining wounded, and with a kindly word of advice from Von Tummy I went on board, and we started.

The voyage was quite uneventful and very pleasant. The wounded enjoyed the fresh air immensely after their long confinement in the close wards of the hospital. Thanks to Von Tummy's influence, a large awning was spread over the deck, which shielded them from the rays of the sun. They had grapes from the prince's vineyard, and tobacco, supplied by the Russian committee, and were fairly comfortable on the whole. The boat stopped at Topchidere, a place about a mile beyond Belgrade. A large concourse of people were awaiting our arrival, for it happened that my convoy was the first that had been sent by water, consequently a good deal of fuss was made about it.

Amongst the lookers-on I noticed a slovenly little personage in a dingy white holland tunic. He wore spectacles and a shabby beard and moustache, and seemed to me to be very seedy and poverty stricken. Thinking that he was probably looking out for a job, I motioned to him to lend a hand to the men who were carrying out the wounded soldiers, and tendered him a *franc*.

Never shall I forget the look of disgust and offended pride with which he declined my well-meant offer.

"Sir," said he to me in French, "do you know who I am?"

I shook my head.

"I am Dr. Yermaylaff Giggleivitch, Chevalier of the Order of St. Michael and St. George, and chief surgeon to His Imperial Majesty the *Czar* of all the Russias." So saying, he gave me another withering glance, and turned away.

When I had delivered my charges into the hands of those appointed to receive them, I proceeded, under the guidance of my two assistants, to an hotel—yclept the Hotel London—remarkable, as I learnt to my discomfort, for the extraordinary number of unsavoury insects which infested its bedrooms. Von Tummy's instructions to me were to return by the boat, which would leave Belgrade at seven the following morning. So, after strolling about and amusing myself in various ways for the rest of the day, I turned in about nine o'clock in the evening. My two assistants had left me early in the day, and gone to visit their sweethearts, under promise to return early and to be up in time for the boat, and I had arranged with the landlord to call us all at five the next morning.

I was somewhat tired when I went to bed, and threw myself on the mattress with that satisfaction which one feels after a long and fatiguing day. But I was doomed to get no sleep that night. Just as I was dozing off, a burning bite on the face aroused me, followed by another on the hand, and another on the foot. Springing up and striking a light, I discovered that I was assailed by legions of insects that crawled and insects that hopped; in fact, in imminent danger of being devoured alive. They came marching down the walls in battalions, and they dropped on to me from the ceiling. I spent the whole night in doing battle with my adversaries—destroying them by scores on the wall, on the coverlet, and on the floor; nor did the carnage cease until four o'clock in the morning. Then I began to dress, and whilst sitting down for a moment, had the misfortune to fall fast asleep.

Now had the landlord done his duty and called me, as he promised, at five, all would have been well. As it was, I slept on until eight o'clock, and of course lost the boat. My two assistants, who might have called me, and did not do so, alleged in excuse that their respect for me prevented them from disturbing my repose. In reality, the scamps wanted another day's holiday at Belgrade. There was nothing for it but to wait until the next day, as any other kind of conveyance to

Semendria was unprocurable. From what I had seen of Von Tummy's disposition, I expected that this unfortunate mischance would get me into a scrape, and so it proved; but I anticipate.

Whilst I was at breakfast, a party of twelve or fourteen Russian officers came into the coffee-room, making a prodigious clanking with their sabres, and occupied most of the vacant tables. I looked at them with considerable interest. They were of all ages and sizes—from six feet two inches to five feet nothing—and apparently of every rank, from the polished noble to the unlettered boor. One group, in particular, attracted my attention. It consisted of three persons. The senior member of the party was a well-made man of medium height, with finely-cut features, blue eyes, and a heavy, blonde moustache, and completely bald. His air was commanding, and by the respect shown him by his companions, he was evidently a personage of some importance.

Of his companions one was a very tall, fair-haired young man, with one of the handsomest faces I have ever seen, and the other was a slightly-made, pleasant-looking man of average height, and about twenty-eight years of age. They drank champagne freely, and seemed in a very jovial mood. Whilst gazing at the group, I became aware that someone was dodging about me in a very odd manner, and looking up, I saw a little Russian officer, with a face like a monkey, dancing backwards and forwards behind me. He had a heavy scimitar at his side and a revolver in his belt, and was pointing with an expression of intense contempt at the red cross on my coat sleeve. By-and-by I saw that this singular demonstration meant to indicate to me his opinion that men with the cross on their arms were cowards; for, after pointing to the cross with a grimace and a sniff, he pretended to run away in a great fright. Presently he advanced boldly up to me with a menacing air, and drew his revolver. Not understanding his object, and not liking his rudeness, I drew mine, and watched him closely, fully determined to use it if necessary.

What might have happened I do not know. Fortunately the bald-headed gentleman with the big moustache said something to him in a sharp, authoritative tone of voice, and he slunk away, when the tall, handsome young fellow came forward, and making me a polite bow, said in French:—

"Permit me, sir, to apologise in the name of the Russians here present for that fellow's rudeness!"

I replied that no apology was necessary; whereupon he made me another polite bow, and we shook hands cordially. The Russian courteously invited me to drink a glass of wine with him and his friends. I accepted the invitation, and as I approached their table, both the bald-headed officer and the slim young man with the agreeable countenance rose and treated me to a friendly shake of the hand. They informed me that they were officers of the Russian Imperial Guard, and were going as volunteers to the front, and would leave Belgrade next morning for Semendria, by boat, *en route* for Deligrad. I told them we should be fellow-passengers as far as Semendria, at which they seemed very pleased. After the wine we had coffee and cigarettes, and all became very sociable.

Several of the other Russians joined in the conversation. I observed, however, that they always treated the bald-headed individual with great deference, and I noticed also, with some pride, that my *gutta-percha* boots attracted considerable attention and several approving smiles; at least, they appeared to me to be so. Two of the Russians, however, took exception to them. One of them told me that my boots, though possibly good in theory, were not practical; the other, a rough-looking fellow of gigantic stature, with a shock head of yellow hair and a shaggy moustache, offered me, through the medium of an interpreter (for he could speak no language but his own), another pair of boots, expressing at the same time the utmost disgust for my favourite *gutta-perchas*.

I was a little bit hurt at his apparent inability to appreciate their merit, so I requested the interpreter (one of the Imperial Guard officers) politely to decline his kind offer for me. My refusal apparently offended this singular person very much, for he frowned fiercely, and said something in an angry tone.

"Sir," said the interpreter to me, "he is much disappointed at your declining his offer, and trusts you will reconsider the matter."

I replied that I thanked him very much, but having plenty of boots of my own, it was quite unnecessary for me to deprive him of a pair of his. At this the shockheaded gentleman waxed exceedingly wrath, and darting a fierce look at me, struck the table a blow with his clenched fist.

"Sir," said the Imperial Guardsman, "I think that perhaps it would be prudent of you to accept his offer, otherwise he may want to fight you."

"Bless my soul!" said I, laughing; "if he looks at it in that light, I'll accept his offer at once;" and walking up to him, I nodded my head at him, and extended my hand in token of friendship. Before taking

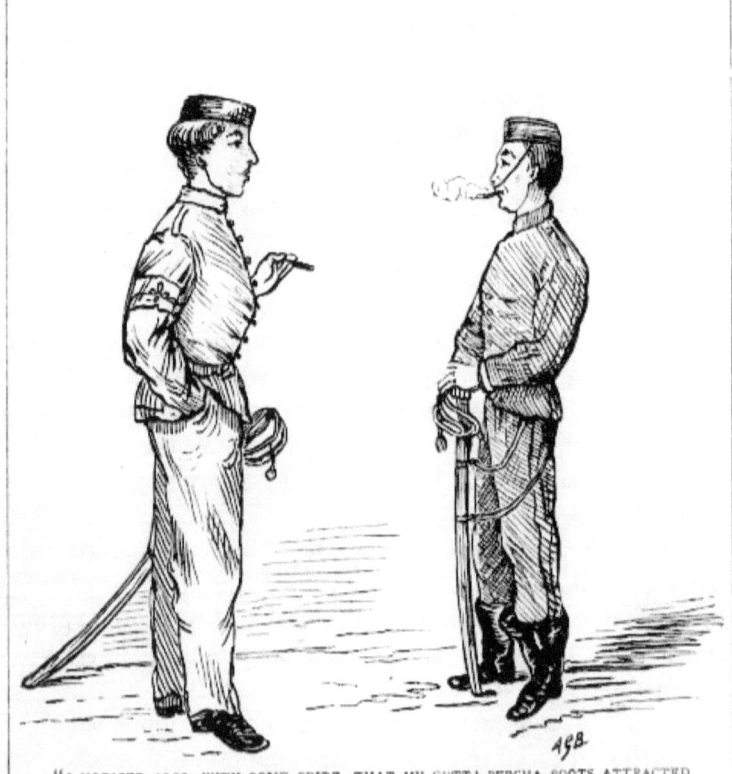

"I NOTICED ALSO, WITH SOME PRIDE, THAT MY GUTTA-PERCHA BOOTS ATTRACTED CONSIDERABLE ATTENTION."

my hand, this susceptible giant appealed to the guardsman, and then seizing my hand in his enormous paw, squeezed it almost into a jelly, pushed me into a chair, and dashed out of the room. In a minute or two he returned with a pair of top boots under his arm, and kneeling down, whipped off my beloved india-rubbers, and put his own on my feet in their stead. Then sitting down and leaning his elbows on the table he supported his chin on his hands, and taking a good look at me, told me that I was very like a dear friend of his, who had been killed in battle, *à propos* of which he said he would like to ask me a question.

"Some time ago, I was engaged in a battle with the Turkomans. We were greatly outnumbered, and for five hours were exposed to a terrible fire. For the first four hours I felt calm and cool, as a soldier ought to feel under fire, but after that I became, all at once, terribly frightened. I want to know how it was that I should all at once lose my presence of mind."

Having delivered himself of this question, the burly dragoon officer—for such he proved to be—rested his chin on his hands again, and looked at me with a wistful earnestness of expression that indicated the anxiety with which he awaited my answer.

For the moment I was fairly puzzled. Then I asked him if he had a wife and children. He replied with ecstatic energy, "Yes, yes, yes!" and kissing his hand fervently, placed it first about two feet from the ground, then he kissed it again and placed it a foot higher, then again, raising it a foot higher still, which I understood to mean that he had a wife and three children of the sizes indicated.

"Well then, sir," said I, "I think your conduct on that battlefield can be easily explained. During the first four hours you thought only of your duty, and consequently feared nothing, but in the fifth hour you remembered your wife and children, and that thought unnerved you!"

No sooner had my reply been explained to the dragoon, than he sprang up with much energy, upsetting his chair and nearly capsizing the table, and then folding me in his arms, smothered my face with kisses, exclaiming that I had taken a great load off his mind, for he had fretted about his conduct on that occasion ever since. Then, summoning the waiter, he ordered a bottle of champagne, and filled a glass tankard up to the brim for me, and one for himself, and clashing his glass against mine, tossed off his wine at a single draught. I had already had one tumblerful of champagne, and consequently could drink very little of the wine, which greatly astonished and disappointed him, but he was pacified when I explained that I scarcely ever took wine at home.

"Why," said he, in a tone of surprise, "in Russia I drink a bottle of brandy and five bottles of wine every day."

In the afternoon, the young officer who had remarked that my boots were unpractical, and whose name was Mouravioff, proposed that we should go for a walk, and a party, consisting of five or six of the Russians and myself, went in the direction of the arsenal. On our way we happened to pass the palace. Princess Natalie was at the time lying ill there, and an edict had been issued forbidding people either to drive or ride past. The princess was exceedingly popular, and the good people of Belgrade, in their anxiety for her recovery, carried out the edict to the letter, and when passing the palace used to speak in whispers and walk on tiptoe.

I was not aware of this at first, and consequently was somewhat surprised and amused to see scores of people—soldiers, civilians, and women—whispering together and walking about as lightly as possible, like nurses in a sick-room, but when I knew the cause, this popular demonstration of sympathy touched me considerably, and heightened my respect for the Servian character. Suddenly the silence was broken by the clattering of a horse's hoofs and the yelping of a cur! Who should appear upon the scene, mounted upon a large chestnut horse, but Colonel Bragg! He sat his horse pretty well, but from his fiery complexion, and the way he swore at the dog, which bayed furiously at his horse's heels, I fancy he must have been intoxicated. That, at least, is a charitable supposition!

The cur yelped and snapped at the horse, making it rear and plunge in a way that threatened to unseat the gallant colonel, who, livid with rage, cursed until he was hoarse.

For fully five minutes a frightful war of sounds continued—the dog growling and barking, the colonel roaring and swearing, and the horse kicking and striking sparks from the rough pavement with his hoofs. Suddenly the terrible Bragg changed his tactics, and drawing his sabre made a vigorous down cut at the dog. The blow was well aimed; the dog's head rolled on the stones. Then sheathing his weapon, the colonel trotted along, twirling his moustache with an air of triumphant ferocity on his truculent face. Undeterred, however, by the awful fate of the cur, a presumptuous *gendarme* took upon himself the enforcement of the edict in the colonel's case, and fearlessly confronting him, forbade him to ride further in that direction.

"Get out of my way, you idiot! What's the —— matter with you?" said the colonel, contemptuously, putting on a tremendous expression,

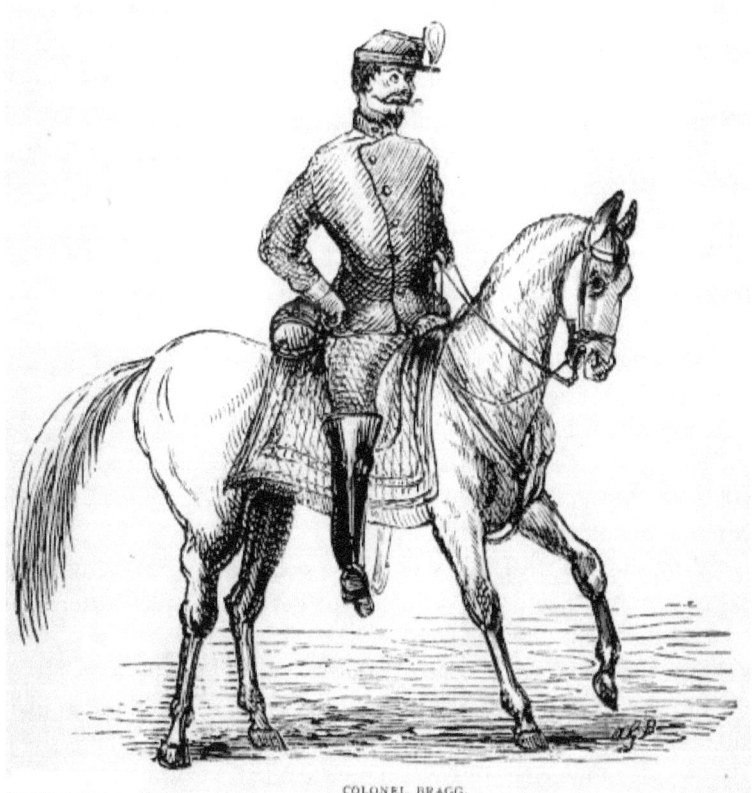

COLONEL BRAGG.

and endeavouring to spur his horse past the bold *gendarme*. The "bold *gendarme*," however, laid hold of the bridle.

"Will you take your hand off my bridle?" shouted the colonel.

The *gendarme* stood firm, whereupon, uttering one of his choicest oaths, the colonel struck him on the face, and making his horse rear at the same time, succeeded in shaking him off. Then invoking a lot of the most bizarre and recherche maledictions I ever heard on his discomfited adversary, the twice triumphant Bragg rode off.

"Do English officers usually behave like that?" asked Mouravioff, sarcastically.

"Never," replied I, indignantly; "they are gentlemen. As for this Colonel Bragg, I believe he is an American adventurer. I am quite certain he is not an English officer."

When we got out into the open country, we threw ourselves on the grass beneath a shady tree, and refreshed ourselves with a nip from our flasks and a whiff of tobacco smoke.

"M. Wright," said the irrepressible Mouravioff, "what will England do when Russia declares war against her?"

"She will probably fight," said I.

"How can she fight us? She has only 100,000 men, we have 3,000,000. Moreover, her soldiers, though they are brave, cannot stand extremes of cold and heat like ours."

"Why, sir," replied I, "they did very well in the Crimea, where it was cold enough, and they contrive to get on in India, where it is rather warm."

"Still, sir, the fact remains that you have only 100,000 men."

"On the contrary, we have a great many more: 120,000 regulars, 150,000 militia, and 200,000 volunteers; besides," said I, "there are all our sailors, numbering 180,000. These sailors," I continued, waxing warm in defence of our national prowess, "are all armed with pistols and cutlasses like this (pointing to the one I wore); and they have a peculiar kind of guard, called the hanging guard, which I will show you, which renders them invincible as swordsmen. This," said I, drawing my cutlass, and putting myself into my very best hanging-guard position, "is how British sailors fight!" and I looked round to see what effect my formidable attitude produced upon the Muscovites. They were all smiling, doubtless with admiration.

"If English soldiers fight like that," said Mouravioff, in an altered tone, "they must indeed be invincible!"

****

On our return to the Hotel London, we separated for the night, under promise to meet again at five o'clock the next morning, and I retired to bed—but, alas! not to sleep, for fresh swarms of insects, as if to avenge their deceased comrades, kept me awake until three in the morning, when having slaughtered the greater part of my tormentors, I at last managed to snatch some repose.

CHAPTER 9

Von Tummy Blows Me Up

Bang! bang! bang! Thump! thump! thump! Bang! thump! bang! thump! bang! These were the sounds which aroused me the next morning; the landlord and the Russians were hammering at the door.

"Hulloh, Mr. Englishman!" said one of the Russians, when at length I appeared, "you sleep pretty soundly."

"I daresay," said I, rubbing my eyes. "I am very tired; I have hardly slept a wink through insects."

"Bah, *monsieur*," said another, "you will not make a good campaigner if you cannot put up with a few fleas."

"I suppose one can get used to all things in time," replied I, a little bit nettled; "but at present I must say I am not quite used to the disgusting vermin one meets with in this place."

"Certainly, certainly," replied the Russian; "but meanwhile breakfast is ready, and the steamboat starts at seven o'clock."

I dressed in a trice, and went down into the coffee-room, where my assistants and the Russians were assembled at the breakfast table. I sat down, and soon had occasion to ask the Russian next me to pass me the salt. To my surprise, however, he absolutely refused, and I had to rise and get it for myself. The young officer who had apologised to me on the preceding day for his countryman's rudeness explained, that amongst Russians of a certain class a superstition exists, that passing salt to comparative strangers leads to a quarrel.

After breakfast the Russians called for champagne, and concluded their last meal at Belgrade, before going to the front, by toasting the *Czar* and singing their national anthem. We then all proceeded to the riverside, and embarked in good time. We were favoured again with the most lovely weather. After a pleasant voyage of a few hours the boat drew up at the Semendria landing-place.

I was so charmed with the companionship and courtesy of the

Russians that I invited them to the rooms that Hiems and I held in common. Ten of them, including the tall young officer who first spoke to me, his bold friend Mouravioff, and the dragoon who gave me the boots, accepted my invitation, and I was preparing to leave with them, when the terrible Von Tummy planted his substantial corporation in front of me, and fixing his piercing eyes upon me, said, with a dark frown,

"*Well, sir!*"

So sharply did he speak and so stern were his looks, that for the moment I was dumfounded. The Russians, however, were standing round looking on.

With a bland smile, therefore, I extended my right hand, and said in accents of hearty cordiality:—

"Ah, baron! How d'ye do?"

My impudence surprised the baron; for a moment he looked at me in speechless indignation. Then stamping one of his ponderous feet on the deck he asked me what the —— I meant by not returning yesterday.

"It was an accident, sir," replied I. "I had the misfortune to lose the boat."

"It's a lie, sir! You wanted to lose the boat!" roared the angry baron. "Be off to your quarters, sir. I'll talk to you by-and-by!"

"I am not in the habit of telling lies," I replied, imprudently.

"How dare you answer me, you impudent English jackanapes!" thundered Von Tummy, shaking his fist in my face.

"And how dare you call me jackanapes, you twopenny-halfpenny Austrian baron!" screamed I, beside myself with passion.

Just then Hiems, who had heard this dialogue with much alarm, came to my rescue, and putting his hand over my mouth, attempted to drag me away, saying:—

"Don't be a fool, old fellow; you're spoiling all your chances!"

"I'll dismiss you from the service," roared Von Tummy.

"Dismiss me, and be hanged!" shouted I, succeeding, after a desperate struggle, in tearing Hiems' hand from my mouth; but this was all I could say, for the next moment my friend carried me bodily away. Once removed from the baron's irritating presence, I recovered my equanimity. The Russians were full of sympathy for me, and when I told them the baron had called me a jackanapes, which I explained to them meant a conceited, insignificant, monkey-like fellow, their friendly indignation knew no bounds.

"Resign your post as surgeon at this hospital, *monsieur*," said the bald-headed gentleman, "and come with us to the front."

"Yes, yes, come with us to the front!" cried the other Russians in chorus.

Matters had gone so far, that in spite of Hiems' remonstrances and disappointment, I decided to accept their invitation, and told them that I would be glad to cast in my lot with theirs, and accompany them as a volunteer. My decision was hailed with great applause. Even Hiems reluctantly admitted that after what had taken place it would be impossible for me to remain under Von Tummy; so, I wrote the latter a letter, regretting my hasty conduct, and sending him, at the same time, my resignation as assistant surgeon at Semendria. To this I received no response.

We spent the rest of the afternoon in the most festive manner—drinking success and rapid promotion to one another; and all separated for the night in the highest spirits, except poor Hiems, who took my approaching departure very much to heart, and would not be comforted, in spite of all my efforts to console him.

CHAPTER 10

An Unpleasant Ride

The next morning, as I was sitting at breakfast with Hiems, Mouravioff and another Russian came to the door and told me that the waggons that were to convey us to Deligrad were waiting at the Lion Hotel. I had already packed up my small stock of wearing apparel in my knapsack and a large travelling bag. The former I strapped on to my shoulders, the latter my good-natured landlord assisted me to carry. Hiems accompanied me to the hotel, and we walked there in silence, for now that the moment for parting had come, we both felt heavy-hearted. I noticed that the bald-headed officer—instead of sharing a waggon with two or three others, like the rest of us—had a well-appointed carriage, and started a few minutes before us.

Our waggons were of the very roughest description, more like large hencoops with the tops off, on wheels, than travelling conveyances. They boasted of neither springs nor seats, the place of the latter being supplied by bundles of rushes. Three of us were stowed in each of these vehicles, mine being the last of the train. A large crowd assembled by the hotel to witness our departure. Just before we started, Drs. Ibaum and Stephanovitch appeared upon the scene, and wished me "God speed "with much heartiness and fervour; then Hiems gave me a last squeeze of the hand and "God bless you," and we were off, amidst a waving of handkerchiefs and *fezzes*, and a shout of "*Jivio*" from the crowd. My companions in the car were Mouravioff and the handsome young officer who first spoke to me, and whose name I learned was Savrimovitch. Both were officers of the Russian Imperial Guard.

We were rather silent for the first half-hour or so. Probably we were all of us thinking of home and home friends; at least I know I was. But the broiling heat of the sun and the terrific jolting of the car were fatal to sentimental contemplation. Our coachman was a tall, narrow-chested, round-shouldered individual, who sat in front

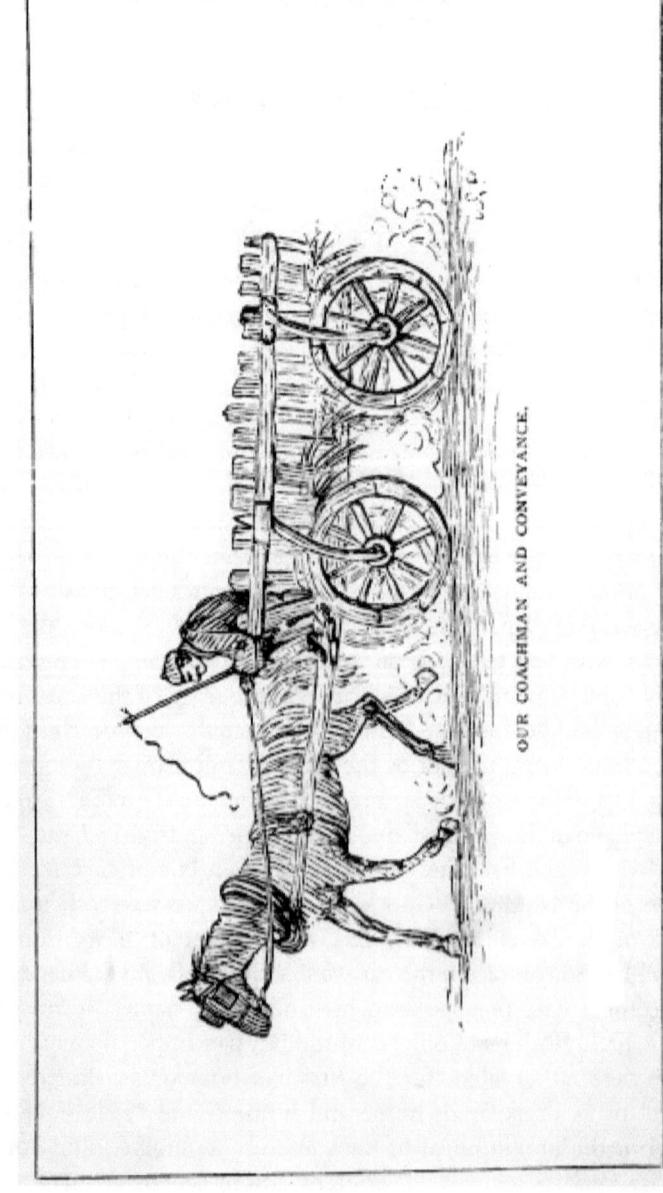

OUR COACHMAN AND CONVEYANCE.

of us with his head on a level with his knees, and taking no notice of anything or anybody, devoted all his energies to humming a wearisomely monotonous ditty in an utterly disagreeable *falsetto*. Our horse's appearance was strangely in keeping with that of his driver. He was, without exception, the very scraggiest and most dejected looking specimen that I ever saw, and his pace was the slowest of slow jog trots.

The road along which we were driving was crossed every few hundred yards by a drain about a foot deep and eighteen inches wide, into which the trunk of a tree had been rolled to enable vehicles to pass. The casual Servian wayside authorities apparently made no effort to select trees of the same size as the trenches; some were too big, and projected six inches above the level of the roadway, others were too small.

Our coachman's method of getting over these trenches was peculiar. When within twenty or thirty yards of one of them, he would shout out something, which I suppose meant "Hold on," urge his horse into a gallop, and go straight at it. The result, as may be conceived, was extremely shocking to the occupants.

Our first experience of one of these trenches may be better imagined than described. The waggon struck the obstacle with a crash, and bounded over it with a smash and a bump, shooting me a foot or so into the air, and bringing the back of my head into such violent contact with the side of the car, that for the moment I was stunned. My companions fared no better. When I came to, they were lying—one on the top of the other—at the bottom of the car, and struggling to get up. The only one of us who seemed not to have suffered was the coachman. He was sitting just as before, humming precisely the same ditty, and our Rosinante had relapsed into the same jog-trot again.

We requested this musical Jehu to be more careful the next time he took us over one of these trenches. He stopped his humming for a moment, and without turning his head, replied that he would, and then droned away again at his ditty as monotonously as ever. His idea of being more careful, however, was to go over the next trench with a little extra spurt, so that we got as badly shaken as before. This was too much for our equanimity, so as soon as we had got over this second bruising, we held a brief council of war, which ended in our pulling coachee off his seat, and bundling him into a corner of the car with one or two gentle thumps, by way of reprisal for the knocking about he had inflicted on us.

My two companions then desired me to drive, remarking that all Englishmen could ride and drive. Now it unfortunately happened that I could do neither, having been brought up in London with no opportunity of learning. However, I had seen people drive often enough to know something about the *modus operandi*, and being most desirous of maintaining the honour of my country, I, with many secret misgivings, but with much outward show of cheerfulness, took the reins. For some time, fortune favoured me. Savrimovitch and Mouravioff, thinking all was right, entered into a little *tête-à-tête* conversation, without troubling themselves about me. The next few trenches, too, were provided with trunks of about the right size, and the road was nearly straight. True, I failed to keep the cart in the middle of the road, still, by constantly working at the reins, I succeeded in keeping the horse out of the hedge on either side.

At last, we came to a sharp turn. By pulling strongly at the near side rein I got the horse round the corner in grand style, but unluckily forgot to loosen the rein, so the stupid old creature ran right into the hedge. The wheel ran up the bank, the waggon turned over, pitching us all into the road, and upsetting the horse as well. For a minute we all lay in the dust without attempting to move—I, because I was so much astonished at what had taken place, the Russians because they were a good deal shaken, and because our crafty Servian coachman, with an eye to saving himself, had contrived to fall on the top of them.

Then we were suddenly roused to action by our venerable steed, which, possessed with an unwonted spirit of friskiness, began to kick so vigorously that it threatened soon to make matchwood of the waggon. I was on my feet in a moment, and running to the horse's head forced it to the ground again and sat on it, after the manner of London cabmen in similar emergencies. Neither Mouravioff nor Savrimovitch were much hurt, and shaking off the coachman, who was reclining comfortably on the top of them, they came to my assistance.

The coachman did not offer to help us, but sat down in the middle of the road, sobbing and wringing his hands in a most dismal and lackadaisical manner, and praying his "dear Gospodin" horse not to kick his cart quite into little bits. However, we managed to right the cart and set the horse on its legs again, and I resigned the reins to Savrimovitch, who proved an excellent driver, and we soon found ourselves in Jagodina—a large straggling town of about 10,000 inhabitants. Here we joined the rest of our party. Jagodina has acquired some local celebrity from its manufacture of wooden flasks and water-bottles. Some of these are very quaint and pretty. I became the possessor of one, under rather singular circumstances.

We had started again, and were driving through the outskirts of the town, when an old peasant came running after us in great distress, and asked if any of our party was a doctor. He was referred to me, and I ascertained that his grandchild was in a fit. On following him into a cottage hard by, I saw an old woman, holding on her lap a fine boy, about a year old, in strong convulsions. I lanced the child's gums, which were much swollen, and putting him into a warm bath, had the satisfaction of seeing him come round. Before I left, the old couple blessed me with touching fervour, and begged me so hard to accept a wooden bottle that they had made themselves, that I felt constrained to take it.

The road between Jagodina and Paratchin, the next large town that we stopped at, is very good. It runs through a beautiful and fertile tract of country, covered with vast groves of plum trees, apple orchards, and vineyards. The scenery, moreover, became more picturesque as we went on. The ground undulated considerably, whilst the horizon was bounded by a lofty range of blue mountains. Between us and them, and at a considerably lower level than the road, was a beautifully wooded and well-watered plain. As the evening advanced the weather became very close and sultry, and a severe thunderstorm broke upon us before we reached Paratchin.

It was about half-past ten and pitch dark when we arrived, and we were all wet and very uncomfortable. The two or three hotels in the place were full, for a body of cavalry and two battalions of infantry had entered the town earlier in the evening, and they seemed to have taken up all the available accommodation. To add to our misery, the rain began to fall again in torrents. As a last resource we went to the Commissary of Police, and requested him to find us quarters. That worthy, however, shook his head, and said he was afraid it was impossible, but he would do the best he could, and sent a *gendarme* to take us to all the likely places. The *gendarme* proved a humbug. He walked us about fruitlessly for half an hour, and then quietly gave us the slip, leaving us more wet and miserable than ever.

Under these circumstances we began to make up our minds to pass the night as well as we could in our cart, and with that object we made tracks for the market-place, where we had left it in charge of our Servian coachman. But lo! when we got there, both cart and driver had vanished! We now became desperate, and going into the coffee-room of the nearest hotel, we ordered some supper, intending to remain in the room all night. The place was crowded with Servian officers and soldiers talking, eating, drinking, singing, smoking, gambling, and sleeping. The uproar was tremendous, and the atmosphere, composed of steam from their wet clothing and tobacco smoke, particularly dense.

We succeeded, however, in getting a corner to ourselves and making a first-rate supper. Then we strolled outside, to smoke a cigarette before going to sleep. On the way out, I noticed a door which had been left ajar. Curiosity impelled me to push it wide open, and I beheld a large, well-lit room with—oh, rapturous spectacle!—twenty comfortable-looking beds ranged round it. None of them were tenanted. My mind was made up at once, and I resolved at all hazards to sleep in one of them. True, they were engaged, as was evident from caps, swords, cloaks, and revolver cases laid on them, but that was a minor consideration. Running after Mouravioff and Sarvimovitch, I led them back to this room. They also went into ecstasies and appropriated beds. I tore off my sopping wet and clinging garments in the twinkling of an eye, and clapped on some dry things out of my knapsack, and jumping into the bed I had selected, removed the late owner's sword, revolver, etc., tucked myself under the coverlet, and wishing my comrades goodnight, was asleep in no time.

How long I had been asleep I don't know, but I was roused by someone giving me a thump and dragging me on to the floor. Looking up, I became aware that the hideous little Russian who had insulted me in Belgrade was standing over me, grinning with rage, and cursing me in his guttural language with fierce volubility. Infuriated at this treatment, which was not perhaps altogether unjustifiable under the circumstances, I sprang to my feet and hit the Muscovite a blow on the nose that sent him reeling to the opposite side of the room. In a second his sabre flashed out of its sheath, and I had just time to put my eyeglass in my eye and raise my cutlass, when he aimed a desperate cut at my head.

In my hurry, I quite forgot the hanging guard, and put up my weapon anyhow, and such was the force of his blow that it nearly struck it out of my hand, and made my fingers tingle for some minutes afterwards. I could see from the way the fellow handled his sword that he knew more about fencing than I did, still the blow on his nose had made his eyes water, and interfered with his sword play so much, that he had to stop every now and then to wipe away the tears. By nimbly jumping about, and by the lucky interposition every now and then of my cutlass between myself and the enemy, I contrived to avoid his cuts and thrusts; and, indeed, if my eyeglass would have stopped in my eye, I think I should soon have vanquished him, but each time I made up my mind to try to disarm him, the eyeglass fell out. Nevertheless, I managed to strike several vigorous blows at him, which I flatter myself he had some difficulty in parrying.

At length, by a lucky chance, I snatched up my knapsack with my left hand, hurled it with such skill and dexterity at my adversary, that it struck him full in the chest, momentarily deprived him of breath, and jerked his sword out of his grasp. Then, without giving him time to recover himself, I closed with him, and we rolled over on the floor together. Meanwhile the noise of the combat brought a crowd of armed men out of the coffee-room, and also awoke Savrimovitch and Mouravioff, who hurried to my assistance.

"Hulloh!" said Mouravioff, rather sarcastically, "do English sailors fight with knapsacks as well as cutlasses?"

"Yes," replied I, triumphantly; "they always knock their enemies over, and are not very particular how they do it!"

Savrimovitch strode up to my late opponent, whose name, by the way, was Pauloff, and gave him a sharp reprimand for molesting me. Pauloff replied by a defiant scowl, and began haranguing the soldiers and detailing his grievances to them, and some seemed half disposed to take his part. Savrimovitch, however, soon put an end to the quarrel. Speaking in a loud, authoritative tone, he ordered the soldiers to arrest that "drunken fellow (pointing to Pauloff) for assaulting this good English doctor."

My friend's fine presence and commanding manner acted like magic on the Servians. The infuriated Pauloff was collared, and in spite of his frantic struggles and remonstrances, marched off to the guard-room. Peace being thus restored, the soldiers cleared out of the room again, we returned to our beds, and slept tranquilly the rest of the night.

Chapter 11

Prince Obolenski

The first thing next morning, we went to the marketplace in quest of our lost conveyance. To our great delight we found it, but just on the point of starting without us. Our friends welcomed us with a cheer, and the caravan pulled up whilst we took our places. Then we bid goodbye to Paratchin, and trundled off towards the front again. It was a lovely morning, and we were all in excellent spirits, for we expected to reach Deligrad early in the evening. We whiled away the time in planning all sorts of desperate expeditions and adventures.

Savrimovitch proposed that we should provide ourselves with horses, and act as mounted scouts—for the army—whenever an opportunity offered. I suggested that we should imitate the example of Athos, Porthos, and D'Arlagnan of the *Mousquetaires*, provision a cottage in the midst of the Turkish lines, and defend it for six months against the whole of the hostile army. My suggestion was received with shouts of approving laughter. Mouravioff patted me on the back, and said I was undoubtedly a military genius of the highest order. The handsome Savrimovitch said, with a smile, "But supposing they bring cannon against your cottage!" to which I replied, that our defence then would be all the more creditable. He smiled again, and shaking me warmly by the hand, said that I was a "brave!"

When we were still some distance from Deligrad, we heard the distant booming of cannon for the first time. This excited us all so much, that we gave a loud cheer, which was caught up by our friends in the other waggons, and the drivers whipped up their tired horses, and we bounded along in fine style. Soon after this a party of horsemen approached us, led by an officer in whom I recognised, to my surprise, the bald-headed Russian I had met at the restaurant with Savrimovitch.

"See," said Mouravioff, "here comes the prince!"

"The prince!" said I, in astonishment, "what prince?"

"Why, Prince Obolenski, of course."

"You don't mean to say," said I, "that that gentleman is a prince?"

"Certainly, I do!"

"Goodness me!" I exclaimed in dismay; "I trust he was not offended at the cool way in which I spoke to him."

"Not he," replied Savrimovitch, "he is very good-natured."

Meanwhile the *cortège* had come up to the leading waggon, which stopped, and its occupants stood up and saluted the prince.

As he approached us, we did the same.

The prince reined up at our waggon, and shook hands very kindly with all three of us.

"Ah, M. Wright," said he, "I am very pleased to see you. I have been talking about you to Dr. Giggleivitch."

"Dr. Giggleivitch?" repeated I, in alarm.

"Yes," rejoined the prince, "Yermaylaff Giggleivitch. We travelled from Semendria together. Do you know him?"

"Well," said I, "I cannot exactly say that I know him, but I met him once under rather embarrassing circumstances;" and I narrated my little adventure with him at Belgrade.

The prince laughed heartily, and then said, "That explains it all. Yermaylaff Giggleivitch looked anything but pleased when I told him you were coming, and absolutely refused to give you a surgeon's commission as surgeon under him (I looked very blank at this), but you need not let that trouble you. I can offer you, if you like, the rank of lieutenant in one of our best brigades here—the Medvedovski's Brigade—where you will have plenty of opportunities both of practising your profession and of fighting."

I was overwhelmed with joy and gratitude at this. Even had he given me the chance, I doubt whether I could have found words in which to thank him; but without waiting, he shook hands with us again, and trotted off with his followers.

When we reached the camp, we were directed to headquarters, which were held at a large cottage close to the road. We left our waggons and formed into line. Presently three or four officers came out; we all stood at attention. I was particularly anxious to create a good impression, and threw my shoulders well back and held myself as rigidly as possible.

"That officer with the imperial moustache and beard is General Tchernaieff," said Savrimovitch to me in a whisper. Without turning

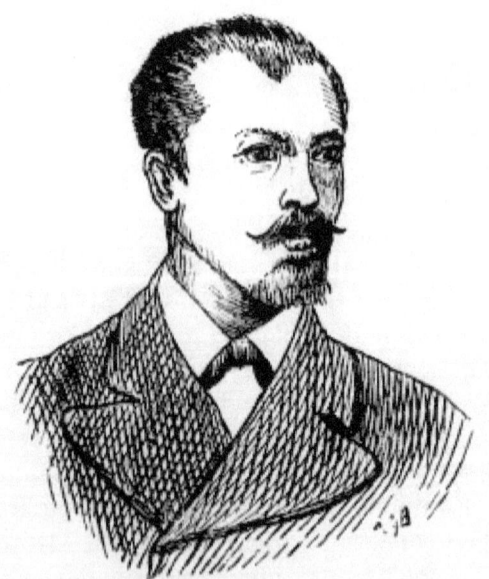

GENERAL TCHERNAIEFF, FROM A PHOTOGRAPH BY YOVANOVITCH OF BELGRADE.

my head, I looked at this renowned soldier out of the corners of my eyes with greater interest.

Before coming to us, the general spoke to two or three men who were standing near in a group.

"By Jove," continued Savrimovitch, still whispering, "the general's in a great rage about something! Do you notice the way in which he puffs out his cheeks and sucks them in again? He always does that when he's angry. I expect these men are asking for leave of absence, a thing he hates."

The general, who was a sallow-faced man of medium height, and nowise remarkable in personal appearance, was indeed puffing out his cheeks in a very odd manner. Presently, and without returning their salute, he turned his back on the unfortunates who had excited his wrath, and came towards us.

"If he is pleased with us," said Savrimovitch, "he will beat a kind of devil's tattoo with his finger against the side of his leg."

I watched him carefully as he walked deliberately up to our line, and noticed, first, the angry shade fade away from his face. As he passed from man to man and asked each one where he came from and what service he had seen, his fingers began to play at first slowly, then more quickly, and finally, when he spoke to Savrimovitch, his satisfaction appeared to reach its climax. He looked rather doubtfully at me, and I thought I could discern just the suspicion of an inflation of the cheeks when he heard I was an Englishman; but as I answered all his questions satisfactorily, this indication of displeasure passed away, and before he left me, I had the satisfaction of seeing his fingers gently ambling up and down his continuations.

Four of us—namely Savrimovitch, Mouravioff, the big dragoon officer who gave me the boots, and whose name was Nicolaitch, and myself—were told that we were to join the Medvedovski Brigade, so without losing time we set out for its headquarters.

Deligrad itself is—or rather was at that time—an insignificant hamlet, numbering a normal population of perhaps a couple of hundred, but the camp, which surrounded it on all sides, contained from thirty to forty thousand men. The position was naturally strong, and had been fortified by trenches, rifle pits, and earthworks, mounting upwards of one hundred guns of every calibre and of all kinds. There were old smooth bores and new Krupps, little six pounders and huge sixty pounders. The plain in front of the camp was, moreover, Studded with little pits containing sharp stakes for the benefit of the enemy's cavalry. The trees, too, in the vicinity had been felled, stripped of their leaves and twigs, and, with their branches sharpened, disposed as an abattis to further hamper the movements of an attacking force.

The position of the Medvedovski Brigade lay about half a mile to the right and rear of the general's headquarters.

The Medvedovski Brigade—so called from its commander, Colonel Medvedovski, an officer of the Russian Imperial Guard—was also known as the Russian Brigade, from the nationality of many of its officers.

Colonel Medvedovski, a dark, stern-looking man, with a short, well-trimmed moustache and beard, bade us welcome to his brigade in a short, and doubtless pithy, oration in Russian, of which, unfortunately, I failed to understand a single word.

"You are a medical student!" said the colonel to me in French, at the end of his harangue.

"I am, sir," replied I.

"May I ask why you elect to serve as a combatant instead of following up your own profession?"

"Because I wish to see some fighting, sir."

The colonel gave me a keen glance, and said, with a smile:—

"You are evidently an original, sir. May I trouble you to hand me your passport and other papers? Thank you; you must entrust them to my keeping until you leave the camp. Do not think, sir, that we suspect your *bona fides* in any way; we adopt the same precaution with all volunteers coming here. Meantime, I am very glad to receive an Englishman into my brigade, and if I can be of any service to you whilst you are with us, you have but to speak to me, and I will do what I can for you."

Standing behind the colonel was a singular-looking individual, apparently about thirty-five years of age. His hair was of an extremely light colour, his complexion florid and weather-beaten. He had a feeble white moustache, and a little tuft of hair on either side of his chin, one of which was bright red, the other of a pale straw-colour. His features were flat, his right eye grey, and his left blue. In spite of the peculiarity of his appearance, his expression was pleasing.

This was Count Réné, who had the reputation of being one of the bravest of all the gallant Russians then in Servia.

I had just thanked Colonel Medvedovski for his kindness, and was turning to leave the tent with my companions, when Count Réné came up to me and shook me by the hand.

"You are to join my battalion—the fourth. Permit me to offer you a hearty welcome to it. You are the only Englishman in the whole brigade, therefore I shall expect great things of you, for I have heard much of English courage!"

The count's words set my ambition in a blaze; my heart beat wildly, and I felt the blood mount to my face. I, however, restrained my feelings until I had bid him *adieu*, and merely replied that I should be proud and happy to do the best I could for the honour of the battalion. I inwardly resolved, however, to do something desperately valiant to maintain my reputation as a brave Englishman. The idea that occurred to me at the moment was to send a challenge to the officers of the Turkish Army, defying any of them to meet me in single combat.

With a feeling of proud elation, I imagined myself posing in the hanging-guard attitude before the assembled Servian and Turkish hosts, and after a terrible encounter vanquishing the hostile champion, and then saving his life by a brilliant surgical operation. The fame of my glorious deeds, I rapturously thought, would not be confined to Servia, but would extend all over Europe to England—and then, who knows what might happen? Many a man has passed along a less creditable avenue to Royal patronage! I rubbed my hands, and laughed with glee at the thought!

"Why, how now, M. Wright," said Savrimovitch, banteringly, "what are you laughing at? Have you been drinking champagne on the sly?"

"No," replied I, somewhat vexed that my elation should be deemed of the vinous sort; "I am simply very glad that we shall so soon have an opportunity of distinguishing ourselves."

"Pooh, is that all?" said Savrimovitch. "I thought you were a little bit screwed, and was hoping you had brought a bottle or two of Heidsick with you."

"I daresay, M. Wright, that you will not feel quite so festive when you really have seen some fighting," said Mouravioff, dryly.

CHAPTER 12

A Mysterious Resemblance

The brigade of which I was now a member was about 2,000 strong, and was encamped on what had once been a field of maize. Here and there lines of stiff, stubbly stumps still stuck out of the ground. The camp was very picturesque. It was composed of hundreds of booths, arranged in rows, and intersected at regular intervals by broad thoroughfares. These booths were ingeniously constructed of green boughs, interlaced, and supported by one or two stout upright pieces of timber. Some of them were like little huts, and afforded very complete shelter, and others were entirely opened on one side, like arbours, and to one of these latter we were directed.

It already contained two occupants—Count Tiesenhausen and Baron Kleist—both of them Courlanders. They proved to be old acquaintances of Savrimovitch and Mouravioff, to whom they gave a very warm and hearty welcome. They also received Nicolaitch and myself very politely, and we were soon all on the very best of terms. Count Tiesenhausen was a handsome, blonde little man, who encased his legs in a huge pair of cavalry boots, and smothered his face under a Servian military cap, which was many sizes too large for him, and came down to his eyes and brows. Baron Kleist, a tall, gaunt man, with very strongly-marked aquiline features, and a sandy-coloured beard and moustache, suffered a good deal from ague, and always wore an overcoat with its collar turned up. He divided his spare time between sleeping and smoking, and for the greater part of it I think he was to be seen squatted on his heels puffing at a cigarette. But both Kleist and Tiesenhausen were brave soldiers, and amiable and accomplished gentlemen.

It was now late in the afternoon. We had eaten nothing but a biscuit or two and a few grapes since we left Paratchin. We were glad, therefore, when the count summoned our mess servant, who was quite a character in his way, to prepare supper. Imagine a funny mannikin, with a pair of very roguish-looking, twinkling black eyes, the smallest and snubbiest of small snub noses, and a gigantic pair of moustaches. The creature, whose name was Jenko, at once cut some thick slices from a large piece of mutton, put them on a long spit, and proceeded to grill them over a large wood fire which smouldered in front of our hut.

We all lent a willing hand in one way or another. Tiesenhausen and Mouravioff walked over to Deligrad, and bought some wine and spirits at one of the numerous provision stalls which had sprung up round the camp; Nicolaitch occupied himself in superintending the baking of some potatoes; Kleist roasted coffeeberries in a frying-pan; and Savrimovitch and I pounded the same, he with the butt end of his revolver, and I with the heel of a drinking horn. When we had finished breaking up the coffee-berries, we put the fragments into a pot containing about half a gallon of water. The resulting fluid was of a pale straw colour, and tasted very strongly of wood and smoke, and feebly, very feebly, of coffee.

The meat was terribly tough, having been killed that morning, and the black commissariat bread of the consistency of putty, and about as digestible. Still, in spite of these little drawbacks, we all ate very heartily, and formed an exceedingly merry little party. As the evening advanced and the stars began to twinkle overhead, hundreds of huge fires were lit throughout the camp, round which groups of armed men sat or reclined, their faces and accoutrements, illumined with vivid distinctness by the leaping flames. I looked with delight on the scene, and said to myself, "Yes, this is real warfare, and no mistake about it!"

Whilst indulging in warlike musing, a voice struck my ear so singularly like that of Marie Miloikovitch that it sent a thrill right through me. It came from a group of three officers who were walking towards our hut. I could not make out their faces in the gloom, until the light of the fire fell on them. Then I saw with amazement that one bore so astonishing a resemblance to the charming Bulgarian who had captivated my heart at Semendria, that I started and exclaimed, "Hulloh!"

All three turned their faces towards me, and I fancied that the young officer who was so like Marie changed colour when he saw me. But it might have been only my fancy, or a fitful shadow cast by the flickering flames. Anyway, they resumed their conversation, and passed on without taking further notice.

The likeness was most amazing.

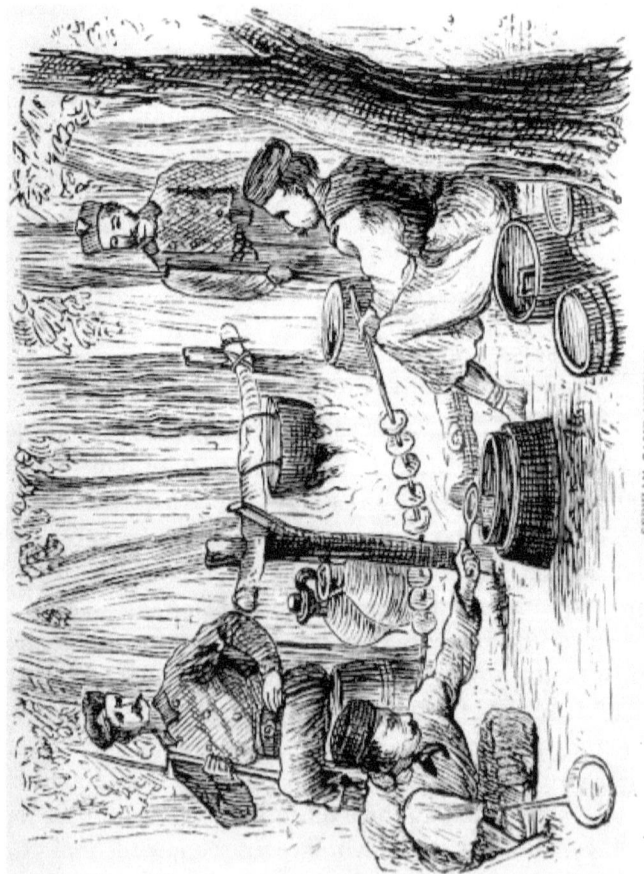
SERVIAN CAMP KITCHEN.

"Still," thought I, "I must be mistaken. It is all but impossible that the beautiful and accomplished Marie should have cast aside the feelings of her sex and donned a soldier's uniform."

Then I recalled her strange conduct during our memorable walk at Semendria when she discharged my revolver, and I came to the conclusion that it might be she after all. I was agitated and perplexed, and resolved to follow the cause of my mental confusion and ask if he was Marie, and had actually started off, when the absurdity of putting such a question to a man brought me back to my senses—and—our fireside.

"Why! what's the matter with you, M. Wright?" said Savrimovitch, slapping me on the back. "You're not ill, I hope?"

"Ill," replied I, looking at him vacantly; "no, I'm not ill!"

"I'm glad to hear that," said my friend, "for you've been muttering to yourself, starting and staring about you, like a man with *delirium tremens*, for the last fifteen minutes. Come to the hut, and be a little more sociable."

At ten o'clock we all turned in for the night; *i.e.*, we lay down on the ground in the clothes we wore. I had no overcoat, so Savrimovitch good-naturedly insisted on spreading a portion of his over me.

My companions were soon fast asleep, but the novelty of the situation and the exciting events of the day—especially the incident I have just described—kept me awake a long time, and when at length I fell asleep my rest was disturbed by all kinds of strange dreams.

The bugle roused us next morning at half-past five, and in a few minutes, we were all wide awake and astir. Most of the Servian bugle calls are tuneful—the *réveille* especially. It begins with a quick and lively strain, and ends with a long, melancholy wail. Half-a-dozen buglers were sounding it in different parts of the camp, so that the whole air was ringing with melodious and inspiring sounds. Though I got up with as much show of alacrity as the others, I felt both stiff and chilly, for the morning was cold and the dew falling heavily. I excited some surprise and laughter by stripping to the waist to wash myself. The mannikin, Jenko, could not understand the proceeding at all.

When I shouted to him for *"voda"* (water) he brought some in an earthenware pitcher of classical shape, and poured about ten drops on to my hand.

"What's the good of that, you little duffer?" said I. "I want you to pour some over my head and back," and stooping down, I motioned to him to do so.

With a nod and smile of intelligence, the little man dropped about four minims more on to my back, and then turned to depart. I stopped him angrily, and appealed to Mouravioff, who was standing near, to explain to him What I wanted.

"I think Jenko understands what you want, M. Wright, but our water supply is brought from some distance, and we are consequently compelled to use it as sparingly as possible."

"Good gracious me!" said I in dismay; "but we shall get very dirty if we are allowed only fourteen minims of water *per diem* for our ablutions!"

"My dear M. Wright, that is one of the disagreeable exigencies of campaigning. In Turkestan I have been very thankful sometimes to have enough water to drink."

"And I've wasted my fourteen minims!" said I, with a groan.

"Oh, well!" laughed Count Tiesenhausen, who just then came up to us barefooted, with his top boots under his arm, "I daresay Jenko can find a drop or two more at the bottom of his pitcher!"

The imp, Jenko, did contrive to squeeze out about a couple of scruples more, and these I caught on a corner of my pocket-handkerchief, and with it polished up my visage as well as I could. At about six o'clock we sat down to a breakfast of hot coffee-water (I won't tell a falsehood and call it coffee!), black bread, grilled mutton, biscuits, and sheep's-milk cheese. This last was white, friable, and rather palatable, though intensely salt.

At seven the whole battalion turned out for drill. The men were a motley crew. They had no uniforms, and everyone was dressed in the costume of the class to which he belonged. At first, I drilled in the ranks, partly because I thought I should so learn the words of command, and partly *pour encourager les autres*. On this occasion I recollect that my right-hand man was a dapper little patriot, in a grey civilian suit, while my left-hand man was a huge, stupid-looking peasant, wearing a short jacket over a loose linen garment, bound round the waist by a broad sash, baggy knickerbocker trousers, and a *fez* without a tassel. I wore my black volunteer suit.

Nearly all the Russian officers had bought regular military uniforms at Belgrade.

About a fortnight after my arrival, however, at the camp, Prince Obolenski generously supplied the whole brigade with a smart, serviceable uniform and overcoat at his own expense.

Had I known the peril of drilling in the ranks with raw recruits, I think my zeal, great as it was, would not have nerved me to undergo such a trial.

The drill was of the most elementary description. We were simply put through our facings; made to stand at attention, present, shoulder, slope, and trail arms, and form fours, but everything was very badly done.

This is not to be wondered at, for the men had been hurried into the ranks from the desk and the plough, but I was not prepared for the extent of their ignorance. To make matters worse, the bayonets remained fixed throughout the drill, and some of the recruits, in spite of orders to the contrary, had their rifles loaded—notably the burly idiot on my left. This interesting individual distinguished himself by doing everything wrong. At the word "Attention!" he grounded his rifle with horrible force on my toes; in forming fours he was my rear rank man, and gave me a nasty prod in the back with his bayonet, and had it not providentially struck against my waist belt, the wound might have been serious.

As it was, I got off with a painful scratch, and finally the charge in his rifle exploded, and was within an ace of blowing my head off. This was the climax. Count Tiesenhausen sternly ordered him to fall out of the ranks, gave him a good cuffing, which he took with stolid meekness, and put him under arrest. I was afterwards told that he and two or three other dangerous incompetents had been relegated to the awkward squad.

After drill, Savrimovitch and Count Tiesenhausen introduced me to several officers of the battalion, who invited us to dine with them. We accepted the invitation, and accompanied them to their quarters, which were in what had once been a farmyard.

Chapter 13

A Trip to Jubovac

This farmyard was surrounded by a low wall and had a wide entrance, on either side of which stood a wooden post. To each of these was tied a man, stripped to the waist, and bound hand and foot, with a placard hanging from his neck, on which was written a sentence in Servian characters.

"Hulloh!" said I, "what is the meaning of this?"

"One of them has been guilty of stealing, the other of gross insubordination," said one of our hosts, Major Bernadski, a fine-looking old Russian, "and they are to be flogged this evening."

I asked if they were Russians or Servians.

"The thief, I am sorry to say, is a Russian, the other is a Sclav. Some of our men are very angry that a Russian should be treated like that, and have asked me to intercede with the colonel for him. But I shall do nothing of the kind; the rascal deserves his sentence well. Did you ever see such a villainous face?"

Looking closely at the unhappy man, I recognised, to my unbounded astonishment, my acquaintance, Pauloff, the man whom I had vanquished in the bedroom at Paratchin a day or two before. He evidently recognised me, too, for he darted a very evil look at me out of his wicked little eyes.

I felt so sorry for the poor fellow that I persuaded Savrimovitch and Count Tiesenhausen to try to get his sentence remitted. I am happy to say their intercession proved so far successful, that he escaped the flogging.

Dinner that night was quite a banquet. We had mutton broth, beef tea, made with Liebig's Extract, grilled and haricot mutton, potatoes and rice, wine and smoked coffee-water—the latter, by the way, tasting a little more of coffee, and a little less of smoke, than that of our own manufacture.

After dinner we disposed ourselves comfortably on the straw with which the yard was littered, filled our glasses, lit our cigarettes, and began to chat.

"Pardon me for asking you such a question, M. Wright," said Bernadski, politely clinking his glass against mine, "but what will you do when Russia declares war against England?"

"I would ask the general for a flag of truce, and go over to the Turks," replied I. The Russians laughed.

"Our general would never allow you to do that, after having seen our positions. He would probably send you to Belgrade, and detain you there on parole," said one of them.

"Well, I should think that very shabby treatment," said I, rather indignantly; "but it is to be hoped that there will be no necessity for war between our countries."

"It is to be hoped not; still a war with England would be very popular with us, because your government so openly support our enemies the Turks!"

"What will England do when we have conquered India?" said Baron Kleist, solemnly, from behind his rampart of coat collar, and blowing at the same time a huge cloud of tobacco smoke from his nostrils.

"Russia never *will* conquer India," replied I, amused at his cool cheek.

"What! Do you mean to say they don't believe in England that we are to get India?" said Bernadski.

"Certainly!" said I. "We don't doubt that you would like to get India, but we are quite sure that you will never have it."

"Well," said Bernadski, "you must be either blind or infatuated, that is all I can say. Do you not see how rapidly we are approaching your frontiers?"

"Yes, we notice that," replied I.

"Then what is there to prevent us from attacking you and driving you out, as soon as we are ready?" said the Russian.

"Simply the fact that you are not, and never will be, strong enough." My reply was received with a shout of laughter.

"Not strong enough!" said Bernadski, echoing my words as if he had not heard them aright.

"No, not strong enough," repeated I. "I doubt if you would be able to conquer and hold Afghanistan, much less India."

Another shout of laughter followed this reply.

"Why," said Mouravioff, confidently, "I would undertake to conquer Afghanistan with one regiment of infantry and a single squadron of Cossacks; and give me 20,000 of my old Khivan comrades, I would undertake to make the whole of India mine."

"And I am equally willing to undertake," said I warmly, "that if you had ten, or even twenty times the number of men you mention, you would not succeed, for the whole manhood of England would rise in arms to prevent you!"

"M. Wright," said Baron Kleist, very solemnly indeed, "if you do not believe that we are to conquer India, you cannot believe in the Bible!"

"I believe in the Bible," said I, "but I cannot see what that has to do with a Russian conquest of India."

"I will tell you," replied the baron. "In the eleventh chapter of Daniel it says that the king of the north shall fight against the king of the south, and shall conquer him, and take his possessions and the rich and glorious land from him. Now, you cannot deny that Russia, the great northern power, is the king of the north, and England, with India, is the king of the south. Ergo, we shall conquer you, and take India, the rich and glorious land referred to, from you. Is not that clear enough?"

The Russians greeted the baron's rendering of this portion of the Scriptures with loud applause, and turned to me for my reply.

I said that if the prophecy had any reference to the conquest of India, it had probably been fulfilled when England conquered India. At that time, England might well claim to be the king of the north and India the king of the south.

My answer was received with a groan of disapprobation, and one of my audiences said that my interpretation of the policy was a very strained one.

"Sir," said another officer, "the possession of India is part of Russia's destiny!"

"How so?" I asked.

"Russia, at present," said he, "is not a rich nation; it is absolutely necessary for her to acquire wealth. India, with her incalculable treasures, offers herself an easy prey to us, therefore we shall take her."

"Your reason does not seem to be a very good one, and, moreover, leads you to a wrong conclusion," said I, enthusiastically; "for I am convinced that it is England's destiny to civilize and Christianise India, and so long as we do our duty by her, so long shall we keep her. It is quite possible, I admit, that we may not have done all that we might in this direction, but I think that we have done much more than you or any of the other powers would have done under the circumstances."

"Well, well, my dear sir," said M. Bernadski, giving me a pat on the back, "wait a bit, and we shall see!"

"Yes," said I, "we shall see!"

On the way back to our quarters I mentioned to Savrimovitch and Count Tiesenhausen my idea of sending a challenge to the Turkish officers, but they told me that my scheme was out of the question, and impracticable; at which I was greatly disappointed. I was somewhat comforted, however, when they told me that we should soon be attacking the Turks, and that then I should not be wanting in opportunities in which to display my courage.

That night I lay awake for a long time thinking over different schemes for distinguishing myself I was not satisfied with the prospect of merely taking part in a general engagement.

"Thousands and thousands of men," thought I, "will do the same, and I shall be no more distinguished than they. No," I argued, "as I am the only Englishman in the brigade, it behoves me to perform some remarkable feat!"

But what on earth this was to be I could not, for a long time, conceive. Suddenly, I remembered my plan of occupying a cottage in the Turkish lines.

"I'll propose that to Savrimovitch and Mouravioff tomorrow. Hurrah!" and I was meditating with great delight on this magnificent and warlike adventure when Morpheus slyly stole me away from the contemplation of Mars, and dropped me into the land of dreams. In other words, I fell asleep.

The next morning, I suggested to Savrimovitch that he and I should go on a reconnoitring expedition, and if we found a suitable cottage within the enemy's lines, or within a reasonable distance of them, we should occupy it forthwith.

Savrimovitch talked the matter over with Mouravioff, and the latter said he would very much like to accompany us in the reconnoitring expedition, but he feared that if we did occupy a cottage in the Turkish lines the occupation would be permanent.

"No, no," said I, "there's no object in our permanently occupying the place; six months will be quite long enough."

Both my friends, for no reason that I could see, laughed heartily at this, and Mouravioff said that I was indeed a remarkable military genius; at which I felt flattered, although I tried not to show it. As soon as we had breakfasted, we asked Count Réné's leave to go on our reconnoitring expedition; but he, after giving us a kindly greeting, referred us to Colonel Medvedovski. We accordingly repaired to our brigadier's quarters, and found him standing in front of his tent, perusing some despatches.

"Well, gentlemen," said he, returning our salute, "what can I do for you?"

"We wish for a day's leave of absence from the camp, sir. We want to see the enemy's lines!" said Savrimovitch.

"You want to go on a reconnoitring expedition, in fact," observed the colonel.

"Precisely so, sir," said Savrimovitch.

"Then I am sorry to say I cannot give you leave. However," continued he, seeing our disappointment, "I want some letters conveyed to the commander of the Krusevac Brigade, which is stationed at Jubovac, close to the Turkish position. If you like to take them you will have an opportunity of seeing something of the enemy, only mind you don't get into any mischief. If you will be good enough to come into my tent for a minute, I will give you the documents.

We followed him into his tent, which, by the way, was the only bit of canvas in the whole of our camp. Colonel Medvedovski desired us to be seated, pointing to some boxes and camp stools, offered us some wine, and then rapidly penned and handed us a note, which, together with a bundle of papers, he asked us to give to Colonel Philipovitch.

"Jubovac," said he, "is nearly twenty miles from here, so you shall have a waggon." Turning to an orderly who stood by the door of the tent, he said some words to him in Russian. The man immediately disappeared: then he wished us "good day!" and told us the waggon would be at our quarters in a few minutes.

We thanked the colonel heartily, and hurried back again to our hut, our hearts beating high with excitement and pleasure.

Our comrades were not a little jealous when they learned that we were going to Jubovac. They, however, good-naturedly wished us *bon voyage* and a pleasant time of it. We took with us a supply of biscuits, some Liebig's Extract, some spirits and water, our revolvers, a rifle apiece, and some ammunition. My friends tried to dissuade me from taking my cutlass with me, saying it would be a useless encumbrance, but I really could not bear to part with it.

How could I figure in the hanging-guard position, thought I, without a cutlass?

I also took with me a few drugs, some lint, bandages, etc., and a small amputating case. As I felt the edge of the knives, I reflected complacently on the inestimable advantages humanity derives from surgical science. The wounded Turk, said I to myself, that falls into my hands may well consider himself a fortunate individual! My incisions shall be boldly and skilfully made, and I flatter myself that his stumps will be perfect pictures!

Scarcely were our preparations completed when the waggon came rumbling up, and bidding our friends *au revoir*, we got into it, and in another minute were being jolted over the uneven ground *en route* for Jubovac.

We had a good driver, a good horse, a good road, a beautiful day, and lovely scenery. It is not surprising, therefore, that we were as jovial as we could be. Some distance from Deligrad we crossed the Morava by a bridge of boats. We passed several inns, but were so eager to push on that we would not stop until we had covered about twelve miles. Then, as the horse began to show signs of fatigue, we halted at a little wayside place, gave him a feed and a drink, of which he was badly in want, as the sun was terrifically hot, and partook of a little refreshment ourselves.

About one o'clock we were off again. We had gone a considerable distance further on our way, when we suddenly heard the distant report of a rifle, then another, and another, then a volley, followed by a smart and continuous fusillade. Excited beyond measure by these martial sounds, we made our driver urge on the horse to its utmost speed, and eagerly inspected our weapons, to see that they were in readiness. As we hurried along, the din was increased by the boom of cannon. The sound seemed to come from our left front, but partly from the hilly nature of the ground, and partly from the distance, we failed to see even the smoke of the firing. Presently we were challenged by a sentinel, and coming to a standstill were surrounded by an armed party, and conducted into the camp of the Krusevac Brigade. Here we found all the men under arms.

As we drove past their ranks. Colonel Philipovitch, the commanding officer of the brigade, rode up. He was a tall, stout man, with a stubbly ginger-coloured moustache and beard, and a very good-natured face. A Servian, and a native of Belgrade in the piping times of peace, he carried out a flourishing business as general merchant, which probably accounted for his sleek and comfortable appearance, and now at the call of duty he had donned the "horrid panoply of

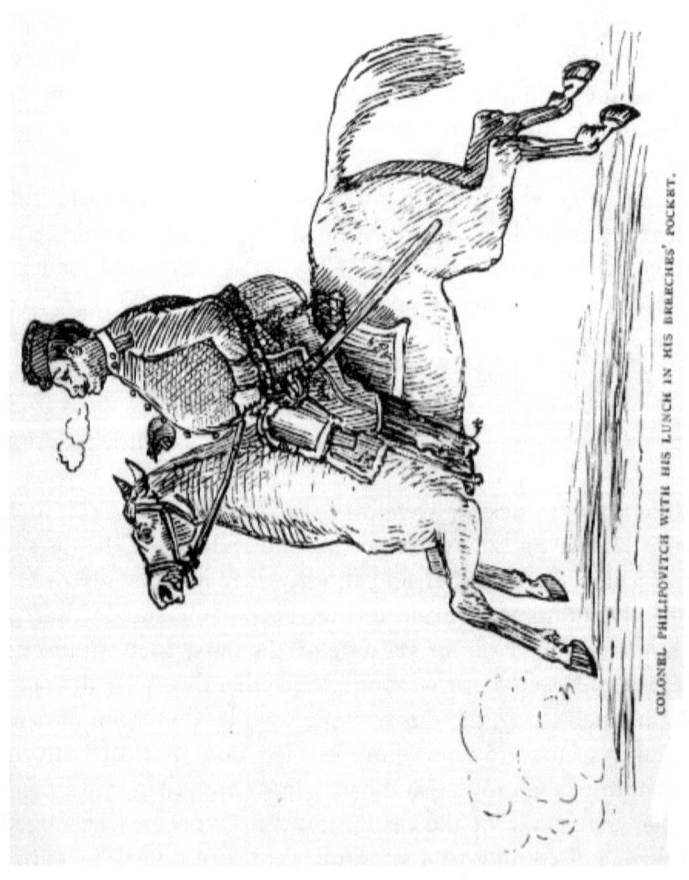

COLONEL PHILIPOVITCH WITH HIS LUNCH IN HIS BREECHES' POCKET.

war," and was transformed into a stout—a very stout—soldier. His cap, which was far too small for him, was cocked very much on one side of his head, and between his lips he held a cigarette, at which he sucked with a smacking noise. As he read the letters we gave him, he would look at us ever and *anon* with a friendly smile and a nod, and then go on with his reading again. All at once he flung the reins to one of the soldiers, and scrambling out of his saddle with a considerable amount of agility for his size, shouted out:—

"Ah! an Englishman! an Englishman!" and rushed up to us with outstretched arms. "Which, which," said he, with affectionate eagerness, "is the Englishman? Which is my English brother?"

I modestly replied that I was an Englishman.

Scarcely were the words out of my mouth, when I was enveloped in his huge embrace, and I verily believe he would have kissed me had I not averted my face.

Such was the energy of his greeting that he turned me round, so that, on looking over his shoulder, I found myself facing my friends. I could not resist the temptation of improving the situation and of making a really striking tableau, so I wagged my head about behind the back of the all-unconscious colonel, and indulged in a few of my choicest grimaces, with the effect of sending his staff and Savrimovitch and Mouravioff into convulsions of laughter. I blamed myself very much afterwards for this ill-timed jesting, of which, luckily, Colonel Philipovitch remained in entire ignorance.

We then asked the cause of the firing.

"General Horvatovics (Horvatovitch) has been making a reconnaissance of the enemy's position at Greviatz," said one of the officers.

"How far off is that?" we asked.

"Four miles," was the reply.

"Then you will not have any fighting today," said Savrimovitch, in a tone of disappointment.

"No, unless they attack us, which is not likely, as we are very strong here," said the officer.

"Captain Ilia Ilianovitch, dismiss the men. There is no occasion for us to remain longer under arms," exclaimed the colonel; then turning to us, he added, "Now, my friends, come to my quarters and have some dinner with me, for I am sure you must be hungry."

We readily accepted this hospitable invitation, and following our host into his tent, soon had the satisfaction of seeing a magnificent banquet spread before us. It was very obvious, that even in the midst of the horrors of war the gallant colonel did not forget the creature comforts of peace. There was a cold fowl, some pork cutlets, a ham, sardines, caviar, and oh, ye gods! a couple of Rehoboams of champagne. Our long and dusty drive gave zest to our appetites.

Colonel Philipovitch, moreover, was an excellent host, and took care that we did ample justice to his hospitality; he would not suffer our glasses to remain empty for a moment, and when at length our appetites were stayed he produced cigars, and we enjoyed a blissful half-hour's smoke.

"Colonel," said Savrimovitch, when he was half through his cigar, "how far off is the enemy from here?"

"Well," said Philipovitch, "his nearest pickets are stationed about a mile off, and he is in force on a range of hills about a mile further back. I will show you his batteries if you like, gentlemen."

We replied eagerly that we should like to see them, so our host rose, took down a field-glass that hung from the tent-post, and asking us to accompany him, walked out.

The camp of the Krusevac Brigade was situated on the side of a hill, to the brow of which the stout colonel laboriously, and with much puffing and groaning, endeavoured to mount. When at length we reached the top, we saw beneath us a valley about three thousand yards in breadth, bounded on the opposite side by a range of hills similar to the one we stood on. The intervening space was, for the most part, covered with forest

"There," said he, pointing across the valley to one of the opposite hills—"there are the Turkish batteries!"

The batteries were so cleverly masked that at first, I could not make out where they were, but after a long look with the glass I succeeded in discerning them.

"Which position is the best," said I, "ours or theirs?"

"Theirs," said Savrimovitch; "it commands this altogether. By Jove! they are firing at us; look there!"

Just as he spoke a puff of white smoke leapt forth from the battery, and the next moment I heard, for the first time in my life, the screaming of a shell as it whistled through the air.

"Lie down, boys!" sung out Colonel Philipovitch, throwing himself down on the ground.

The noise of the shell was extremely disagreeable, and I felt a strong inclination to follow the colonel's example, but as Savrimovitch and Mouravioff refused to budge, I felt bound to remain standing as well.

The missile, luckily, went over our heads, and exploded with a loud but harmless crash a good way behind us.

"Foolish boys, foolish boys!" said the colonel, as he got up again; "you are not wise; you want to be killed for nothing! Ah, ah! I am angry with you!" and he shook his head reproachfully at us, and then patted us affectionately on the back. Probably disgusted with the failure of his shot, the enemy did not fire at us again, and we continued our survey without further molestation.

About half a mile from the foot of the hill was a clearing of about four hundred acres in extent. In this secluded spot a group of cottages had stood before the war; now, only, one remained intact, the others having been knocked into shapeless heaps of ruins. The only signs of life that we could see were two or three curling wreaths of smoke that ascended from the outskirt of the forest on the other side of the clearing.

"That smoke," said Colonel Philipovitch, "comes from the Turkish outposts in the forest."

The sight of the ruins and the horrible noise made by the shell in its flight and explosion had greatly shaken my faith in the feasibility of a six months' occupation of a cottage in the Turkish lines, but I was ashamed to withdraw from my proposal, so pointing to the little building in the clearing, I proposed that we should straightway occupy it. My two friends nodded and smiled, and addressing Colonel Philipovitch, informed him of our wish.

For a long time, our kind-hearted host would not hear of it.

"We should be going," he said, "to certain death. The Turks would infallibly cut us to pieces;" and he tried to frighten us by relating, with rolling eyes and working fingers, stories of the atrocities committed by *bashi-bazouks*—that they gave no quarter, sparing neither age nor sex, and that one of their favourite methods of disposing of prisoners was to chop them into little bits and afterwards roast them alive.

We were, however, resolute, and succeeded at last in gaining the colonel's permission to pass a night in the cottage.

I did not feel so joyful and enthusiastic as I ought to have done; possibly the blood-curdling earnestness with which Colonel Philipovitch had alluded to the black doings of the bloodthirsty *bashi-bazouks* had acted as a damper to my spirits. Still, I contrived to assume an appearance of considerable glee and martial alacrity, and proposed in a frisky tone that we should start at once.

The stout colonel, however, insisted that we should drink a farewell glass with him, and lay in a stock of provisions.

"If you *must* go," said he, sadly, "take plenty to eat and drink with you. It is hard," and here he spoke with an air of the profoundest conviction, "to be valiant and fight well on an empty stomach."

We all agreed that there was much sense in what he said, and accompanying him to his quarters, we gratefully accepted at his hands a bottle of *raki*, some cold meat, bread, a tin of *pâté de foie gras*, and a bundle of cigars.

It was about four o'clock when we set out. Colonel Philipovitch walked a short distance, and showed us a zigzag trench, probably part of a rifle-pit, which ran down the hill to the outskirts of the forest.

"Walk down that trench, dear friends," said he, embracing us as affectionately as if he had known us for twenty years, "and you are less likely to be seen by the Turks. I do wish you would let me dissuade you from going on this mad errand, but I see it is no use talking to you about it. Well, well. I only hope you'll come to no harm, and mind, if you are found out, to make at once for the trench, and I will do what I can for you. Goodbye!"

"Goodbye, colonel!" we shouted as we leaped into the trench.

He waved his hand, and for some seconds stood gazing at us with an expression of deep concern in his fat but pleasant face: then a sudden turn in our pathway hid him from our view.

Chapter 14

A Lovely Evening

We walked down the steep and narrow path in single file. Mouravioff led the way, Savrimovitch came next, and I brought up the rear. We carried our loaded rifles in our hands, unfastened our revolver cases, and brought them well round to the front of our belts, in order to be handy, if required. None of us felt much inclined to talk, so that for some distance the only sounds we heard were the snapping of twigs under our feet, the hum of insects, and the note of birds in the woods hard by.

"How is it," said I all at once to Savrimovitch, "that the Turks don't put their outpost into that comfortable little cottage instead of keeping them in the open air?"

"For the very simple reason," replied he, "that we should knock it into pieces in two minutes with our cannon."

"Oh!" said I, mentally casting a glance at my scheme of a six months' occupation, to which this reply dealt a staggering blow.

"And similarly," continued he, "the Turkish guns render it impossible for us to occupy it openly."

My favourite plan was now completely demolished and pulverised.

On emerging from the trench, we entered the forest which clothed the hill on this side right down to its base, and extended as far as the heights occupied by the Turks. A few minutes' brisk walking under the trees, whose shade gave welcome relief from the burning sun, brought us to the edge of the clearing, and within two hundred yards of the cottage. We now walked from our cover, and scanned the forest held by the enemy. Everything was as still as death. We held brief discussions whether one of us should enter it first, or all three advance together. We decided upon the latter course. We left the shadow of the trees, therefore, and walking boldly across the clearing got to the cottage without being perceived by the enemy.

The place looked cheerless and uninviting. The walls were of hardened mud, and a roughly-constructed door swung loosely on its hinges, and the thatched roof was in a dilapidated condition. There were but two rooms, each with a small aperture for a window. The room in the front of the hovel had apparently been used as a kitchen, and in it we found a large heap of grain, a three-legged milking stool, and the fragment of a distaff. The back-room was perfectly empty.

By this time, it was about five o'clock, so we agreed to keep guard alternately until the following morning, by watching three hours each; Savrimovitch to take the first watch, Mouravioff the second, I the third, and so on. We decided also to use the back-room which looked towards the Turks as our watch-room. The enemy's advanced post was only two hundred yards off.

We next proposed to make ourselves as comfortable as circumstances would permit. The evening was excessively close. We divested ourselves of our belts and accoutrements, and unbuttoned our tunics; indeed, the Russians, who seemed to feel the heat more than I did, tore open the front of their shirts as well. I observed that each of them wore a gold locket round his neck. Thinking that they were love tokens, I made some chaffing remark about them, but Savrimovitch gravely informed me that I was mistaken, and handed me his locket, which contained a beautifully executed picture of the Madonna. Mouravioff, who was an avowed sceptic in matters of religion, flippantly remarked that he only wore his charm to oblige a lady relative, who believed that it would render him invulnerable to Turkish bullets.

For some time Mouravioff and I chatted pleasantly about various topics. Suddenly an exclamation from the watch-room startled us.

"Hulloh, Savrimovitch! Do you see anything?" cried Mouravioff.

"No," replied the other, "but I can hear the Turks. Listen a moment, they are singing." We kept silence for a minute or two, and heard our enemies indulging in a wild but monotonous chant, or rather howling, the burden of which seemed to be—

"*Ya! Allah! Hoo Allah!*"

We thought at first that this might presage an attack, and seized our weapons; but as time went on, and they made no signs of advancing, we became reassured, and prepared and ate our evening meal. At eight o'clock Mouravioff mounted guard in place of Savrimovitch. The moon was now shedding a flood of silvery light upon our cottage, the adjacent forests, the hills beyond; the sky was studded with innumerable stars, which shone and twinkled with a brilliancy far exceeding anything seen in the heavier atmosphere of England. From a tree close by a night-bird was filling the air with liquid notes of great sweetness and purity; and while two armies were encamped within a mile of us, only waiting for an opportunity to rush at one another, the whole scene around seemed to breathe nothing but peace.

My thoughts wandered thousands of miles away—first to my parents and brothers and sister in Calcutta, and then away to the beautiful Bulgarian, who had captivated my heart at Semendria, and whose presence seemed to haunt me even in the camp. Once the thought presented itself to me that I might never see them again, but it was immediately and ignominiously expelled, and replaced by a bright vision of their delight when they should hear of my extraordinary achievements as medical Field Marshal, and see the long lists of illustrious personages, from emperors down to mere generals, who had been or were about to be benefited by my skilfully wielded scalpel. Savrimovitch was sitting near the fire, with his face buried in his hands, and was apparently lost in a gloomy reverie, "A *ducat* for your dreams, my boy," said I, laying my hand on his shoulder. "They seem to be dismal."

"They are not very lively," he replied, raising his handsome face, which wore an unusually sad expression. "I have somehow a presentiment that I shall never return from this war. I had a strange dream the other night, which I cannot forget!"

"Pooh," said I, as cheerily as I could, "podophyllin for presentiments! Digestible food for dreams! Colonel Philipovitch's champagne and camping out have disagreed with you. Nothing is more inducive to gloomy forebodings than pork and *pâté de foie gras*. Tell me your horrible dream, and I will try and interpret it for you."

"Thank you," replied he, quietly, "I had rather not speak about it, but," and here he gave a slight shudder, "I believe I had my warning."

"Well, well," said I, "let's change the subject. Suppose we talk about love."

"You will think me a doleful subject, M. Wright," replied he, forcing a smile, "but even love is a painful subject to me."

"How's that?" asked I, with a sympathetic frown; "have the fair but fickle angels treated you badly?"

"No, no," said he, laughing slightly. "On the contrary, I have received nothing but kindness at their hands, and I am entirely devoted to their service."

"You perplex me," said I. "How then can it be painful to you to talk of love?"

"Because I happen to be desperately, but hopelessly, attached to a lady who can never return my affection."

"My dear M. Savrimovitch," said I, quickly, "I am a month or two older than you, and have seen much, very much, of the ways of the world. Permit me, therefore, to tell you that there need be no such thing as hopeless love in this world. Have you ever made any proposal to your lady-love?"

"No," replied he.

"Then," said I, "I have great hopes for you. The very next time you meet the lady, make her a declaration of love; never mind if your first attempt is unsuccessful. The poet wrote the beautiful lines:—

If at first you don't succeed.
Try, try, try again;

.... chiefly, I believe, for the encouragement of desponding lovers. I don't believe there ever was a maiden who could refuse twenty successive matrimonial proposals from the same pertinacious suitor."

"My dear M. Wright," said he, "you don't know what you are talking about! The lady in question is a Russian grand duchess, and since I last had the honour of seeing her, she has been married."

"Phew!" whistled I, in amazement, "a grand duchess, and married! That does make a difference. I am afraid your case really is hopeless," and I shook my head despondently, "unless you like to wait until Her Imperial Highness is a widow. But how, in the name of goodness, came you to fall in love with a grand duchess?"

"It happened in this wise," said he. "The *Czar* annually gives a ball in the Winter Palace to the officers of the Guard, when the lady members of the Imperial family honour the officers by dancing with some of them. Russian Court etiquette forbids any officer to ask a grand duchess to dance with him, so the Imperial lady indicates to the Lord Chamberlain the officer she chooses for her partner, and he straightway introduces the lucky guardsman. Well, on two occasions I had the supreme felicity, or rather the terrible misfortune, of dancing with the same princess, with the result that I have been hopelessly and despairingly in love with her ever since."

At this juncture we heard a peculiar whining noise close outside, accompanied by a scratching at the door.

We all sprang to our feet at once. Mouravioff and Savrimovitch seized their revolvers, and I whipped my trusty cutlass out of its sheath.

"Deuced odd sound that!" said I, in some alarm. "What on earth can it be?"

"I'll soon see," said Savrimovitch, and striding to the door he quickly swung it open. Lo, there was nothing to be seen! But we heard a sound as if something or somebody were scuttling away in a great hurry. Mouravioff stepped outside and looked around. All was as still as death. "There's *diablerie* in this," said Savrimovitch, looking slightly scared, and probably thinking of his presentiments; and I must confess that I, too, felt half-inclined to ascribe the sounds to something supernatural.

"*Diablerie*, pooh! A dog or a donkey more likely; at any rate, it doesn't matter to us what it is, so long as it is not a Turk," said the matter-of-fact Mouravioff.

"Let's leave the door slightly open," said I, "and we'll watch for it, whatever it is; Savrimovitch and I on this side, and you through the window on the opposite side of the cottage."

They agreed to this, and we commenced our watch, not without a good deal of dread and some curiosity on my part, for it occurred to me that the late occupants of the place might have been murdered by *bashi-bazouks*, and that their shades were hovering around us. We listened for some minutes in breathless silence for the slightest sound. The night-bird had stopped his song, and we could hear nothing but the sighing of the wind in the forest leaves. Suddenly Mouravioff gave a loud laugh, and exclaimed:—

"*Parbleu!* Here comes your devil! Here comes your fiend! Look, Savrimovitch! look, M. Wright! Ah! he's going round to your door—look!"

We put our heads outside the door, and just as we did so a large black dog rounded the corner of the building, and came straight up to the door. As soon as it saw us, however, it scurried away to some distance, and sitting on its haunches set up a most melancholy howling.

Mouravioff and I looked at one another, and burst out laughing at this unromantic elucidation of the mystery. To my surprise, however, I noticed that Savrimovitch was pale and agitated.

"How peculiarly that dog howls!" said he, with a shiver. "Does it not seem to you that there is something weird and unnatural in the sound?"

"Why, Savrimovitch," said Mouravioff, "what nonsense is this? You are as pale as a ghost, and shaking like an aspen. Are you ill?"

"No, it's nothing, thanks; a little dizziness, no more. There, I'm all right now," said he, drawing himself up to his full height, "and fit for anything. You may laugh if you like, but I tell you candidly I would rather have seen twenty Turks just then than that dog. Whenever a misfortune is about to befall our family, a hound like that makes its appearance, and howls as that one is doing." Savrimovitch's explanation made a considerable impression upon me, but Mouravioff laughed aloud.

"Stuff and nonsense," said he, "that dog's no demon. I am surprised that a *stout* soldier should be (I trust I shan't offend you) so absurdly superstitious. Here, M. Wright, kindly pass the spirits round, and let us have a glass apiece. Let me pour you out a bumper, Savrimovitch you're in a fanciful mood tonight, and need a tonic; low spirits require a pick-me-up! We'll keep our spirits up by pouring spirits down!"

The usually cynical Mouravioff was in high spirits this evening, and displayed an amount of kindliness and good-humour for which I had not given him credit. At eleven o'clock I mounted guard, and my two friends rolled themselves up in their overcoats and went to sleep.

Nothing happened during my three hours' watch. I had great difficulty in keeping myself awake, and was very glad when it was time to rouse Savrimovitch and relegate my duties to him. Then I threw myself on to the heap of grain and almost immediately fell asleep. I had perhaps been asleep for an hour, when a violent blow on the side and a loud scuffling noise awoke me. Starting up, I beheld a man struggling desperately with Savrimovitch, who held him fast by the throat.

The Russian was a powerful young man, but no match for his opponent, who seemed possessed of Herculean strength, and whose uniform and swarthy complexion proclaimed him a Turk. Before we could rush to our friend's assistance the combatants fell with a crash to the ground, the intruder uppermost, and brandishing a formidable Circassian knife in his hand. He had no time to use it, however, for Mouravioff struck him a terrible blow on the head with his clubbed rifle, and he rolled over senseless. To our unspeakable relief Savrimovitch rose to his feet uninjured, vowing that he had tripped over some inequality on the floor.

After this sudden and unexpected attack, we all kept on the alert with our weapons in our hands for some time, but the Turks in the opposite woods showed no signs of moving, and the stillness of the night was unbroken. In answer to our eager queries, Savrimovitch said that he had kept a sharp look-out on the Turkish side, and that our prisoner must have skirted the clearing and approached the hut from behind, and that when they met the Turk seemed as much surprised as he had been. This explanation reassured us, and led us to the conclusion that the Turk had been in the habit of helping himself to the maize that lay in the hut.

Having satisfied myself that we were not going to be attacked just then, I left the two Russians to watch and prepare breakfast, and proceeded with feelings of the liveliest enthusiasm to examine the injuries of our captive. He was still comatose, and his breathing was stertorous. I discovered, with sensations of sympathy and satisfaction, that he had sustained a depressed fracture of the skull, and that an immediate operation was necessary. I will not harrow the feelings of my non-professional readers by describing the measures I adopted, but will content myself with saying that I succeeded, not without considerable difficulty, in elevating the depressed piece of bone. The condition was at once greatly improved.

"Bravo, doctor!" exclaimed Mouravioff, "but what are you going to do now?" (I had produced my beloved amputating case and a pair of bullet forceps.) "You are surely not going to cut off his head?"

To this ridiculous question I replied with the gravity of tone a medical man should always adopt when speaking to a layman on professional subjects, that I could see no necessity for removing his head, and that I was merely about to institute a search for old gun-shot wounds, as it was quite possible that my patient might have a bullet in him which required extraction.

"I should have thought, doctor," said Savrimovitch (I noticed with much gratification that they called me doctor now), "that he struggled much too vigorously for that."

"My dear Savrimovitch," replied I, ripping up the prisoner's garments and exploring his limbs, "fear and excitement often inspire the weakest and the completely disabled with remarkable strength. We have a saying in England which is doubtless intended to be illustrative of this fact, but which, of course, is not to be interpreted literally, that King Charles I. walked and talked half an hour after his head was cut off; and I myself have seen fowls leap into the air and run about for some seconds after decapitation."

The sceptical Mouravioff laughed loudly, and even the courteous Savrimovitch looked incredulous, but I was far too much interested in the work I had in hand to take any notice of either of them.

To my disappointment I found no old bullet wound on the prisoner, but my desire to confer further surgical blessings on our barbarian captive was not altogether thwarted. I perceived that he had a small *epitheliomatous* ulcer on the lower lip. I decided there and then on its removal, and explaining the malignant nature of the lesion to the Russians, cut away the affected part, without the slightest objection from my patient.

Perhaps I ought to add that he remained insensible the whole time, but if he had been conscious, no reasonable person could suppose but that he would have submitted cheerfully—nay, gladly—to an operation fraught with such advantage to himself. I then dressed his lip, and putting my head out of the window, sniffed up the fresh morning air, and gave myself up to the complacent mental gratification which is the proper reward of every good deed. In very truth, I had heaped coals of fire on my adversary's head!

It was now nearly four o'clock; the grey dawn was giving place to the brighter light of day, and a crimson flush suffused the eastern sky. I watched the changing of the tints and brightening of the light with much pleasure, when suddenly the flash of musketry sparkled forth from the opposite trees, and I had just time to withdraw my head, when a bullet whistled through the window and knocked a large piece of dry mud and plaster from the wall of the apartment. Half-a-dozen Turks issued from the wood and advanced towards us at a run, headed by an officer, who held a revolver in one hand and brandished a gleaming sabre in the other.

The whole thing was so sudden that I was thoroughly scared; however, I thrust the muzzle of my rifle through the window, and taking a hurried aim at the leader of the party, pulled the trigger. The report of my piece was followed immediately by the loud *bang-bang!* of the rifles of my friends, who had rushed outside at the first alarm. When the smoke cleared away, the Turkish officer, evidently severely wounded, was being raised from the ground by a couple of his men, and the others were retreating to the forest at the double. Our triumph was very short-lived. Bugles rang out and shouts resounded from various parts of the forest, showing that the other Turkish outposts and pickets had taken the alarm, and that more men were hastening to attack us.

"M. Alfred, M. Wright!" shouted Mouravioff and Savrimovitch, entering the cottage, "come away, come away; we've no time to lose! In two minutes, the place will be surrounded!" I was reluctant to leave my patient, who still lay helpless on the ground, though he was now showing signs of returning animation (I had quite discarded the notion of standing a six months' siege in the cottage); but the enemy now reopened fire on us from the wood, and the bullets whistled about the place so unpleasantly that I was glad to hurry away. By keep-

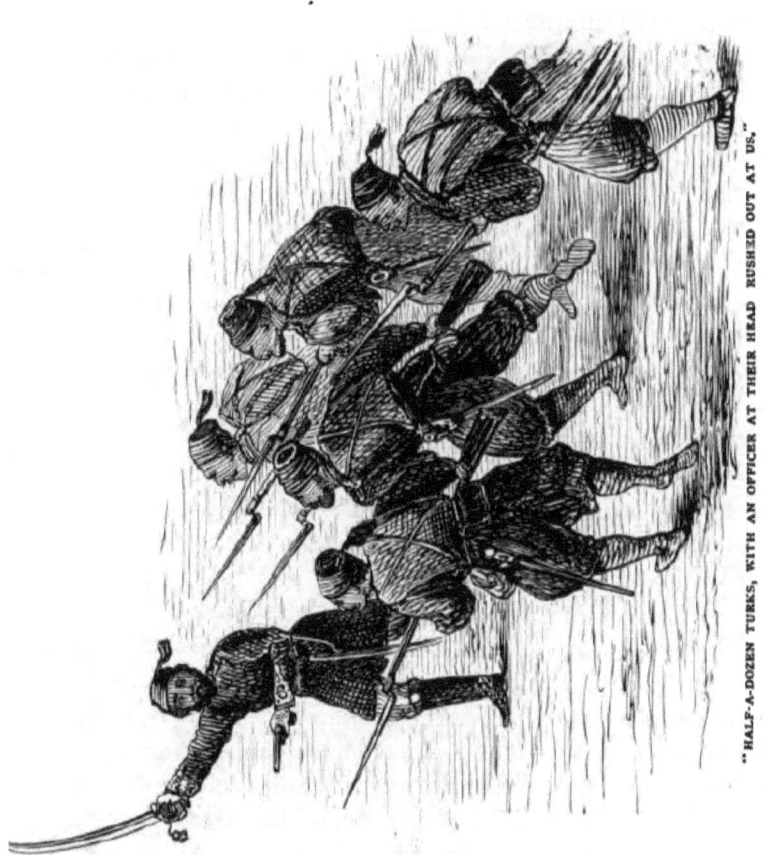

"HALF-A-DOZEN TURKS, WITH AN OFFICER AT THEIR HEAD RUSHED OUT AT US."

ing the little building between ourselves and the enemy we succeeded in getting a good way off before we were discovered.

But presently a loud shout proclaimed to us that we had been seen, and that we should have to run the gauntlet. We hurried up the hillside, under a smart rifle fire, towards the Servian camp, and fortunately reached the trench uninjured when we met a body of Servian soldiers hastening downwards, headed by fat Colonel Philipovitch, who was in a very excited state and much out of breath. He saw us, and gave a loud halloo of surprise and delight.

"Or—or, dear frents! dear frents! I thought you was killed, and all dead; now I am glad ever so much more—ha! Ha!" exclaimed he, and flinging down his drawn sabre he embraced all three of us, one after the other, most vigorously, sobbing and laughing alternately. When he became a little calmer, he told us that he had not slept a wink all night, and that at the sound of the firing he took it for granted that we had been surprised and killed, and was coming down to recover our bodies and avenge our deaths. Then stepping back a pace or two, he scanned us from head to foot, and eagerly asked if any of us had been hurt. We assured him that we were all right, on the strength of which he gave each of us another suffocating hug, and then marched back with us to his quarters.

On the way we related our adventures, which, simple as they were, filled him with astonishment and admiration. When Savrimovitch—who, being the best linguist amongst us, acted as our spokesman—told him of the strange scratching noise heard outside the hut and of the mysterious dog, his fat face turned pale, and his stubbly hair stood on end with superstitious awe. When he heard of the capture of our prisoner, he broke forth into a torrent of sympathetic and enthusiastic *braves* and *bravissimos!* He was much disgusted with my attempt to set the wounded Turk to rights again, and rolling his eyes about in a manner that was frightful to behold, drew his hand significantly across his throat, as much as to say that I should have done much better if I had made an end of him (the prisoner) instead.

On our arrival at the colonel's tent, we found a really sumptuous breakfast spread, which we attacked with keen relish, and immediately after the meal we prepared to start for Deligrad again. Our kind entertainer was most anxious that we should prolong our stay with him, but this, we explained to him, was quite impossible, and taking a really affecting leave of this warm-hearted soul, we got into our cart and trundled off to our own camp.

CHAPTER 15

Strange Conduct of Savrimovitch

We reached the Medvedovski camp the same afternoon, and found it in an unwonted state of excitement. A gorgeous silken banner, the handiwork of some Russian ladies sympathetic with the Servian cause, and which had been consecrated by the Metropolitan of Moscow, had just arrived, and General Tchernaieff was coming to present it formally to the brigade.

The whole brigade was under arms, and we had hardly time to fall into our battalion. The troops were marched to a large open space a few hundred yards to the right of the camp, and formed into an immense hollow square. General Tchernaieff then rode up, surrounded by his staff, and dismounting, entered the square, where he was received by Colonel Medvedovski, some of the other officers of the brigade, and three priests.

Amongst the general's staff a stout, sleek-looking young man was pointed out to me as the Roumanian prince, Ghika, and I also saw for the first time that well-known English or rather Scottish soldier of fortune. Colonel McIvor. One of the priests opened the proceedings with a long prayer, during which the soldiers crossed themselves incessantly. Holy water was then sprinkled on the banner, and General Tchernaieff, taking it from the priests, made a speech to the brigade, and presented it to Colonel Medvedovski, who in turn handed it to one of his officers. Then the whole brigade was marched in single file past the priest, beside whom was a small altar with a cross on it, and each man as he passed was touched on the lips and forehead with a spray of hyssop dipped in holy water.

This ceremony lasted an immense time, and the priest's arms must have fairly ached by the time it was over. I witnessed these proceedings with the greatest interest and enthusiasm. Here was a magnificent opportunity of distinguishing myself. I resolved on the spot to ask for the proud privilege of carrying the banner the first time we went into action! Thousands of men would go into battle, but only one could be the standard-bearer at a time.

"This," thought I, "will distinguish me above my fellows, and maintain my reputation as a brave Englishman!"

When the ceremony was over, I mentioned my scheme to Savrimovitch. He heartily approved of it, so the next morning I went to the colonel for the purpose of preferring my 'request to him.

"Well, sir," said he on seeing me, "what can I do for you?"

"I have come, sir," replied I, "to ask if you will let me carry the standard that was presented to us yesterday into action the first time we are engaged."

The colonel looked very pleased, but for a moment said nothing; then he observed that if I would call again the next day at noon, he would give me an answer. Delays of any description are very disagreeable to me, so I felt slightly disappointed at the reply, still I saluted with a good grace and went away.

On the following day I presented myself at the appointed hour, and with my heart full of hope and expectation. The colonel received me most graciously, and beside him were Count René and Prince Obolenski, both of whom shook hands with me with kind cordiality.

"Well, sir," said the brigadier, "your request has pleased us very much; it shows us that you are actuated by a loyal and worthy spirit. Nevertheless, this brigade is, *par excellence*, the Russian brigade, therefore we think it better that a Russian should carry the colours."

I suppose my face displayed the disappointment I felt, for the colonel continued:—

"I am very sorry to refuse your request, but never fear, you will soon have plenty of opportunities of showing what stuff you are made of!"

I walked back dolefully enough, and confided my trouble to Savrimovitch, who seemed, however, to be brooding over some trouble of his own, and was less sympathetic than usual.

The heat that afternoon was intense, and Savrimovitch, Mouravioff, and I were silently smoking under the shelter of our hut, when a bullet whistled between us, and passed out through the leafy wall behind. We started to our feet and rushed outside.

A number of soldiers were standing or sitting about engaged in cleaning their rifles, cooking, etc. Mouravioff demanded furiously who had fired the shot.

A heavy, stupid-looking fellow was pointed out as the culprit, whereupon our friend strode up to him, and seizing him by the collar, asked him sternly what he meant by discharging a loaded rifle in camp. The soldier sulkily answered that he had only fired his piece in the air, and did not know there was any harm in that, whereupon the rough-and-ready Mouravioff replied:—

"Idiot! Don't you know that when you send a bullet into the air it is likely to come down again, like this?" and striking him on the head with his clenched fist, knocked him over.

This severe treatment caused some murmuring amongst the soldiers, who were already beginning to tire of Russian discipline. A sinister rumour that many Russian officers had been treacherously slain in battle by some of their own men, whose ill-will they had incurred, was current in camp, and it was undoubtedly true that Russian officers frequently treated the Servians with great harshness, but considering the rawness and inaptitude of the material they had to deal with, and the absolute necessity of enforcing discipline, I do not think that the kicks and cuffs I often saw them bestow on their men were unmerited.

Again, although the unwarlike Serbs murmured at being dragooned into discipline, they seemed very soon to regain their equanimity. They are naturally too good-natured and easy-going a race to be vindictive, and therefore I believe that the heavy losses among the Russians were due to their reckless valour and not to Servian treachery. Nevertheless, many Russians I met firmly believed this rumour, in spite of the indignant denial of it given by the Servians.

As the days passed by, I noticed with pain that my friend Savrimovitch became more and more reserved and melancholy, and that every now and then he would fly on the slightest provocation, or even without any at all, into the most ungovernable fury. On one occasion he took offence at something Count Tiesenhausen said to him, and calling him a German coward, drew his revolver, and would certainly have shot him if I had not disarmed him.

Another time he came up to me and asked me to give him enough opium to make away with himself. On these occasions he looked and behaved like a madman. He said that he was tired of life, and wished to die. Of course, I refused his request. For a minute or two he pressed me earnestly, nay, coaxingly, to give him the opium, and when I persisted in my refusal, he laid his hand on his sword, and with flushed face and flashing eyes told me he would compel me to give him what he wanted. Up to this time I had tried to laugh him out of the idea, but his furious and menacing attitude made me serious.

"My dear friend," said I, looking him steadily in the face, "you will not get a grain of opium from me. If you wish to die, you will soon have abundant opportunities of satisfying your desire when we go into action. If you were to poison yourself now, it might be said that you were afraid to face the Turks. Is it not far better to fall like a brave soldier than to die of poison like a rat?"

At the end of my speech the wild glare left Savrimovitch's eyes and the crimson flush died out of his cheeks. He threw down his sword, and embracing me called me his English brother, and begged me to forgive his frenzied petulance, then passing his hand across his forehead he said, "When these whirlwinds of fury seize my mind, I feel like a tiger or a madman, and lose all self-control. Two or three years ago I received this sabre wound," and he showed me a scar on the side of his head concealed by his hair, "and I have never been the same since. Lately, though, I have become more irritable and excitable than ever, and I wish, like a dear good fellow, you would look after me. You have a strange influence over me, and may be the means of preventing me from doing some irreparable mischief."

Then we kissed after the Russian fashion, vowed eternal friendship, and agreed henceforth to call one another by our Christian names of Alfred and Alexis.

Alexis' favourite topic of conversation was India. He was never tired of asking questions about that marvellous country, or hearing stories of encounters with tigers, elephants, and wild boars in the jungles; of adventures with crocodiles and venomous snakes, and fights with pirates by land and sea, of which I had learned any number from my Anglo-Indian uncles and aunts.

My tales fired his imagination to such a degree that he resolved to go for a tour in India after the war was over, and asked me to accompany him, which I agreed to do. I now noticed, with gratification, an improvement in my friend's mental condition. Both his fits of depression and his outbreaks of temper became less intense and less frequent. This satisfactory result was partly due to the fact that I contrived in various ways to divert his attention from himself, and also because he made a real effort to exercise more self-control.

His state of mind was never such as to incapacitate him from attending to his duties, indeed, everything that he had to do was well and thoroughly done, and it was only during his idle moments, and when he was interfered with, that he behaved strangely. Still, his conduct was at times very unaccountable, sufficiently so to justify the belief that his reason was within a measurable distance of becoming permanently impaired.

He attributed his condition to the sabre wound he had received on his head, and that had, in all probability, a great deal to do with it. *Apropos* of this wound, I asked him one day how he received it, and the following was his account:—

"I went out as a volunteer with General Kaufmann's army during the late campaign against the Turcomans. One bitterly cold winter's day, when the plains were thickly covered with snow, I accompanied a detachment of fifty Cossacks on a reconnoitring expedition. As we were returning, snow began to fall heavily, and the consequence was we came unawares upon a large body of the enemy. They were all of them mounted and were headed by a chief on a magnificent black horse. As soon as they saw us, they raised a fierce shout and dashed at us at a gallop. So swift was their approach that my men had just time to give them a volley from their carbines and to level their lances, when they swept upon us like a whirlwind, and surrounded us on all sides, cutting, thrusting, and hewing at us with the fury of demons.

"Though my men were outnumbered, ten to one, they fought with desperate valour, for they knew that no quarter would be given them. As if by mutual consent, the chief on the black horse and I singled each other out, but the press was so great that after we had exchanged a cut or two, we were separated. Twice we succeeded in cutting our way through the Turcoman host, only to find ourselves surrounded again, and our condition began to look hopeless indeed. Numbers of the enemy, it is true, had fallen, but we had also lost heavily, and could ill afford to do so.

"My sword arm became so tired that I could hardly raise it, and all my men were suffering either from wounds or exhaustion. Still, we fought on, hoping against hope, that the discharge of our carbines might be heard from our camp and assistance be sent to us. Whilst I was defending myself against another man, the Turcoman chief attacked me again, and aimed a terrible cut at my head. I saw it coming, and tried to parry it, but ineffectually. My guard was beaten down, and the blow descended on me, inflicting the wound you see, and knocking me from my saddle. The chief was about to finish me off with another stroke, when one of my men ran him through the body with his lance.

"I recollect nothing more about the affair, except that I found myself in our camp hospital the next day, with my head aching terribly, and covered with dressings and bandages; our firing, it seems, had been heard, and a rescue sent, but only just in time, for my little band had been reduced to fifteen men, not one of whom was unwounded."

Some days after this conversation we got leave to go to Paratchin. My friend was very fond of riding, and tried hard to borrow a couple of horses for the occasion. However, he was unsuccessful, and was grievously disappointed thereat I expressed much sympathy with him, but really felt much relieved, for I was by no means a good horseman. However, we managed to borrow a dingy-looking, but comfortable open carriage, which actually boasted of good springs, and left the camp in it one morning, amidst the envious remarks of our brother officers and the admiring criticisms of the men. When we were about four miles from Paratchin, we were overtaken by three officers on horseback, one of whom proved to be the young man who bore so striking a resemblance to Marie! He looked into our carriage as he passed, and as our eyes met, he blushed to his temples, and hurriedly returning our salutation, turned his face away, and putting spurs to his horse galloped off.

"What a shy-looking young fellow that is!" said Savrimovitch. "He looks more like a girl than a man, doesn't he? Still, he rides well."

"I've seen him before somewhere," said I.

"Do you know anything about him?"

"Nothing," was the reply.

On arriving at Paratchin, we told the driver to go to the best hotel, and he took us to one called the *Kneas Serbski* (Servian prince.)

We went into the coffee-room, which was crowded with Servian soldiers and officers, feeding and smoking, and ordered a substantial dinner. Whilst we were waiting for it to be served, who should I see, extended on a bench by the wall, but my distinguished Belgrade acquaintance, Colonel Bragg, of dog-slaying and swearing celebrity!

Although I was not one of that hero's admirers, I was concerned to see that he looked pale and miserable, and leaving my seat for a moment, I went up to the colonel, and saluting him, expressed a hope that he was well.

"Who the —— are you? Ah, I know! The little doctor who came to see me in a pair of d——d stupid india-rubber boots; I hope you are better than I am. I'm d——d bad I can tell you!"

"What is the matter, sir?" said I. "Perhaps I can do something for you?"

"I don't know what's the matter, doctor," said he, "but I've been d——d ill this last ten days. Rheumatism, gout, or some kind of fever or another. It was a confounded shame to send me to the front; I'm not fit for it."

"Let's look at your tongue," said I.

"No, I shan't," said he, "what good will that do? All I want is to keep quiet." Then raising himself on his elbow, and drawing me closer to him, he said in a whisper, "I say, doctor, couldn't you give me a certificate to the effect that I am too ill to go to the front? I'm d——d fond of fighting," here he gave a sickly smile, "but I'm not fit to go. These mulligrubs, you know, are the very devil; they are playing old Harry with me." Before I could reply a loud and wrathful exclamation from Savrimovitch startled me. Turning round I saw him, his face crimson with fury, seize a wine bottle by the neck and fling it with all his force at the head of one of the waiters. The bottle struck the man on the back of the head and smashed into a thousand pieces, deluging him with its contents, and sending a shower of wine and pieces of glass over several of the tables.

Immediately the whole place became a pandemonium. Everyone sprang to his feet, tables were overturned, and plates and dishes fell clattering and smashing on to the floor. Swords leaped from their scabbards, and the air resounded with oaths and imprecations, and in place of a party of merry fellows enjoying their dinners, one could see nothing but angry faces and bristling weapons and general confusion.

In the middle of all this turmoil stood Savrimovitch, sword in hand, defying the tempest he had raised with angry, scornful contempt and jibing temper.

Though I inwardly cursed his hasty temper, it was impossible for me to leave him in this pickle, so quickly drawing my cutlass I placed myself alongside of him, and looked terrific things at the wrathful mob that surrounded us.

For about a second, we faced one another; then, as if with one accord, they rushed at us. I was overwhelmed with a storm of blows, knocked down, and my sword forced out of my hand. I recollect struggling desperately to get up and receiving another blow on the head. After that a faint, giddy feeling came over me, and I lost consciousness. When I came to, it was to find myself in a darkened room, with a very vague idea of what had taken place or of where I was. In the middle of my speculations on these two points, I was disturbed by the flash of a light and the sound of footsteps entering the room, and looking up saw the young Bulgarian officer who so much reminded me of Marie, accompanied by Doctor Yermaylaff Giggleivitch.

A half-muttered exclamation from me brought the young officer to my bedside, with clasped hands and a look of the most anxious interest in his face.

"I am so glad, sir," said he, "to find you better. I trust that you are not suffering much pain."

Convinced that this young man was no other than Marie, I foolishly said:—

"I am ever so much better already, and if you will only come and see me every day, Marie, I shall soon be well again."

But I had not finished the sentence before I saw the mistake I had made. The young officer drew himself up stiffly, and said with a frown:—

"My name, sir, is Milosch Darvorin;" and then turning to the doctor, added, "I thought that he was better, but he is still delirious. Had we not better leave him?"

Agonised at the thought of having offended one to please whom I would have given worlds, I exclaimed:—

"Yes, I am delirious; I don't know what I am saying. I assure you, sir, that I am a miserable fool, who having but little sense to begin with has now lost that little. I trust, therefore (here I cast an imploring glance at the young officer), that you will not take offence at anything I may have said." At this pathetic appeal both the doctor and the young officer laughed; the former, however, suddenly checking his merriment, came to the side of the bed and said drily:—

"I quite agree with you, sir, as to your having no sense, and unless you keep perfectly quiet, you'll have no life either. Not another word, sir; your recovery and my reputation, which I have staked upon it, depend on your having complete rest and keeping silence." With these words Dr. Giggleivitch and his companion left the room, and I was again alone and in darkness.

Chapter 16

Good News

My mind was still in a considerable muddle, and when I was left to myself, I pondered hazily over what Marie or rather Milosch Darvorin and that confounded Dr. Giggleivitch had said to me, when all at once I began to wonder what had become of Savrimovitch. When I last saw him, he was fighting desperately by my side, and after that my recollection failed me.

I was afraid he might be dead, and felt terribly uneasy and anxious about him. Luckily, however, for my peace of mind, Dr. Giggleivitch came into my room again, and I seized the opportunity and asked him about my friend.

"I told you not to talk just now, sir," said he, sternly, and without answering my question.

"Yes, I know you did, doctor, but I must know; for Heaven's sake tell me what has become of Alexis Savrimovitch, and I promise I won't talk anymore."

"He's alive, and doing very well; drink this;" and he gave me a filthy draught of some sort, and walked out of the room again.

My mind was relieved, and when I awoke next morning I felt refreshed and much better. But I had received such a mauling that I could not leave my bed for a week. I had three nasty scalp wounds and a sabre cut across my forehead, which I am afraid will permanently mar my beauty. I was not allowed to see Savrimovitch for some while, but one day he stalked into my room, looking very pale and handsome, and with his left arm in a sling. I was sitting up in bed, a still more dilapidated-looking object.

"My dear Alfred," said he, in a voice full of emotion, "can you forgive me for having brought all this trouble upon you?"

"My dear boy," said I, quite distressed to see him so moved, "you have nothing to reproach yourself with. The Servians are the most quarrelsome and cantankerous set of fellows I ever came across."

"No, it was my fault entirely," said he. "I ought not to have got into such a rage with the waiter, but I had called on the fellow twenty times to serve us, and he paid no attention, and went on attending to everybody else first—at least, so it seemed to me. Then I got angry, and spoke sharply to him, and he had the audacity to tell me I must wait my turn! Confound the fellow's impudence! I feel warm when I think of it;" and the peppery Alexis stamped his foot and got into quite a passion at the recollection of it.

"Well," said I, "and what happened then?"

"Why, I lost my temper, and threw a bottle of wine at him, which smashed into a thousand pieces, and flew all over the Servians, who were all on the grin, and made them laugh the wrong side of their mouths."

"And then?"

"Then they made a great show of jumping to their feet and drawing their swords, so I called them a lot of cowardly Turkish slaves, and told them to come on if they dared. And the rest you know "

"But what happened after I was cut down?"

"Cut down! You weren't cut down at all; you were knocked down with a chair, and I shared the same ignominious fate; the same blackguard did for us both. He smashed my sword blade into twenty pieces, and broke my arm with the same disgusting weapon. I wish I had the chair-wielding scoundrel here, and my sword at his throat, I'd teach him a lesson!"

The entry of a servant with our dinner put an agreeable end to the conversation. I was not sorry, for Savrimovitch was getting so excited that I almost feared another outbreak on his part.

After this we were allowed to share the same room, and both made rapid strides towards recovery. Every now and then we received a visit from some of our brother officers at the camp, and one day the Count Réné came to see us.

"Ah, young fire-eaters!" he said, after shaking hands with us, "this sort of thing won't do at all; you will be giving the brigade quite a bad name. The colonel was very vexed when he heard of your little escapade here. Tell me all about it."

When the count heard our story, he twirled his little shadowy yellow moustache, and said that he did not think we were altogether to blame, "only," he added, "I really do think that an Englishman and a Russian ought to have given a better account of those Servians. By the way, M. Wright," he went on to say, "I have a newspaper here which contains an extract which may probably interest you; "and with his eyes twinkling with merriment he took from his pocket an English newspaper and handed it to me. It was a copy of the Daily Courier, in which was the following paragraph:—

Fiendish Servian Atrocity.—It is my painful duty to have to record the following fiendish outrage which was perpetrated by a party of Servian marauders on a wounded Turkish soldier. I can vouch for the truth of the incident. On the — inst. the Turkish advanced posts near Jubovac discovered that a cottage close to their position was in the hands of the Servians. Captain Hussein Avni, and half a company of the—battalion, instantly attacked and drove out the enemy, not, however, without loss, for the gallant captain was severely wounded in the leg. On entering the cottage, the soldiers found the senseless body of one of their comrades stretched on the floor. The poor fellow was most shockingly mutilated. Not content with slicing off his upper lip, the barbarians had committed the atrocity of drilling a hole in his skull. The indignation excited throughout the army by this piece of devilment is extreme, and we hear that Adul Kerim has sent a *parlementaire*, with a strongly-worded remonstrance on the subject to the Servian headquarters.

This atrocious paragraph overwhelmed me with consternation and dismay. I had hoped and expected that my careful treatment of our Turkish captive's wounds would have gained me no little *kudos*, instead of which it was looked upon as a blood-curdling instance of *bashi-bazoukism,* and I was described as a diabolical monster.

The paper fell from my hands, and I gazed alternately at the count and Alexis in utter bewilderment. My friends did not sympathise with me. On the contrary, they burst into an uncontrollable fit of laughter, which completed my discomfiture and mortification.

"Confound it all! What are you laughing at?" cried I, beside myself with rage. My anger increased their merriment, and they laughed until the tears ran down their cheeks. I felt a strong inclination to quarrel with them for their ill-timed hilarity, but I reflected in time that laughter is a physiological process, which as often as not takes place quite independent of the will. Something tickles that part of the nervous organisation which corresponds with the fancy, and a peculiar stimulus is reflected to the diaphragm, and causes it to move spasmodically, in such a way that the air is jerked from the larynx with an asinine *ha! ha! hee! hee! hau! hau!* sound. The thought that I had set these doughty Russian warriors braying like a couple of asses more than atoned for the want of sympathy they had shown me. I folded my arms, and awaited their return to gravity with the most perfect equanimity. Of course, they were profuse in their apologies, which, however, I assured them were quite unnecessary, for their laughter had afforded me the greatest possible amusement.

Before he went. Count Réné informed us that he had some grand news.

"What is it?" we asked.

"Next week the brigade is to join Horvatovitch's army. That means that we shall have some fighting directly, for Horvatovitch is a fighting fellow. What do you say to that, boys?"

At this delightful piece of intelligence, we both gave a loud hurrah. Alexis fell on the count's neck and kissed him, and I executed a war-like and spirited *pas seul* on the floor of the ward.

Our enthusiasm greatly pleased the count, and he bade us *adieu* with a sweet smile on his weather-beaten countenance.

CHAPTER 17

We dispose of a Pig

The count's invigorating news, combined with Dr. Giggleivitch's skilful treatment and disagreeable prescriptions, soon completed my restoration to health, so that within a week of the visit of the former we were back again at Deligrad.

The day after our return our brigade received orders to march to Jubovac, when we occupied the ground that Colonel Philipovitch's men had held, and we were consequently in full view of that never-to-be-forgotten cottage of hateful memory. For the first few days at Jubovac the weather was terribly bad. The sun was invisible, and the rain came down in torrents, and mud and slush prevailed everywhere. Sometimes on waking in the morning, I found myself half smothered in a pool of water which had collected in the depression made by my weight in the soft soil. To add to my discomfort, Savrimovitch, who up to this time had shared his waterproof with me, was appointed adjutant to the brigade, and now seldom slept in our part of the camp.

It is not very surprising, therefore, that I began to suffer from ague. Several of the Russians, however, regarded my seediness as a proof of their theory that Englishmen might be brave, but had no stamina, and one of them had the assurance to tell me so to my face. I determined, if possible, to cure myself straight away, and with that object in view I stirred a whole teaspoonful of quinine into a wineglass full of *raki*, and tossed the mixture off. Heavens! what a bitter draught it was, and what a headache it gave me! However, it answered its purpose, and cured me for the time being of ague.

Besides the wet, we had every now and then to put up with very short commons in the way of provisions, due, I suppose, to some temporary breakdown in the Commissariat Department. More than once the only dinner I got during the day was a piece of bread and a roasted onion, supplemented with a dessert of acorns and wild honey, luxuries

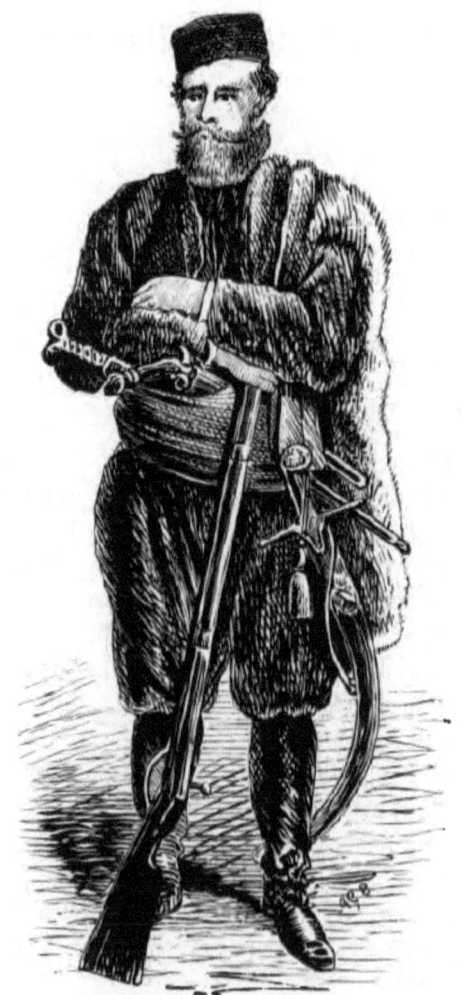

A BULGARIAN VOLUNTEER.

with which the oak forest surrounding us abounded. As if to tantalise us, the peasants used to drive their herds of swine into these forests, where the herbage and fallen berries supplied them with plenty of fattening food.

For the protection of these precious pigs Colonel Horvatovitch had issued the most stringent regulations. They were private property—so went his decree—and the troops were forbidden to touch them, under the severest pains and penalties. In spite of these threats, of which, at the time, I knew nothing, pigs were mysteriously murdered and pork surreptitiously devoured almost every day in some part or other of the camp.

The peasants became clamorous about their slaughtered swine, and Horvatovitch, in a rage, instituted pig-protecting patrols, and vowed that he would hang the first pigsticker who fell into his clutches.

One day, when we had been particularly badly off for food, Savrimovitch, Mouravioff, and I went for a stroll into the woods. We were all very hungry, and I, at least, was in blissful ignorance of the commander's pig-protecting *pronunciamento*. We were sauntering along quietly under the shade of the trees, when the grunting of a porker greeted our ears. We exchanged significant glances, my friends, doubtless, thinking of the regulations, whilst I smacked my lips in anticipation of a delicious meal of roast pork with crackling.

The next moment a luscious spectacle burst upon our enraptured gaze! Two fat pigs, in the very pink of condition for eating, and with the curliest of tails, trotted into view, and with a series of happy and contented grunts, commenced muzzling and guzzling amongst the roots and berries that lay about them. The prospect of crackling overcame me! In the twinkling of an eye, I had raised my rifle to my shoulder, and sent a bullet through the head of the nearest. I sprang forward with a shout of triumph to secure my prey, and laughingly called on Alexis and Mouravioff to assist me, but neither of them stirred.

"Heavens, M. Wright!" said Alexis, "what have you done?"

"Have you not heard fire-eating Horvatovitch's proclamation of death to the pig-slayer?" said Mouravioff.

"Murder!" said I. "You don't mean to say that it is forbidden to kill pigs?"

"I should rather think it is," was the reply.

"Well, but what would you have me do?" said I, in an agony. "We surely must not leave that lovely carcase there to waste?"

"Well, no," said my friends, who also cast longing glances at it. "It would be a pity to waste it."

"Wait a bit," said Mouravioff. "I'll tell you what will be the best thing to do. Issue invitations to all the officers you know to a supper party this evening; get as many others in the same hunt with yourself, and you'll find it will end all right. The general won't like to punish a score of officers just on the eve of a battle."

The idea seemed to me a good one, so I agreed to adopt it. Meanwhile we covered the beautiful body with leaves in a most artful manner, so that no one would suspect there was a dead pig there, and on our return to camp we directed the handy Yenko to the spot, and commissioned him to cut up the pig and bring it back piece-meal. The astute mannikin succeeded in doing this without being discovered, and we then issued our invitations. About twenty Russian officers, including Counts Tiesenhausen, Réné, and Baron Kleist accepted, and we made a most excellent supper and spent a most enjoyable evening.

The next morning, however, whilst I was performing the usual apology for a toilet, an officer, with a guard of soldiers at his back, came up to the tent, and politely requested me to accompany him to the headquarters. I asked him if he would be good enough to wait while I beautified myself for the occasion. He consented, so I made Yenko give my boots, which had not been off my feet for nearly a week, a good greasing (blacking was an unknown luxury in the camp), and put a respectable-looking piece of pink twine to my eyeglass in place of the original black silk cord which had been reduced by hard wear to a disreputable little chain of knots about eighteen inches in length.

Moreover, bad weather and rough usage having caused the shedding of most of my buttons, I deemed it advisable to make my pantaloons secure with some stout string, and then distributed my scanty allowance of water for washing as judiciously as possible over my face and hands. These arrangements completed, I bade a dignified farewell to the friends who crowded around, and signifying my readiness to depart to the officer, drew myself up to my full height and strode off with them, erect and calm.

Close to headquarters we passed a party of soldiers leading away two prisoners, whose hands were pinioned behind their backs.

"Hulloh!" said I to my guide, "what have those fellows been up to?"

"Killing pigs, *monsieur*," was the reply.

"And what's their punishment to be?" inquired I, wincing slightly.

"I believe they are to be hanged, *monsieur*," said the officer, blandly;

"but I am not sure, or it is possible that they will be shot."

"Confound it all!" exclaimed I, much startled; "you don't really mean that?"

"Yes, *monsieur*, that is what I have heard," said the officer. "The general is determined to make examples of the next pig-killers he catches, but here we are!"

The headquarters were established in a large barn, which at this moment was thronged with officers, some of whom were seated at a table, and seemed to constitute the court martial, whilst others were merely lookers-on. At the head of the table stood a heavily-bearded man of immense stature, fully six feet six in height. His strongly marked but handsome features were flushed, and his blue eyes glittered with anger as I entered, and I noticed with concern that he utterly ignored my salute.

This indignant giant was General Horvatovitch, the biggest and bravest man in the Servian Army, and a very stern disciplinarian.

I saw that I was in a desperate scrape, but I cannot say that I felt very much dismayed; on the contrary, the unique and critical position in which I was placed seemed to offer me an excellent opportunity of distinguishing myself, of which I resolved to take full advantage. For a few moments the conclave of officers maintained a low-voiced conversation amongst themselves, in Servian or Russian, of which I understood nothing, and I availed myself of the interval to prepare for what was coming. In the first place, I arranged myself in an attitude that I thought was dignified, easy, and respectful, and assumed an extremely affable expression of countenance. I contrived also to examine the piece of string, and the button which supported my pantaloons. I thought they "gave" a little, but to my relief they seemed to be all right. Then I waited calmly for the general to speak.

"What is your name, sir?" said he at last.

"Your Highness," said I (I addressed him as Highness partly to display my pleasant humour, and partly out of compliment to his great height), "my name is Alfred Wright."

"You are an Englishman?" quoth he.

"I am proud and happy to say that I am, Your Highness," said I.

"You are charged, sir, with shooting a pig, the property of Jovan Jovanovitch, and stealing its carcase, whereby you have been guilty of disobedience of orders—a crime which, in time of war, is punishable by death—and also of looting. What have you to say in reply?"

"Your Highness——" replied I.

"Why, in the fiend's name, do you call me 'Your Highness,' man?"

"Because Your Highness is such a great man," replied I, with pleasant significance.

"Pooh! what does he mean?" said he, turning angrily to some of the officers beside him.

These officers, however, seemed as dense at perceiving the exquisite humour of the joke as he was himself, and shook their heads.

"Your Highness," continued I, with grave and emphatic solemnity, and drawing myself up as well as the tetherings of my nether garments would allow me, "I am deeply grieved if in anything I have done I have given offence, but I pray you to believe that I have always felt the most benevolent wishes and the best intentions towards the people of this country. When I knew them to be hard pressed by the Turks, I flew *vi et armis* to their rescue, and when again I beheld my brethren in arms suffering the pangs of hunger, I, at great personal risk and inconvenience, slew a pig and provided them with food."

"Saints preserve us!" exclaimed Horvatovitch, banging the table with his fist with angry impatience, "what is the man chattering about?"

"This is all very fine, sir," said another officer, "but be good enough to keep to the point."

I was a little surprised at the general's discourteous interruption, but replied,

"That is the point, sir."

"Do you mean to tell me," cried the general, "that you think it right to disobey orders in the teeth of the enemy, and kill another man's cattle?"

"Your Highness will pardon me," replied I, politely, "if I have failed to regard the matter from the same elevated point of view as yourself." I then went on to say that I had never heard of the order, and that I did not know that the pig was anyone's property, it looked to me like a young wild boar. This statement was received with a loud and rude burst of laughter.

I drew myself up to my full height, and looking defiantly round, was about to launch forth into an impassioned and eloquent attack on my ill-bred persecutors, when to my utter and irretrievable confusion the strain caused by my upright position proved too much for the wretched button that supported my pantaloons, and it gave way, and they immediately became so uncomfortably loose that I required all my wits to keep them together.

Fortunately for me, Counts Réné and Tiesenhausen came to my aid at the critical moment, and bore witness in very flattering terms to my character and capacity as a medical officer. Their remarks were vehemently seconded and applauded by Savrimovitch, Baron Kleist, Prince Obolenski, and other Russians present, and ultimately the general let me off with a slight reprimand and a recommendation to restrict my abilities for the future to the slaughtering of Turks instead of Servian swine.

On leaving His Highness's presence I was escorted to my quarters by a large party of friends, who overwhelmed me with kind and enthusiastic congratulations, and the evening was spent in uproarious festivity.

We did not separate until a vast quantity of weak wine, weaker tea, and still weaker coffee had been consumed, and the hands of our watches indicated the near approach of midnight.

CHAPTER 18

The Attack

When our party had broken up, Alexis Savrimovitch came up to me and said, "There is mischief in the wind, Alfred; we shall have a battle tomorrow. Just after your trial was over an orderly galloped up to Horvatovitch with despatches from General Tchernaieff, and immediately afterwards there was a grand hurrying and scurrying about of the commanding officers!"

"I hope we shall go under fire together!" said I.

"Well spoken, dear friend," replied Alexis, pressing my hand. "If my duties as *aide-de-camp* do not call me elsewhere, it will be as you say."

For a moment he was silent, then turning to me again, he said in a low voice:—

"Let us say a prayer together, Alfred. I have a strong presentiment that tomorrow will be a fatal day for me, and I would ask the Almighty to enable me to do my duty well and bravely as a good Russian should."

"If it is a fatal day for you, it shall also be fatal for me," I replied, speaking with real emotion; "but I cannot believe that either of us will fall yet—indeed, I feel convinced that we shall both be spared to lead good and useful lives."

"Maybe I am wrong," said Alexis, gravely, "but something tells me to prepare for death."

We then knelt down, and each in turn offered up a short petition to Heaven to watch over and protect us throughout the coming day, and to enable us to die, if need be, as brave Christian soldiers should. Then, as the night was rather chilly, for there was an east wind blowing, we stirred up the fire, threw a few more logs on it, and lay down in convenient proximity, to share the one waterproof we possessed between us. We endeavoured to go to sleep. Alexis, however, was restless and uneasy, and could not settle down. A few minutes after we had wished each other *bon repos* he gave so violent a start that he roused me immediately. I saw that he was sitting up, and staring, with an expression of intense alarm, at some object on my right. Following the direction of his eyes, I was just in time to see what looked like a black dog scurry away into the darkness with a dismal howl.

"The omen! the harbinger of death!" exclaimed Alexis in an awestruck tone.

"Nonsense, Alexis!" said I; "it is simply a starving black cur that has been attracted by the smell of our supper."

Savrimovitch shook his head gloomily. In a second or two he said, "I tell you, Alfred, I believe that to be a supernatural appearance, to warn me of my death. Such an apparition has always been seen before a Savrimovitch dies, and I am the only surviving son of an only son; but," continued he, resolutely setting his teeth together, "if the archfiend himself were to appear and roar my doom in my ears, he should not hinder me from doing my duty tomorrow! What do you think," said he, rising to his feet and stretching himself, "of a cigarette and a cup of coffee? I shan't sleep at all tonight!"

"With all my heart," said I, rising too. Now, though I do not consider myself to be at all superstitious, and have no faith in ghost stories, yet the air of conviction with which Alexis spoke, the darkness of the night, and the silence around us, broken only by the moaning of the east wind among the trees, awed me, and I shivered with fear.

However, cigarettes and coffee soon dispersed these uncomfortable sensations, and in a few minutes, we were chatting pleasantly together. Then we carefully inspected the condition of our weapons, oiled the locks of our revolvers, and tried the edges of our blades.

After this I became terribly weary, and gradually and unconsciously dropped off to sleep. I know that I intended to keep awake the rest of the night, and shall regret to my dying day that I failed in my endeavour. That was our last evening together! Savrimovitch's forebodings of the coming day were, alas! only too thoroughly realised.

When I had been asleep I daresay about a couple of hours, I was roused by someone shaking me and saying:—

"*Levez-vous, monsieur, nous allons attaquer les Turcs!*"

I sat up immediately, and rubbing my eyes, looked around. It was still quite dark, but by the flickering firelight I could perceive that the whole camp was astir. Savrimovitch was lying beside me, fairly tired out at last like myself, so I awoke him. He sprang to his feet in a second, all life and activity, without a trace of the anxiety and apprehensions which he had displayed on the previous evening on his handsome face.

As it was the intention of Horvatovitch, if possible, to surprise the Turks, strict silence was kept in the camp. No bugles were sounded; no talking was allowed in the ranks. Even the officers spoke to one another in an undertone. To me the sight of so many hundreds of armed men, assembling noiselessly together in the cold, dark morning to do battle for their country, was deeply impressive.

Just before marching, the commanding officer of each battalion read out a short and pithy speech from Colonel Medvedovski.

He trusted the soldiers would do their duty that day in a manner worthy of their country and the great Sclav race.

"The first man," we heard, "that lays his hand on a Turkish cannon shall receive forty *ducats* reward, and the cross of the Takovo; but the coward and runaway is hereby sentenced to death." I have omitted to state that on going to the place where I had left my rifle on the preceding evening, I found, to my unspeakable dismay, that it had disappeared! Some patriotic scamp, who had damaged or lost his own, had appropriated it.

Whilst I was searching for it the order came to march; seeing, therefore, a rifle that apparently had no owner lying on the ground, I snatched it up and took my place beside Baron Kleist and Mouravioff. Alexis Savrimovitch was close by, mounted on a magnificent bay charger, and right noble he looked as he reined in and checked the ardour of the spirited creature.

Whilst the other battalions were moving off, and we were waiting our turn to follow, he suddenly beckoned me to him, and putting his arm round my neck gave me a kiss, and slipped the locket I had seen him wear and a paper with an address on it into my hand, saying:—

"If I fall, beloved friend, send the locket to the address on the paper. *Adieu!*" and he rode off into the gloom.

A minute after we formed fours, and the order was given to march. Knowing that the Turkish position was distant only two miles or thereabouts, I expected that we should very soon have been at them. But hour after hour we plodded on, until we must have covered quite fifteen miles.

I afterwards understood that the object of this wide detour was to make an attack upon the Turks, simultaneously in flank and rear. The road we followed lay across a very hilly and thickly wooded country, indeed, the whole way, we were either climbing hills or descending into valleys, or passing through forests.

Soon after we started day began to break, and the sunrise that followed was a superb and gorgeous spectacle. The whole eastern sky was a sea of crimson and gold, in which floated a number of island-like cloudlets of the most lovely tints. The tops and ridges of the mountains were capped and streaked with radiant light, and the foliage, on which sparkled myriads of diamond-like dewdrops, looked so temptingly fresh and beautiful that my heart thrilled with delight as I gazed on the enchanting scene. As we surmounted the crest of a hill, I observed with satisfaction that we formed part of a very large force. As far as the eye could reach in front and rear, the sun glittered on the bayonets of our column as it wound its way right athwart the landscape.

About this time, it occurred to me to look at my rifle, which was a Peabody. To my great disgust I found that the lever which jerks open the breech was broken. The weapon was consequently useless, so I threw it into a tumbril and trudged along, armed only with my cutlass, revolver, and surgical instruments. The cutlass rather impeded my movements by flapping against my legs, so I unhooked it from my belt, tucked it under my arm, and got on much better.

Suddenly, soon after sunrise, we heard a rattling musketry fire far away on our left.

"Bravo!" exclaimed Baron Kleist, "there goes Tchernaieff! He's tackling the Turks in front, and we are to take them on the rear, and smash them up entirely!"

"Do you think we shall beat them easily?" asked I.

"Bah, I should think so!" said Bernadski, who happened to be close by; "it will be a walk over for us. They'll run like rabbits!"

"They won't show much fight then," said I, rather disappointed.

"They'll be massacred if they do," replied he. "We shall beat them as easily as we used to beat the Turcomans in Asia; they are all the same lot."

Meanwhile the sound of the firing increased until it swelled into a roar as rapid and incessant as the rolling of kettledrums, and the thunder of artillery now added to the din as gun after gun boomed in quick succession. The field of action was completely hidden from our view by a range of hills, but above these thick clouds of white smoke began to rise.

"How many men do you suppose are engaged now?" I asked.

"About 60,000" replied Von Kleist. "Tchernaieff has 30,000 and the Turks as many, and they are pounding away at one another with about 120 cannon!"

"The Turks are not running away yet!" said I, hopefully, because I still longed to see a little fighting.

"No, but they will directly," replied Bernadski. "They are firing as hard as they can to keep their spirits up, always a last resource of bad troops. By St. Michael, we'll make mincemeat of them if they have not bolted by the time we arrive!"

"And how many of us may there be?" I asked.

"About 20,000 and 40 guns."

"By Jove, it won't be a bad battle!" I exclaimed enthusiastically, as I thought with pride of the yarns I would spin to my friends at the hospital and my comrades in the 37th Middlesex.

For quite two hours after the firing had begun we continued marching steadily in a line, parallel with the range of hills which shielded us from the battle. The column then turned rather sharply to the left and entered a thick forest

By this time some of the Servians showed signs of getting fagged, and began to lag behind; and though I was fresh enough myself, still the boots I was wearing, those Mihailoff gave me, galled my ankles, and I stopped once or twice to ease them.

"Hulloh, Mr. Englishman!" shouted a young Russian, seeing me do this, "tired already! You Britons knock up very easily!"

"I am no more tired than you are," retorted I, indignantly; and to show him that I meant what I said, I leapt over the trunk of a fallen tree that lay a little on the side of the path; "I'll bet you half a *ducat* that you won't do that, my boy!"

The young Muscovite accepted the wager. He was both taller and more powerfully built than I, but much less nimble, and in attempting the leap, he caught his heel against the bark of the tree and fell heavily, whereat I chuckled and offered to pick him up, with many expressions of sympathy, which he received rather petulantly.

The forest extended up the slope of a range of heights, and marching became fatiguing and difficult About half-way up we passed large masses of Servian troops drawn up beside the road. These men greeted us with loud hurrahs, to which our brigade responded with equal enthusiasm. I then ascertained that, being considered desperate dogs and fighting fellows, I presume because of the number of Russians amongst us, we were to have the honour of commencing the attack.

We were now approaching the scene of action. The roar of musketry became louder and louder, and the thunder of artillery sounded nearer every minute. Towards the crest of the heights the forest thinned considerably, but there were still sufficient trees to afford us cover. The top of the hill was a plateau of irregular shape and considerable extent, on a portion of which, about five hundred yards distant, and separated from us by an indentation or ravine shaped like a *cul-de-sac*, heavy firing was going on. That was part of the Turkish position we were to storm.

Preparatory to making the attack, the officers drew their swords and moved up and down the ranks, shouting, "Forward! steady!" I drew my cutlass, too, and lopping down a small branch from an oak, stuck a spray of the leaves in my cap. This little action brought a loud cheer from the Servians who witnessed it, for the oak is their favourite emblem, and I had unconsciously paid them a compliment.

To the front, half-hidden by the trees, were eight or ten pieces of Servian artillery. It must have been terribly hard work to get them into that position, but there they were, with gunners standing beside them, ready at the word of command to send a volley of shells at the enemy.

Meanwhile the whole brigade slowly advanced. Several companies were thrown out to line the crest of the heights, and supplement the artillery fire with their musketry.

By this time, it was about half-past ten, and intensely warm.

I noticed several of the timid ones steal out of the ranks, and make off into the forest. Some were caught and brought back, but the majority seemed to make good their escape. Suddenly a horseman, in whom I recognised Savrimovitch, galloped by, and checking his foaming steed for a moment, saluted and said some words to our brigadier, and then dashed off towards the artillery.

Then sheets of flame and vast clouds of smoke burst forth from the guns, as with a crash like thunder a storm of shells was hurled at the Turks. The riflemen let fly a rattling volley, and then kept up a heavy and continuous fire, loading and discharging their pieces as fast as they could. Our drums and bugles now sounded the *pas de charge*. The standard borne by a gallant young Russian named Linden was raised aloft, and the Medvedovski Brigade, in *échelon* formation, dashed forwards at the double, the officers brandishing their bright sabres and waving their caps, and the men hurrahing like mad.

We could see the Turks training round their guns to bear on us, and hurrying up bodies of infantry, whilst an ominous glittering of steel was observable amid the bushes in front. For a minute or two they did not fire a shot. The head of our column advanced two or three hundred yards across the intervening portion of the plateau without suffering a single casualty.

Then a Turkish bugle rang out loud and clear, and immediately after the enemy's position was blotted out by puffs and wreaths and films of smoke; shells screamed through the air, and flamed and exploded about us, and a hail of bullets tore through our ranks, knocking over scores of gallant fellows, and dealing death and wounds broadcast. So deadly was the fire that the front ranks were almost annihilated. Poor young Linden was shot dead, but ere the standard had dropped from his dying hand, the brave Mihailoff seized it and waved it on high. Count Tiesenhausen's horse was killed, and he himself wounded in the thigh. Numbers of other officers whose names I did not know also fell—mortally or desperately wounded. The rain of bullets never slackened, and the column began to waver. At this critical moment my friends, Alexis Savrimovitch, Count Réné, Baron Kleist, Mouravioff, and Bernadski rallied and led them on again, and with loud shouts of "*Jivio Serbski*" we dashed forward once more.

The nearer we got to the enemy the hotter their fire became. Their missiles kept up an incessant humming, buzzing, and hissing about our heads. Again, the men wavered, and this time a number of them, seized with downright panic, fairly turned round and ran away. I must confess to having been considerably scared myself. Like lightning the thought flashed through my brain, "What a fool I am to risk life and limb for men who don't know and don't care anything about me. I'll clear out as quick as I can!" but before I had time to stop myself in my forward rush, Count Réné's words, "You are an Englishman, and we expect great things of you," came to my mind, and with an overwhelming feeling of shame for my cowardly thought, I ran onwards a little faster than before.

The number of mounted officers who were struck down filled me with a great terror for Savrimovitch, and I shouted to him an entreaty to dismount; I think he heard me, for he glanced round. The next moment his cap was pierced by a bullet and swept away, and his horse reared up and sank dead under him.

"I'm all right, friends!" said he, springing to his feet. "See how the Almighty preserves us! *Naprez Zastava Slava!*"

Scarcely were the words out of his mouth than his sword fell with a jerk from his hand, and uttering a painful exclamation, he straightened himself up for a moment and reeled backwards. I ran up to him and caught him in my arms just as he was sinking to the ground.

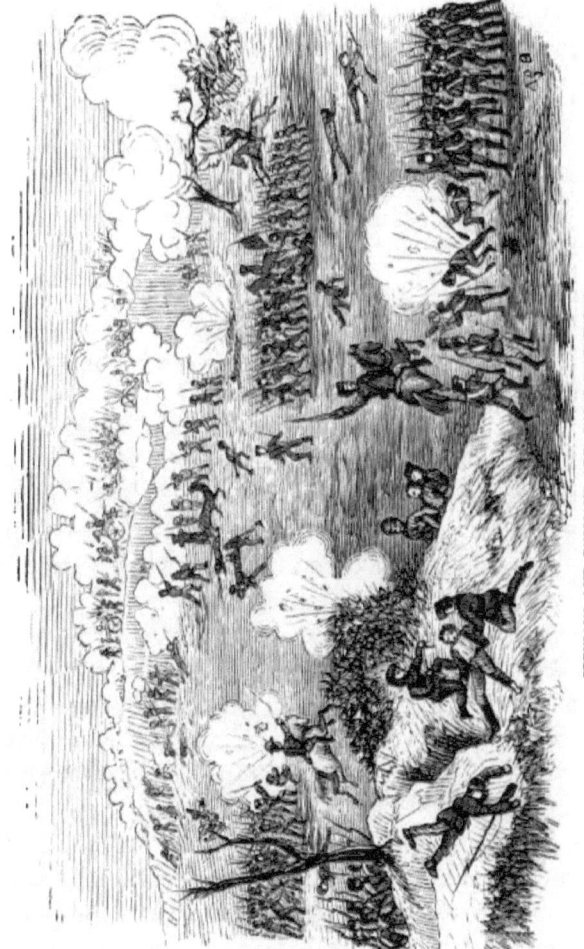

SERVIANS AND RUSSIANS ATTACKING THE TURKS.

"Good God, Alexis!" said I, in an agony of apprehension, "I hope you are not badly wounded."

"I'm done for, Alfred," said he, faintly. "Oh, my arm! Lay me down, there's a good fellow!"

I complied with his request, and then saw that he had received a bullet wound in the shoulder, from which blood was pouring at a terrific rate, his clothes being already saturated. Believing that the axillary artery in one of its large branches had been divided, I ripped up his clothes and attempted to compress the subclavian with my finger, but, alas! my efforts were too late.

The shadow of a smile flitted across his hueless face, his pale lips moved as if he would have spoken, but no sound issued from them. His eloquent blue eyes became fixed and glazed, and with a faint sigh he fell back dead.

For a moment I was scarcely able to realize the fact that my friend was gone. I hoped and trusted that he had only fainted, and I continued to compress the vessel after his circulation had ceased, and to speak to him when his sense of hearing had for ever fled. But it was impossible long to mistake the awful calm and stillness of death, so strange amid the hideous riot and uproar around, and when at length the sad truth forced its way home to my heart, I was utterly overwhelmed with sorrow. The generous and affectionate—if somewhat wayward—disposition of the dead man had made his friendship very dear to me. Soon my grief, however, gave way to a frantic desire for vengeance. Rising from beside the inanimate body, I got a couple of soldiers to help me to move it a little to the left, where it was less likely to be trampled on by the soldiery who were rushing by.

Then, gripping my cutlass firmly and drawing my revolver, I was on the point of dashing forward at the Turks, when a hail from a familiar but discordant voice brought me up sharp.

"*Hilloh, monsieur!* What are you going to do?"

The call came from Dr. Yermaylaff Giggleivitch, who at that moment rode up with a staff of surgeons and dressers and some ambulance waggons. "Don't you think there's plenty of work here for you?"

"Doubtless, sir," said I, looking at the wounded and dying lying thickly around. "There is much to do here, but you have many hands to do it; and there is more to be done over there;" and I pointed to the front, where the fight still raged violently.

"You'll be knocked on the head for a certainty, if you go there, and, moreover, you will not be able to do any useful work."

"I'll take my chance," said I; "I have many friends there. Meanwhile, will you give this poor corpse a place in one of your waggons? It's a shame to leave it here."

"He's quite mad!" I heard Dr. Giggleivitch say to one of his staff. "Our waggons, sir, are for the wounded, and not for the dead," continued he. "However, I'll see what we can do. Who is the dead man?" and he walked his horse up to the spot. "Why, 'tis the other madman. Poor fellow! Take him in, Krabervitch and Yermo. I am very sorry for him—poor, poor boy!"

In spite of the bullets which were still falling pretty thickly about, the medical men set to work with a will amongst the sufferers who strewed the roadway, and I ran on and rejoined my brigade, which, well supported by other Servian troops, had succeeded in driving back the Turkish infantry several hundred yards, and establishing themselves in a part of their position.

We were unable, however, to achieve more than this, and even this success was only temporary. From the trees and bushes in front and on our right flank came a constant blaze and crackle of musketry, and a venomous spitting forth of fire and lead, which told heavily on our already sorely smitten forces.

This fire increased in severity every minute, for the Turks, seeing the importance of recapturing the ground they had lost, brought up strong reinforcements.

Suddenly their fire increased tenfold in violence, due to the fact that they had succeeded in beating back Tchernaieff's attack, and could now devote all their attention to us. Our soldiers were ordered to lie down, but in spite of this precaution they continued to suffer heavy losses. Shells came crashing among the trees about us, smashing down branches, ploughing huge chasms in the ground and filling the air with humming fragments of metal, and the rifle bullets kept up a constant and angry buzzing about our heads. The Russian officers exposed themselves to the fire with marvellous heroism, and as a consequence a large proportion of them were struck down, and their fall had a very bad effect upon the men.

Whilst I was doing the best I could for a poor fellow who had been shot through the lungs, and was choking in his own life blood, I noticed a stalwart young Muscovite, the same I had challenged to leap over the trunk of a tree, standing close to me.

"What is the use of making a target of yourself, sir, in that way?" I asked.

"To encourage the men, surely," said he. "I don't think it can be any encouragement to them to see all their officers killed," replied I. "It will do them much more good to see you lying down and shooting comfortably at the enemy."

"That may do for Englishmen, but does not suit Russians," replied the officer sneeringly. Scarcely were the words out of his mouth when a bullet struck him full in the forehead, and he fell back dead. The Turks now apparently thought us too much demoralised to withstand a bayonet charge. Their fire slackened, and a strong body of their men, bursting from cover, rushed at us with ferocious yells and levelled bayonets.

The word was passed down our line that we were to reserve our fire until they came within thirty paces, and then to let them have it.

Seeing that my patient was dead, and not wishing to be stuck by a Turkish bayonet, I picked up his rifle, and fitting a cartridge into the breech, awaited their approach. On they came, rending the air with loud shouts of "*Allah!*" and a very determined and formidable-looking set of fellows they were—swarthy, wiry, and muscular, with black hair and fiercely gleaming dark eyes. Nearer and nearer, they came, shouting exultantly as they fancied we were afraid to oppose them, whilst our hearts beat high with excitement. At last came the signal to fire, and a deadly hail of lead issued from a thousand rifles, withering their brave ranks and driving them back in wild confusion. Rallied by their officers, however, they came on again, but we had had time to reload, and treated them to another tempest of wounds and death. This time they were past rallying, and ran back to cover.

We were wild with exultation, and shouted Hurrah! again and again; but the Turks are bad to beat, and when they had regained cover, the fire to which we were exposed became terrific. By midday it was evident the Servians would have to retire from the position they had won, but up to this time the men had behaved well. The Turks, however, had been preparing a most disagreeable surprise for us. Hitherto the fighting had been confined entirely to our front and right, and our attention being fully occupied, two Tabors were able to work round to our left, and the rattle of their musketry and the whizzing of their bullets was the first intimation of their presence. This was the turning point of the engagement, for the soldiers now utterly lost heart and fled. Their officers made several brave but useless efforts to lead them to drive back the new-comers, but no; they had had enough of fighting for one day, and had quite made up their minds to run away.

Some of the officers, hoping to check the rush, shot down a few of the first runaways, but all to no purpose. The troops were completely demoralized: they charged past their officers, in many instances bearing them along with them in their rush, and threw away their rifles, belts, and ammunition pouches—everything, indeed, that hindered their flight. A big Servian ran against me and knocked me head over heels. When I picked myself up, which was not till some seconds afterwards, for the frightened vagabond had sent all the breath out of my body, all that I could see of our men were the backs of the hindmost. A few of the officers who had been charged down like myself were lying here and there on the ground.

Meanwhile the Turks continued to advance, and their bullets were singing about us in a way which was decidedly unpleasant.

"Baron," said I, getting up, "if we stay here any longer the Turks will cut our throats."

"*Sacre nom de Dieu!*" he hissed through his teeth; "I'll never run away from this *canaille*."

"You look at it in a wrong light, baron," said I. "We are running after our men, and not away from the Turks. Perhaps we can rally them yet."

"You are right, Mr. Englishman," said he, getting up and beginning to run with me.

"By St. Peter and St. Paul, if ever I catch those pigs of Servians who knocked me down, I'll tan their hides for them!"

"By all means," said I, expecting every minute to feel my back perforated by a bullet; "let's run a little faster!"

The victorious Turks, with characteristic indolence, scarcely pursued our army at all, but contented themselves with sending a lot of shells and bullets after us. Had we been fighting any other disciplined troops, our army might have been annihilated and the campaign ended there and then. However, as far as I am concerned, I am very grateful that they were so apathetic.

It is a very unpleasant thing to face a heavy musketry fire, but it is to my mind far more disagreeable to run away from one. In the first case, your mind is occupied by your duty, your desire ta distinguish yourself, and so on, whilst in the second, your sole thought and desire is to avoid being ignominiously snuffed out and extinguished. Each time that I heard the scream of an approaching shell, I fancied that I was bound to be hit, and felt correspondingly uncomfortable, whereas scores of them had passed comparatively unnoticed by me whilst the action was raging.

The sensations I experienced were shared in apparently a greater degree by many other fugitives. Some of them scrambled along on all fours, like so many rabbits, others, every time a shell flew by, threw themselves on the ground, and crawling along a few paces, rose again and continued their flight. One man, an officer, particularly distinguished himself by the agile way in which, as he ran, he threw himself on his hands and feet and sprang up again. I watched this india-rubber warrior's movements for some time, when a shell burst close to where he happened to be, and he vanished from my view; but reaching the spot where the missile had fallen, I beheld a horrible sight. Three or four dead and fearfully wounded men lay around, and close to them, stretched on his back, with his chin pointing to the sky, was the unfortunate officer, in whom, to my great astonishment, I recognised my acquaintance, Colonel Bragg.

Whilst I was looking at him, the colonel heaved a faint sigh and opened his eyes, so I gave him a drink of water, and asked him if he was wounded, for I could see no hurt

"No, thank God! Doctor, I don't think I'm wounded. Ah! give us a drop more water, so. That's good, but the fact is, I'm infernally sensitive, and have a weak stomach, and when that shell burst and blew a lot of fellows into little bits just by where I was, it upset me, and I fainted."

"Well but, colonel," said I, "you mustn't lie here! The Turks will be here directly, and will cut your head off if they find you."

"For God's sake, then, don't leave me, doctor!" replied he. "Give me your hand, quick!" and he scrambled to his feet. He still seemed rather faint, so Baron Kleist and I supported him between us, until he was steady enough to take care of himself. Presently we overtook a long and dismal train of wounded men, all doing their best to escape. Some were being supported by friends, some limped along painfully with the aid of their rifles or sabres, whilst others again were crawling on their hands and knees.

A very few were on horseback, and these seemed to be suffering terribly from the movements of the animal. Amongst them, grinning with agony, was the brave Mouravioff. He had been shot in the groin, and was supporting himself as well as he could with his hands on the pommel of his saddle. He gave a smile of recognition as he saw Kleist and myself, and begged for a little water. Then we improvised a very respectable litter for him with four rifles tied together with belts and a couple of overcoats, and lifting him gently from his horse, temporar-

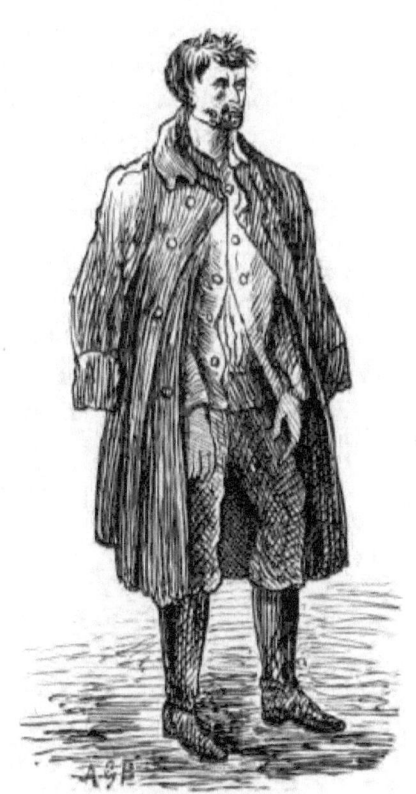

WOUNDED RUSSIAN SOLDIER.

ily dressed his wound, and laid him on our ambulance, greatly to his relief, and made a couple of stout fellows carry him.

But the sight which affected me most was the body of Mihailoff on a stretcher. I thought at first, he was dead. His face was a ghastly colour, his right arm was shattered, and he had received a wound in the abdomen. But though hopelessly injured, he was still alive, and seemed in great pain.

To alleviate his sufferings, which were aggravated by the oscillation of the litter, we gave him some opium, and converting the sheaths of two knives into rough splints, we put his arm up.

He was perfectly conscious, and spoke to Baron Kleist and myself whilst we were dressing his wounds, although every now and then he became very faint. I begged him, through the baron, not to talk, but he said he had something on his mind and must out with it, even though it cost him his life.

"I thank God," said he, speaking in jerks, "that—I have been—able to do my duty today—like a good Russian and a brave soldier—oh! gently, doctor, with my arm! So!—so!—a mouthful of water, doctor. Thank you. Until I was wounded I did not—think once—of my beloved wife and my—angel-children—for fear of flinching. Ah, doctor!" he continued with a sob, "I shall—never—never see—them more—and my sweet wife will break her heart with grief."

Tears trickled down the poor fellow's cheeks as he uttered these touching words. His distress moved both the baron and myself deeply. For a few minutes we walked alongside his stretcher in silence. But suddenly there arose a loud cry of "*Tcherkess! Tcherkess!*" (Circassians), and the name of these bloodthirsty horsemen was now sufficient to strike terror to the hearts of our beaten soldiers. There was a scramble and rush to get away; wounded men were bustled and upset, and, dreadful to relate, the bearers of Mihailoff's stretcher, seized with a sudden panic, dropped their burden and fled. The poor fellow fell heavily, and lay motionless on the ground. Horror-struck, I dropped on my knees beside him, but, alas! the shock proved immediately fatal. A convulsive tremor shook his frame for a second, and then he, too, was added to the long list of our dead.

This alarm, which after all proved a false one, caused the death of several other wounded men. Some were trampled to death, others thrown violently to the ground, and, like Mihailoff, died of the shock; others who still lived were groaning and crying out piteously with pain. Close to us, a waggon containing six wounded soldiers had been upset. The unhappy men were lying on the roadway, piled helplessly one on top of the other, until luckily the energetic Dr. Giggleivitch and some of his assistants appeared on the scene. By their exertions, seconded by the efforts of a number of soldiers, heartily ashamed of their poltroonery and anxious to make amends, the waggon was righted, and the wounded men replaced in it. Then, as we did not wish to leave the dead body of our friend to the mercy of the Turks, we covered it with an overcoat and put it in the waggon also.

Everything possible to alleviate the terrible suffering around us was done by the doctor and his staff.

It was as yet barely one in the afternoon, and the heat was scorching. My water-flask was empty, and I was extremely thirsty, but my thirst must have been nothing in comparison with that of the miserable creatures around me, and the cries of pain were constantly intermingled with agonised supplications for "*Woda! woda!*" (water). Unfortunately, we could get no water, and were powerless to give them a drink. No rations had been served out to the men before starting, probably because the commissariat had broken down again, so that very few of us had eaten anything since the early morning. I remarked to Von Kleist that I was hungry as well as thirsty, when a soldier who understood what I said, saluted and said—

"Vrankovitch, yonder, has some cooked pork." Vrankovitch was not an appetising-looking person, nevertheless the baron and I accosted him and asked him to let us look at his stock of provisions.

"Certainly, *gospodina*," replied the man, and tugged a grimy and very unsavoury-looking piece of flesh from his trouser pocket.

There was a "greenery-yallery" appearance about the morsel that was as good as a meal to me, for it utterly took away my appetite. The baron, however, being an old campaigner, was less particular, and went so far as to sniff at it. The sniff was enough even for him.

"That meat," said he with a horrible grimace, "is tainted and raw. It smells even worse than it looks."

We continued our weary march beside the wounded for several miles, unable to get any water, but greatly refreshed by some sour and half-withered grapes that we gathered from an abandoned and desolate-looking vineyard. These, with some honey which the soldiers found in the forest, were all that we could find for the invalids. So welcome were the grapes to me that I ate a large quantity of them and a good deal of honey, an excess of which I soon had cause to repent. An hour or two after I was seized with a frightful attack of cramp in the stomach; and sat down by the wayside in great pain. The baron was engaged with a wounded comrade, and did not observe my seizure, and the rest of the long procession straggled by without taking any notice of me. The pain became so severe that I was quite doubled up and unable to move, and to ease it, I took a couple of pills containing two grains of opium. These relieved me very much, and about an hour after I had swallowed them, I was able to rise and begin walking again.

Unfortunately, during this rest my limbs had become very stiff and my feet were extremely painful, so after persevering for a few minutes, I took off poor Mihailoff's boots and tried to walk without them. I daresay I managed to creep along for half a mile in this way, at the cost of innumerable pricks and scratches, some of which were really severe. At last, my feet were covered with blood, and in despair I sat down once more with the intention of pulling my boots on again. This, however, was quite impossible, and after two or three useless efforts I gave up the attempt. The fatigue and excitement I had undergone, combined with the effects of the opium, now made me so drowsy, that despite the fear of being captured by the Turks, I fell into a deep and dreamless sleep.

CHAPTER 19

Astounding Horsemanship

It was between four and five o'clock in the afternoon when I fell asleep, and the sun was blazing overhead with undiminished power. I must have slept many hours, but was so tired that I seemed scarcely to have closed my eyes when I was aroused by a vigorous shaking, and saw that I was surrounded by a party of armed men, some of whom held lighted torches which flared fitfully on the breeze. It was now night, and unable to make out whether my captors were Servians or Turks, I put up my eyeglass to see, a movement which elicited much laughter. Then one of them, who was on horseback, said to me.

"*Was machen Sie hier, Herr Englander?*"

"*Ich schlafe,*" replied I.

"Yes, I see that," said my interlocutor, "but how come you to lie here by yourself?" Though I understood the question, I could not muster up sufficient German to reply, so I pointed to my swollen bloodstained feet.

"Good," replied the officer, "we'll give you a horse, and take you along with us. Jovo, get off that horse and let the Englishman take your place! Of course, being an Englishman, you ride, sir?"

"Of course," said I, ashamed to acknowledge that I couldn't.

"Very well then, up with you, and we'll move off again!"

I felt that it was incumbent on me to vault lightly and gracefully into the saddle, and although I was horribly stiff and sore, I determined to make the attempt. Putting both hands on the saddle, and mentally saying, "One, two, three, and away!" I sprang upwards, only, alas! to come down again on the same spot. I repeated this manoeuvre ineffectually two or three times, and at last, much to my annoyance, was compelled to beg assistance on the plea of my lameness. This was readily and courteously accorded by M. Jovo himself, and with his aid I succeeded in climbing on to the animal's back, and I must confess that I never felt more uncomfortable in my life. There were a number of men looking upon me as a wonderful horseman, and expecting to get a lesson in equitation, whilst it was as much as I could do to keep my seat.

Determined not to be upset if I could help it, I shortened the reins and gripped them firmly with both hands, and digging my knees into the creature's ribs, defied him to do his worst; and he did do his worst. He kicked and snorted and reared and curvetted and galloped about like a furious four-legged fiend. He charged in and out of the Servian ranks, and sent the men flying in all directions. He shook and jogged and jolted me about until my internals felt like a quivering mass of jelly, but resolved to distinguish myself, I held on tenaciously. He twisted round, jumped and jibbed, and made me sick and giddy, so at last I let go of the reins and seized him by the mane and neck instead, at which, wonderful to relate, he ceased from his evil ways altogether, and remained quiet and tranquil, though trembling in every limb.

My triumph was hailed by the Servians with shouts of laughter and applause.

"You are certainly an extraordinary horseman, Mr. Englishman!" said the officer, smiling.

I bowed as gracefully to the compliment as my fatigue and breathlessness would allow, and replied "that the horse was an extraordinary animal."

"Do all Englishmen ride like that?" asked he, laughing rather more than I could see any occasion for.

"No, sir," replied I, shortly, "there are very few of my countrymen who cannot ride a great deal better than I." The horse was now evidently on its best behaviour. He walked quietly along beside the soldiers, and I felt quite at my ease, and was able to hold the reins in one hand, plant the other on my hip, just as I believe good horsemen frequently do, and converse at the same time with those about me. After a longish march, throughout which my charger picked his way without the least effort at guidance on my part, uphill and downhill and over some very rough ground, we came in sight of the watchfires of a large camp, and a few minutes afterwards we halted.

I was taken at once to the headquarters of the *commandant* of the brigade, in whom, to my surprise, I recognised that burly warrior, Colonel Philipovitch.

"Or, or, dear boy, dear boy! I am glad, I am glad to see you!" exclaimed he, extending his arms and folding me in his embrace, "You are not dead? You are not kill? Good, good! And your stomick? How

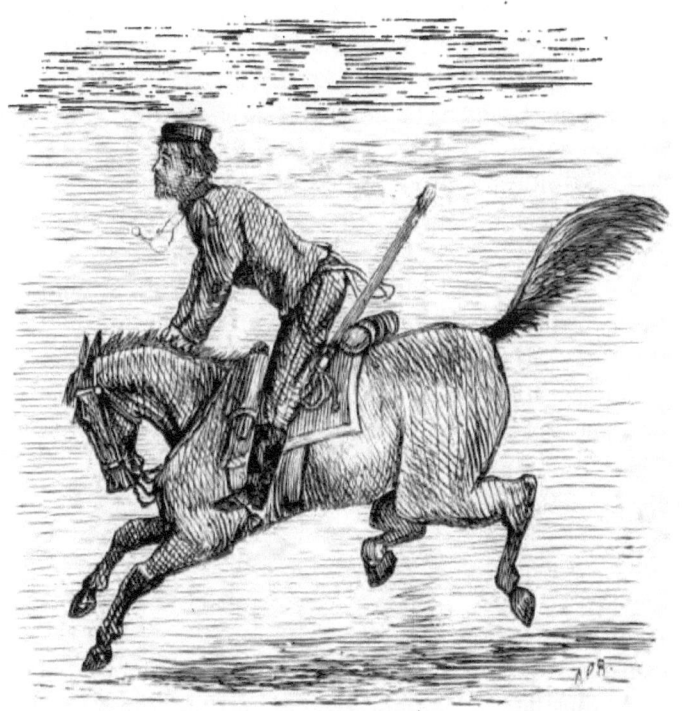

I DISPLAY EXTRAORDINARY HORSEMANSHIP, AND ASTONISH THE SERVIANS.

goes it? *Wie geht's?* Heh!"

I assured the worthy colonel, as soon as I had disengaged myself from his smothering hug, that I was not dead, but that the important portion of my framework to which he had done me the honour to allude was in a shockingly empty condition.

The kind-hearted officer gave a groan of sympathy when he noted my haggard looks, and immediately gave orders for food to be prepared. He then made me take a glass of *sligievitch*, which revived me wonderfully. Then after a cup of Liebig smoking hot, I wrapped myself up in an overcoat which the colonel had left me, and was soon fast asleep.

Early next morning I was disturbed by the crashing report of two pieces of cannon and a rattling fire of musketry. The whole camp was in a state of alarm and uproar. Half-dressed officers were shouting words of command, and men rushing pell-mell hither and thither with arms in their hands. "What's the matter?" exclaimed I to Lieutenant Jovo, as he hurried past me, buckling on his sword.

"A Turkish night attack," replied he, and disappeared.

I strapped on my cutlass and revolver and ran after him, but in about five minutes the firing ceased as abruptly as it had begun. Then Colonel Philipovitch trotted up on horseback with his staff.

"Pooh!" said he, "it's only those wild Montenegrins and Bulgarians. Their camp adjoins ours, and one of their chiefs, Luka Vlahovic, has just died of wounds received yesterday, and this is the way they show their grief!"

"I am glad it's nothing worse," said I. "So am I, my boy. If the Turks had come thus far, they would have eaten us up altogether, I think, before we were awake. Goodnight, go to sleep again." I took the gallant colonel at his word, and lay me down, and actually slept until one in the afternoon.

When I opened my eyes, the colonel was bending over me, his chubby face illumined by a pleasant smile.

"Ha, ha, ha! (the sound seemed to come from the depths of his stomach); you have slept well, dear boy; ho! ho! ho! good, and your poor feet? How is him? Ha, ha! you are fatigue! I am ver dammed busy; good Englisches that, eh? Ha! ha! ver dammed busy, he! he! he! wit mine two tausand childers here. *Grosser famille* is that? two tausand, eh? Ha! ha! ha! (then linking his arm in mine); now shall you come wit me, and we shall have some wine and smoke good tabac, eh?"

"Thank you very much," I replied, "I'll have a mouthful, and then

I must be off to my brigade."

"No, no, no, *nein, nein, nein, ne, ne, ne* (gripping me firmly by the arm), you must not leave me this day, dear boy; your feet is bad, your stomick is bad, your face is bad; pell, very pell. Tomorrow, when you shall be strong, you go if you will, but today, no, no, no;" and he shook his head and pursed up his fat lips and stamped his feet and looked altogether a picture of resolute negation.

"But—" began I, thinking of my wounded friends.

"But," interrupted he, speaking slowly and emphatically, "you cannot go this day. So, I have spoken. What good? What for? When you are ill! Tomorrow you shall have ambulance and good horse and go comfortable, but today I will not let you, and if you say, ' Colonel, I kill you dead,' your friend still say, no, no, no!"

The stout Servian was so resolute that I most unwillingly accepted his hospitality. As soon as he found that he had gained his point he ordered dinner to be served, and introduced me to several of his officers, amongst whom I recognised the leader of the party that caught me napping the evening before.

Lieutenant Jovo, the proprietor of the terrible steed I had so successfully tamed, was there, too. I also had the pleasure of making the acquaintance of a huge Montenegrin chief from the adjoining camp, by name Peko Bolrovitch, who had been invited to share the repast.

"In England," said the colonel, ceasing his attention to his soup for a moment and brandishing his wooden spoon in the air, "you eat rosbif and *Sauer Kraut*, eh?"

"We eat roast beef," said I, "but not *Sauer Kraut*."

"What! you eat not *Sauer Kraut* in England?" rejoined the colonel, his eyes widely dilated with astonishment.

"No," said I.

"Why then do Englanders say when ver angry, 'Ver damm, rosbif and Sauer Kraut? Ver damm, I boxe your heye?'"

I replied that I could not understand why any Englishman should say that unless he were drunk.

"Oho! the Englander only say rosbif and Sauer Kraut when him's drunk!'"

Our conversation was then interpreted to Jovo and the Montenegrin, who received his communication with ejaculations of interest and surprise.

After dinner the colonel beckoned me aside, and said:—

"M. Wright, I will to talk a few with you, sit you down here comfortable; so—good." Then he proceeded to ask me if I would get a medal for him from the English government when I returned home.

"What good will an English medal do you?"

"England," replied Philipovitch, "is rich, rich, and good credit. I am merchant, and when man shall see my Englischer medal, he shall say, ' Oh, see! Philipovitch has Englischer medal, he ver damm respectable, good credit, and rich."

"But on what plea, colonel, am I to claim a medal for you?"

"You shall say," replied he, screwing up his face and wrinkling his brows in a very odd way, "that Philipovitch is a good, good man, that he is Anglo-phil-English lover, eh? That he is good to you and to all Englanders, and that when he have the medal, he will be better still, eh? Will you tell to them that, eh?"

"My dear friend," said I, resignedly, "my influence just now is not so great with our government as it ought to be, and as I hope it will be some day, still, such as it is, I shall have much pleasure in placing it entirely at your service; in other words, I can't promise to get you a medal, but I'll try!"

"Dear boy, dear boy," giving me a grateful hug, "I love you much; you are good friend; I love you!"

We now separated for a while, the colonel and his officers being occupied with military duties, whilst I attended to the hurts of the wounded. These were mostly of a trivial nature, the more severely wounded having been either forwarded to the hospital at Paratchin, or left to the tender mercies of the Turks on the battlefield.

Later on, we assembled again round the camp fire. The evening was dark and stormy; the wind blew in fitful gusts and drove the smoke and sparks into our faces in a very disagreeable manner. It rained, too, off and on, the whole night. The jovial Colonel Philipovitch was, however, equal to the occasion. He had a wonderful supply of good spirits, both mental and alcoholic, and must have possessed an extensive private commissariat department of his own, for he gave us an excellent supper, which included broth and soup and mutton, and even a piece of the prohibited pork.

Nor did his resources end here. Whenever the conversation flagged and the weather became extra depressing, he would produce a marvellous little wooden cigarette holder, with a whistle at one end of it and puffing out his fat cheeks, blow a shrill and soul-inspiring blast thereon, much to our comfort and joy. He had a little clicking machine, too, that he delighted to conceal in the palm of his hand, and when we heard the click, "*Was ist das?*" he would say, putting on an expression of intense surprise, and holding up one 'finger of the disengaged hand, "*Was ist das?* Hear you dat noise? Where comes him from?"

We pretended not to know, whereat the gallant colonel's delight knew no bounds, and he would click away harder than ever.

Although my heart was still sore and sad after the terrible events of the preceding day, I could not help being intensely amused and joining in the fun.

And whilst this roistering revelry was at its height, a soldier presented himself to the colonel, and saluting, announced that two Bulgarski officers. Captain Milosch Davorin and Captain Ilianovitch, wished to see him.

"Show them here, by all means, my son," said the colonel

The soldier departed, and presently returned, accompanied by the mysterious person who had so often puzzled me before, and a slim, graceful young officer, who, in spite of uniform and an apparent roughness of manner, was, I felt convinced, a girl. The soldier's companions were most cordially received by Colonel Philipovitch, and cordially returned his salutations. I should very much have liked to give Captain Milosch Davorin a surreptitious squeeze of the hand, but my self-possession failed me, and I felt and I daresay looked nervous and uncomfortable.

The colonel introduced me to them with a wave of the hand and an unctuous emphasis on my nationality as his *English* friend, Dr. Wright. When our eyes met, Captain Davorin's assumed an expression of frigid reserve, and greeted me with a distant and formal salute. Captain Ilianovitch, on the other hand, gave me a jaunty bow and a friendly shake of the hand. I felt both piqued and hurt. This cold treatment added to my discomfiture, and so humiliated me, that I meanly resolved to say something very sharp and severe if an opportunity offered.

Naturally enough, the events of the preceding day were the sole topics of conversation for the first few minutes. Gradually, however, we drifted to other subjects, and at last the longed-for chance came.

Captain Ilianovitch inquired of me in French if I had lately heard how it fared with my comrade at Semendria. I fixed my eyes on the beardless Milosch Davorin, and speaking slowly and emphatically, replied that "*quelques uns de mes anciens camarades ne sont que des kamaratz.*" Now "*kamaratz*" is Servian for mosquitoes, and surely Milosch Davorin ought to have been cut to the heart by this withering sarcasm! I thought it might bring to mind the happy time when he or she used to crush mosquitoes on my face. But astonishing to relate, he, she, or it, the quasi-captain, showed no outward signs of emotion! Of the others, Captain Ilianovitch alone laughed at the pungent pun! I have no heart to describe the rest of the festivities of that evening, suffice it to say that the so-called Captain Davorin maintained an icy reserve throughout, spoke very little, ate and drank scarcely anything at all, and smoked a cigarette or two so charmingly, that the stern resolve I had almost made never to shake hands with him—that is her—again faded quite out of my mind, and I felt again a weak-minded desire to give her fingers a tender squeeze.

He and his friend retired after they had been about an hour with us. I would have given worlds to escort them to their quarters, but my late rebuff had been too discouraging. We separated with another 15° below zero military salute. When the party broke up, I rolled myself up in an overcoat and lay down near the fire, it must be confessed, in a very miserable frame of mind. I felt penitent and angry with myself. The more I thought about it, the more this last-named form of vexation grew upon me. I saw how impossible it was for Marie—for I felt positive it was she—to acknowledge me under the circumstances, and I resolved to comport myself for the future with greater dignity and discretion.

I kept thinking over these things and making numerous noble and notable resolutions until everybody save the sentries were asleep around me, and all would have been as still as death but for the sighing of the wind and an occasional hiss and crackle from the fire. Suddenly the stillness of the night was broken by a frightful uproar in the camp of the Bulgarians and Montenegrins. I could plainly hear the report of firearms, mingled with shouts, yells, and words of command. At first, I thought it was only some more tomfoolery on the part of these wild volunteers, but the tumult increased instead of subsiding quickly and abruptly as on the preceding evening, whilst the sky was lit up with the crimson and lurid glare of fire. Others in our camp besides myself took the alarm.

Colonel Philipovitch, grumbling vehemently at being disturbed from his well-earned slumber, hurried about hither and thither, and shouted out orders and instructions until he was hoarse. The men quickly fell to arms, and a battalion was despatched under Lieutenant Jovo to assist our allies. Being very anxious and uneasy about Marie, I accompanied this battalion. The night was dark, but the conflagration gave so much light that we were able to advance at the double. As we drew nearer, it became evident that a furious contest was raging. Bullets, too, began to whistle and hiss over our heads very disagreeably. A body of *bashi-bazouks*, taking advantage of the darkness of the night, had attempted to surprise the Bulgarians and Montenegrins, and had so far succeeded as to fire part of their camp.

Fortunately for us, however, they had attacked the Montenegrins first, and these valiant mountaineers, who slept with their arms in their hands, were wide awake in no time, and made a tremendous defence. When we came up, the leaping and roaring flames, the falling huts, the myriad rifle flashes, the struggling figures, the dark shadows of the trees—all this against the obscure background of the night, formed a striking picture.

Without halting us even for a moment. Lieutenant Jovo ordered us to charge the enemy at the point of the bayonet. We went at them with a lusty cheer; at the same time the Bulgarians made a similar advance on our left. This was too much for the bold *bashi-bazouks*, who had merely contemplated comfortably and luxuriously cutting the throats of our friends as they slept, and were, consequently, unprepared to meet with much resistance. Uttering a loud yell of vexation and disgust, they turned their backs on us and fled. This success amazingly stimulated our courage, which had been of the drooping order since the last sanguinary repulse. We pursued them for a few hundred yards in grand style, hurrahing ourselves hoarse, and firing at our discomfited foemen with immense valour and enthusiasm.

Our loss in this gallant charge was one man wounded, a gunshot wound in the leg. The Bulgarians and Montenegrins, however, lost heavily. They had twenty dead, and fifty-seven more or less severely wounded. The enemy lost eighty killed outright, and probably many wounded, who succeeded in escaping. No prisoners were taken. The Montenegrins gave no quarter. Every *bashi-bazouk* who fell into their hands was shot or run through the body and beheaded. The Servians were not allowed to do this, but I saw several Bulgarians bringing back pale and bleeding heads as trophies of their prowess.

After many inquiries, I ascertained, to my intense relief, that Captain Milosch Davorin was unhurt, and had returned to camp with his men. This took a great load off my mind, and I worked away for the rest of the night assisting Dr. Tromboni with the wounded. The doctor was an Italian, and nature had provided him with a very fair bass voice, which he was constantly exercising. He performed all his operations to a deep purring accompaniment, and when he did anything particularly neatly in the way of cutting a flap and so on, he would break out into a thunderous series of "*Tra! la! la! Ho! ho! ho's!*" and, "*Bravissimo!*" etc.

As I can ill bear a noise when operating, I asked him once or twice if he would be kind enough to restrain his musical ardour for a few moments. My request, which was very mildly put, and was by no means intended to be offensive, annoyed the doctor very much, and though he acceded to it, it was with a very ill grace, and we worked much less harmoniously together for the rest of the night.

At 10 a.m., while we were still engaged with our patients, a body of troops, with whom were some surgeons and dressers, marched into camp. The latter immediately came to our assistance, and one of them presented a despatch to Dr. Tromboni from Baron Von Tummy, acquainting him of his appointment as surgeon of the hospital at Uschitza, and requesting him to proceed to his post at once. The officer commanding the troops, an old acquaintance of mine, Nicolai Nicolaitch by name, was quite overwhelmed with astonishment at seeing me. I learned from him that it was generally believed at headquarters that I had either been killed or made prisoner. After heartily congratulating me on my escape, he informed me that a package of letters and telegrams addressed to me lay at the headquarters' post-office.

On hearing this news, I determined to return to my brigade immediately. On my way to Colonel Philipovitch, I saw Captain Milosch Davorin at a considerable distance, riding towards the left of the Bulgarian camp. I made a profound salute, which, to my delight, was promptly and gracefully returned. Colonel Philipovitch was breakfasting when I reached his quarters. He was kind enough to express much regret at hearing of my intended departure. Whilst I was speaking to him Tromboni came in with his despatch in his hand, so we agreed to go together.

"But," said the colonel, addressing himself to me, "the Herr Dr. Tromboni have so good a horse, and you, you have no horse. How can you then go together? What will you make?" This sensible question was rather a poser, and whilst I was cudgelling my brains to think "what I would make," the colonel mysteriously added, "I will tell you what you shall make, my good *English* friend. I have two horse, I want them not. They are not beautiful, no, no, but good, yes, yes. Now I will to give my friend a horse, and when you shall be back in England, you shall tell to the government, and shall say, 'My good Servian friend, Colonel Toma Philipovitch, when I have no horse and will ride, give me a horse. He ver dammed good man, and friend to England,' and they shall, I think, ver like give English medal for me, eh? What think you?"

"I'm afraid, colonel," replied I, "that our government would scarcely bestow a medal on you for giving me a horse."

"Oh! but," exclaimed he, eagerly, "you shall say also that I am very, most good indeed, to all English peoples, and that I loves him, eh?"

I shook my head doubtfully; whereupon a look of the most bitter disappointment came into his face. Suddenly—happy thought!—I recollected an old English Crimean war medal that had somehow come into my possession.

"Colonel," said I, "I can promise you an English government medal, but—" In a moment, before I could get another word out, he had folded me in his arms and was hugging me in a murderously rib-crushing and suffocating fashion.

"Confound it!" gasped I, wriggling out of his grasp, "let me finish what I have to say."

"Yes, yes, *da, da—ya—mein frend, das medal*; is it golden medal or silber?"

"It is silver," replied I.

"Silber, good!" said he, reflectively; "silber is very good!"

"But," said I, "it will not have your name upon it."

"*Nichts! gar nichts.* I care not for that, nothing," he rejoined.

"All right," said I, adroitly slipping aside, and thereby narrowly escaping another overwhelming embrace, "you shall have the medal!"

The colonel then ordered a soldier to bring the not "beautiful but good" horse.

The man presently returned, leading by the bridle the very weediest and seediest, scraggiest and raggedest apology for a horse I ever saw. It was a four-legged phantom, a perambulating mass of skin and bone. So lean was it, that I don't believe a London cat's-meat man would have given half-a-crown for the whole carcase, and I doubt if his flesh would have furnished more than a single meal to a hungry cur. I had seen bad horses before in Servia and elsewhere, but never, never aught like this.

As the fearful and wonderful creature stalked by, there was something so ludicrous in his appearance that I burst into a fit of laughter.

"Ha! ha!" laughed the colonel sympathetically, "you loaf because he have no meat on his bones, ha! ha! I too will loaf—ha! ha! ha!"

Then he told the man to mount and show me its paces. I fully expected to see the skeleton framework collapse under the man's weight, but to my astonishment the charger began to amble easily along in a spectral and dignified manner.

"Well," thought I, "if he'll bear that man's weight, twelve stone if it's a pound, he'll carry my ten stone without difficulty."

"Dear boy," said the colonel, "that good horse I gif him to you; take him, so, so."

However inferior the condition of the horse might be, I hesitated to accept it as a gift from a comparative stranger, but the colonel was so terribly hurt and offended when I ventured to offer him money for it, that I swallowed my scruples, and forbore to press the point. One thing impressed me favourably about the horse; he did not seem to have a spark of friskiness or vice in his nature, and consequently would not be very difficult to manage. About midday we took an affectionate leave of the hospitable Philipovitch and his officers, and mounting our respective steeds (this, thanks to my late equestrian experience, I managed without mishap), we departed.

Dr. Tromboni had not forgiven my inadequate appreciation of his vocal powers; he was cold and uncommunicative. I was sorry to have offended him, but did not at all regret that his taciturnity enabled me to devote all my attention to my beast.

We went along at an uncomfortable bone-shaking jog trot. I kept a careful look out ahead, and held myself in readiness for such a dreadful contingency as an upset, or an attempt on the part of my charger to bolt, but gradually became less and less apprehensive, and ere I had been an hour on horseback felt tolerably at ease.

My companion was the first of us to come to grief. Some portion of his saddle gear—I don't know the name of it—gave way, and, to my surprise and amusement, the saddle slipped round the horse's side, the artistic Tromboni slipped round with it, and came a tremendous cropper on the ground. He disappeared in such a comical manner, and threw me into such convulsions of laughter, that I had great difficulty in preserving my own seat. Seeing, however, that the luckless Italian did not attempt to rise, I began to fear he had injured himself severely, and rapidly dismounting, I hastened to his assistance.

Fortunately, he was more mortified and angry than hurt, and surlily declining my aid, he got up and put his saddle to rights, and then, without saying a word to me, remounted his horse and rode swiftly away. It was my turn to feel mortified and angry now. However, as I did not

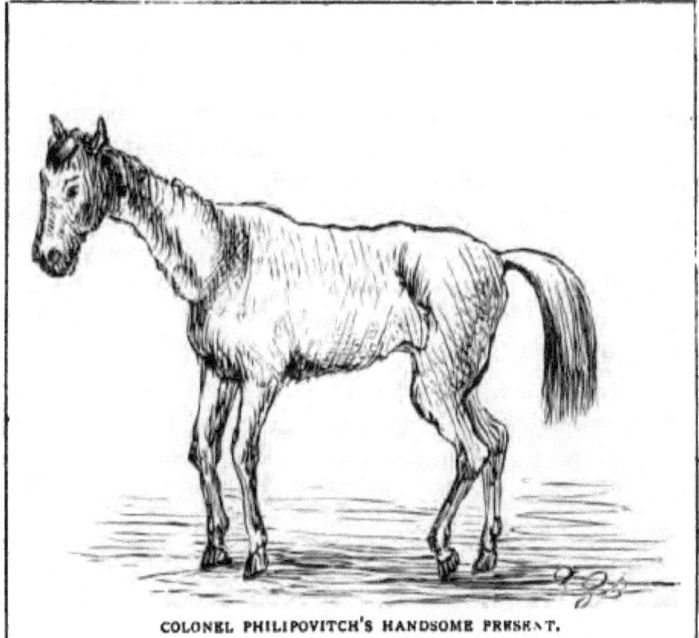

COLONEL PHILIPOVITCH'S HANDSOME PRESENT.

wish to be left in that out-of-the-way spot all by myself, I bottled up my indignation, and calling to my steed, which was quietly grazing a few paces away, I prepared to mount and follow the irate Italian.

I called, I say, to my horse, but, to my surprise and dismay, the confounded creature, in place of whinnying gratefully and trotting up to me, gave a snort, and shambled further off. Dr. Tromboni was rapidly disappearing from view, and I did not know an inch of the way. I hastened after Philipovitch's perverse present, calling coaxingly to him, and trying to beguile him into obedience by such blandishments as handfuls of hay and clover, but to no purpose: The aggravating animal allowed me to come almost within arm's length of him and just as I was beginning to think that I had caught him, he would whisk round, and kicking up his skinny hind legs in a clumsy and impudent fashion, trot to a considerable distance, and then contemplate me with dilated nostrils, and legs wide apart, as much as to say, "I'm not such a fool as I look!"

This disgusting performance was repeated time after time, with the same ill success on my part, and the same insulting kick-up on the part of the animal as he trotted triumphantly away, until I lost patience, and picking up a stone, I hurled it at him with all my force, yelling as I did so, "Pah! take that, you accursed creature, and go to Jericho, or anywhere else you please! Yah! Booh!"

The stone, to my great satisfaction, hit him on his hindquarters, and made him cut his capers in quite another spirit, and then gallop off.

This prompt and summary vindication of my wounded dignity warmed and encouraged my drooping spirits, and I prepared to pursue my journey on foot. But here I was in a difficulty. I did not know the way, and a turn in the wrong direction would as likely as not conduct me straight into the arms of those gentle cutthroats—the *bashi-bazouks*. Of course. Dr. Tromboni had long been out of sight, but while I was chasing my horse, I had been able to follow him a considerable distance with my eyes, and struck out accordingly in the direction he had taken.

The country through which I was passing reminded me somewhat of the Banstead downs in Surrey, as they were eighteen years ago—a desolate stretch of furze-covered, undulating ground. The horizon on one side was bound by a far-off range of hills, which looked blue and purple in the distance; on the other, by a gloomy forest. After walking for three or four miles, the road branched off right and left, and this brought me to a standstill. Not knowing what else to do, and feeling tired, I sat down for a while and refreshed myself, both mentally and physically, by taking a pull at my flask and munching a biscuit.

Whilst I was thus engaged, a waggon filled with wounded men drove up. I stopped it, and explaining that I wished to go to the Medvedovski encampment, asked the driver to give me a lift. He, a surly fellow, shook his head, and saying "Deligrad," whipped up his horses, and drove away along the road to the left. I was very indignant at this discourteous treatment, but, at the same time, it was something to have found out which road led to Deligrad. So, girding up my loins, I plodded on. Presently the sound of wheels was heard again. Looking round, I beheld a light waggon coming along at a rapid pace. There were two men in it.

"These men," said I to myself, "can't pretend they haven't room enough for me."

I stepped out into the roadway and motioned to them to stop. They pulled up at once, but, to my surprise and alarm, one of the men presented a revolver at me, and the other a carbine. "Hulloh!" said I, "what are you up to? I'm a friend—*Ingleski bolnitcho*—English doctor." The two men whispered together for a moment, and I then recognised one of them as Pauloff, my antagonist in the bedroom at Paratchin. The other was a burly Servian, ill-featured enough, but lamb-like in comparison with Pauloff. They signed to me to climb into the cart if I liked.

Under any other circumstances I should have hesitated to travel in such queer company, but I did not think twice of the matter then, and in a moment, I was beside them in the waggon. It would have been better for me if I had been less confiding. In the cart there was a stone bottle containing *raki*, upon which both of the men bestowed more attention than was good for them.

Presently we came in sight of some cottages, which, unlike any I had hitherto seen in those parts, appeared to be inhabited. My companions asked several questions about the route of a meagre little peasant, whose answers I did not understand, and having bought some more *raki*, Pauloff resumed the reins, and we drove off again. Shortly after sunset, which was gloriously beautiful, and as the bright glow was fading from the western sky, we came to a deserted wooden hut by the wayside. It was a weird and desolate-looking spot, and, as I entered the cottage, a vague feeling of distrust and suspicion of my companions came over me.

I determined to keep a sharp look-out, and furtively put my hand to my belt to see that my cutlass was all right and loose in its sheath. The conduct of the two men, which had hitherto been very surly, now, however, changed wonderfully. The Russian became roughly civil, the Servian almost abjectly servile. They made a fire of sticks and dry brushwood, pressed me to take wine with them, and offered me the most comfortable corner. After supper they rolled themselves up in their coats, and, to all appearance, fell fast asleep. I concluded that I had wronged them by my suspicions, and fell asleep, too.

I was dreaming deliciously of home and of Marie, to whom I fancied I was showing the beauties of Box Hill and of Dorking, when the delightful vision was roughly dispelled by an iron grasp on my throat. I awoke with a gasp, and found myself in the grip of the hideous Pauloff. The fellow's eyes gleamed with deadly ferocity, in his teeth he held a long knife, and with his disengaged hand he ransacked my pockets.

Beside me knelt the Servian, who had possessed himself of my revolver, and looked almost as truculent as the Russian. I attempted to remonstrate, whereat Pauloff gave me a most painful prick in the throat with his knife, and, passing his hand significantly across his neck, gave me to understand that he would do for me if I attempted to move or speak. The other villain, who evidently took his cue from Pauloff, thrust the cold muzzle of his revolver against my temple. I was indeed utterly in their power.

The Servian then produced a stout cord, and began to tie me hand and foot in a most elaborate manner. When I first saw the cord, I feared they were about to strangle me, but so eagerly does one cling to life that it was quite a relief to me to find that that was not their immediate object, and that a few minutes' respite was to be allowed me. Although my case seemed almost hopeless, I did not utterly despair; indeed, the terrible danger sharpened my wits. I had been very fond, as a boy, and when a student, of frequenting so-called spiritualistic seances and the entertainments given by the Davenport Brothers, and Maskelyne and Cooke, and had become quite *au fait* at the rope trick.

The knowledge stood me in good stead now. By expanding my chest to the utmost, and holding my arms a certain distance from the trunk, and yet in such a way that my captors had no idea of what I was up to, the fastenings which seemed tight when applied, became loose and removable when I contracted my chest and squeezed my arms to my side. Having made me, as they fancied, thoroughly secure, they left me lying on the ground in a corner of the room, and then sitting down by the fire, they proceeded to help themselves to wine and food, whilst they leisurely examined the contents of my knapsack. To my anguish they took therefrom all my handkerchiefs, and the only shirts and socks I possessed, besides those I was wearing. They next opened my surgical dressing-case, but contemptuously flung it on one side. They took, however, a bottle of quinine and a box of pills. I remember hoping at the time that the latter would punish them, for they were pretty strong ones—Pil. Gambog. Co., B. P. to wit.

Then Pauloff, with a murderous grin on his face, deliberately began to sharpen and feel the edge of his knife, and taking out my own watch, which, by the way he had appropriated, signed to me that in five minutes he was going to give himself the pleasure of cutting my throat. I recollect all this as vividly as if it happened only half an hour ago, instead of more than six years. The hands of the watch pointed to five minutes to one. A horrible feeling of dread came over me as I wondered what the sensation would be like when he plunged the knife into my throat. Still, I tried to look as cool and resolute as possible, and even essayed to smile, which so incensed the cruel scoundrel that he gave me a dreadful kick in the side, and stamped on my mouth with his heel.

At length that terrible five minutes came to an end, and as Pauloff approached me and poised his knife in the air to execute his threat, I hurriedly commended my spirit to God.

It was not, however, my destiny to die then. The Servian suddenly made a suggestion to his companion which evidently met with his approbation, for he burst into a loud laugh, and returning his knife to its sheath, made a brief reply and pointed to the door.

The other went out, and shortly returned with his arms filled with fuel, which he threw on the floor, and then left again for more. Pauloff, who seemed to be inspired with a fiendish malice towards me, thrust a stick in the fire, and went through the pantomime of setting the place ablaze.

The spiteful glee which this devilish Russian displayed in his efforts to terrify me, and the satisfaction with which he gloated over my helplessness and agony, combined with his ape-like appearance, made him look, by the lurid light of the fire, more like an imp of hell than a man. Meanwhile the Servian brought in fresh armfuls of brushwood, and Pauloff was busily occupied in arranging it about the room. Every now and then he paused in his work and chatted at me in Russian. In the meantime, I was not idle. My eyes followed the men in all their movements; my limbs were trying to free themselves from their bonds. The corner of the room where I lay was rather dark, and I succeeded in effecting a good deal of this without attracting their attention.

When the Servian had brought in sufficient firing to satisfy himself and his imperious companion, he proceeded, at the bidding of the latter, to harness the horse to the cart. Presently he announced that this was done. Pauloff then took a brand from the fire, and flourishing it in my face, gave me a parting kick, and set light to the brushwood in two or three places, and rushed out. A second afterwards, the sound of hoofs and wheels told me that they had gone. The brushwood, damp from recent rain, did not burn very readily, but it threw out dense clouds of stifling smoke. Luckily, I had loosed my hands before they left, and was thus enabled to clear myself of the rope sufficiently to crawl about.

I attempted to stand up. The air above was already irrespirable, and I was obliged to keep my head as low down as possible. I crept up to my dressing-case, took out one of the knives, and cut myself clear. Then I snatched up my knapsack and made a rush for the door. Fortunately, it was not fastened, or I must have perished, for the wood was now beginning to crackle and blaze fiercely, and the heat and smoke becoming intolerable. Pushing the door open, with a cry of joy I staggered into the fresh air, and fell to the ground quite exhausted. How delicious the cool night air felt! For some seconds I did not stir, but remained where I lay, drawing into my lungs deep draughts of the pure and balmy atmosphere.

The flames were quickly spreading to every part of the cottage. They soon burst from the window, and seized on the thatched roof Then I pulled myself together, girded on my knapsack, and set out along the road, which was illuminated for a considerable distance by the conflagration. Every now and then I turned round to look at the blaze, and when I was about half a mile off the roof fell in, a bright column of fire shot up into the air for a moment, and then the glow rapidly subsided and faded away.

As I was trudging along with a heart full of gratitude for my preservation, and wondering if I was to meet with any more adventures, I remarked that a rough paling or palisade skirted the road on my left. I was greatly cheered with the hope of approaching a village. The night was pleasant, and the moon shone with great brilliancy, so that I was able to discern objects at a considerable distance. Some way off I noticed something that looked like a gourd or melon stuck on one of the rails of the palisade. It might have been some thirty yards off when it first attracted my attention, and as I walked slowly up to it I puzzled my brains in trying to make out what it could possibly be.

Even when I was quite near, I could not make it out. I put my hand upon it, and found, to my horror, that it was a human head—whether a Turk or a Servian I could not say. The head was that of a young man, and his chin and cheeks were stubbly, as if he had been three or four days without shaving. The palisade ceased to afford me any comfort after that. I shudderingly quickened my pace, and felt thankful when I had placed a considerable interval between myself and the accursed spot. I walked on for several miles, until at last a distant glare in the sky told me that I was approaching an encampment.

Presently I was challenged by a sentry. I was, of course, unable to give the password; the guard turned out, and I was taken before the officer on duty, when I found, to my intense delight, that I was in the Medvedovski camp. I knew the officer well by sight, but not by name, and he recognised me at once.

"Why, M. Wright," said he, in a tone of some surprise, "I thought you were dead, but *milles tonnerres!* you are wounded and ill. Sit down, my dear sir; here, take this drop of *eau-de-vie*. We've another English doctor here now. I'll send for him. *Holà!* Guard there!"

A soldier appeared at the entrance of the hut, and was straightway sent off for the English doctor.

In a minute or two I heard footsteps approaching to the accompaniment of one of Moody and Sankey's hymns, whistled in a most lugubrious fashion; then the English doctor entered.

Looking up, I saw to my amazement my dear old friend Hiems.

"What, Hiems!" said I, speaking thickly, for my lips were swollen and my front teeth loose. If I was astonished, Hiems was almost scared out of his wits. He staggered backwards, and then gasped out, "Wright! Good Heavens! Is it you or your ghost? I thought—we all thought—you were dead. It's been in print, man; your death's been in print!" and he still looked at me doubtfully.

"I am not quite dead yet," replied I, "though I have been next door to it. Come, don't stare at me like that! Don't you know me, old boy?"

"Know you? I should think I did! Ain't you the darling of my heart? Bedad, hurrah!" and he kicked up his heels in a most unprofessional manner.

"And now, my son, let's look at your injuries," suddenly dropping his Hibernicism and assuming a grave tone; "lips lacerated, two teeth loose, any bones broken? Hulloh! what's this? (giving me a punch in the ribs which made me wince); fractured rib, eh?"

"No," replied I, "I don't think the rib is fractured. I got a nasty kick there a few hours ago, and the bruise is tender!"

"Hum!" said he, "draw a long breath— so; that's good—ha! You are not so bad as you might be. We'll put you to rights, my chicken, in no time!"

"Hiems," said I, "why these airs of seniority and superiority? You were not wont to call me chicken and sonny?"

"My dear child," said my irrepressible friend, "if you attempt to command me, I'll put you on gruel and slops for a month. I will, by the powers! Recollect that you are my patient. And now, I'll tell you the news," dropping his voice to a whisper and putting his mouth to my ear; "I'm engaged to be married!" Having uttered these portentous words, he stepped back a pace or two and surveyed me from a distance to see what effect the announcement had produced on me.

"I heartily congratulate you, my dear boy. Who is the lady?"

"But I'll tell you all about it tomorrow, as you must be tired, and require rest."

CHAPTER 20

Letters from Home

The next morning, I narrated my adventures to a numerous assemblage of the brigade officers. Mystery was frequently interrupted by outbursts of indignation against the villain Pauloff, and when I had finished, I was informed that he had been in bad odour for a long time, and had deserted a few days previously.

"He was degraded to the ranks a month ago," said one of my hearers.

"It is a pity he was not shot," said another.

"Shooting is too good for him, the blackguard!" chimed in Hiems. "I'd like to have his head in chancery this minute!"

"We'll catch and hang him yet," said Count Réné. "Parties have been sent out and are searching for him in all directions, and now, doctor, perhaps you had better see the brigadier, who has heard of your arrival. I'll take you to him."

I at once accompanied the count to headquarters, where I was very kindly received by the grim-looking Colonel Medvedovski.

"I am glad to see you, sir," said he, speaking less stiffly than usual. "On what knight errantry have you been lately engaged? Not occupying cottages again in the Turkish lines, eh, or drilling holes in the heads of wounded enemies, or killing young wild boars to supply your suffering comrades with food?" and his fierce little eyes twinkled with merriment as he poked this feeble fun at me. "Take a seat, and let me hear what you have been doing."

Thus invited, I sat down, and told the brigadier everything that had befallen me since the repulse of our grand attack. He listened with quiet attention until I came to the Pauloff episode; when his eyes flashed fire, and striking the table with his clenched fist, he swore a mighty oath that Pauloff should suffer for his crimes. Then congratulating me on my escape, he told me that a bundle of letters awaited me at the camp post-office, and dismissed me. I was curious to see what the bundle of letters, of which I had heard so much, contained, and went straight from head-quarters to the post-office and fetched it.

The first letter I opened had been forwarded to me from the hospital, and was a dun from a tailor, warning me that if a pair of trowsers I had got from him were not paid for by the 1st of August, he would put the matter in his solicitor's hands. It was already September. The next was from one of my brothers in India, telling me that my father was dangerously ill, and had taken it sorely to heart that I had gone on a wild goose chase in Servia instead of pursuing my studies in London. The third was from Messrs. Deville and Impey, solicitors, Chancery Lane, acquainting me with the death of a distant relative, whom I had not seen since I was a child, and whose existence I had almost forgotten, and stating that they had been instructed by the executors to inform me that the deceased had left me a legacy of £1,000.

Another was a circular from Messrs Pigswash, Gripewater, and Slush, wine merchants, directing my attention to the superior quality of their old crusted port at 15s. a dozen. Then a telegram from a cousin to the effect that he had just arrived at Liverpool from America, and asking me to meet him at 11 p.m., the 22nd August, at the Criterion; and lastly, a memorandum from a German lottery agent, asking me to take a one pound ticket in his government guaranteed lottery, in which every ticket was absolutely certain to win a prize, varying in value from £5 to £50,000!

The bad news from India, the desire to see my cousin, and the agreeable prospect of having £1,000 of my own to spend as I pleased, made me resolve to return to England immediately.

Returning to headquarters, I applied to the brigadier for leave, which he was kind enough to accord, and moreover, he introduced me to a Russian officer. Captain Starvemo, who was wounded in the arm, and about to return to Belgrade, and suggested that we should go together.

This arrangement suited us both very well, and it was agreed that we should start early the next morning. I was in a state of the utmost impecuniosity, for the rascally Pauloff had cleared every coin out of my pockets. I was compelled to part with my surgical dressing-case and the few instruments I possessed to raise sufficient money to pay my expenses by the way. The things were eagerly bought up by the Russian surgeons and dressers, and realised the sum of three *napoleons*, of which sum I improvidently expended one-third in bestowing a parting collation on Hiems and some of my Russian intimates.

The next morning, having been duly furnished with letters of recommendation to the Commander-in-chief at Deligrad, we started.

My companion, Captain Starvemo, was an officer in the Russian Marines, and as he could speak English uncommonly well, had been presented with a commission in Colonel Bragg's squadron of cavalry, in order that he might assist the latter, who could speak no language but his own. He was over six feet in height and powerfully built, and though imbued with a strong prejudice against England, confined his dislike to the country and its policy, and not to its people. He was very well informed, and exceedingly courteous and agreeable in manner. Like most of the other Russians I had come in contact with, he was full of the idea that sooner or later they would be at war with us, and when that time did come that we should collapse ignominiously.

"And what would make us collapse, captain?" I asked, as we trundled along the road.

"Starvation," replied he.

"And how are you going to starve us?" I asked again.

"Very easily," said he. "You get nine-tenths of your bread-stuffs from foreign countries, our cruisers would intercept your grainships, and there you are—starved out; can anything be plainer or easier?"

"I fancy it is easier to talk about intercepting our grain-ships than to do it," said I. "What do you think our fleet would be doing all the while?"

"Fighting with ours, or with those of our allies, or reposing harmlessly at the bottom of the sea," replied the captain.

"And who are your allies to be, may I ask?" said I.

"Either France or Italy, or perhaps both of them, France is our natural ally, and Italy your natural enemy. A little Russian diplomacy would secure them both to us. The former sees in us a power capable of restoring Alsace and Lorraine to her, the latter sees in you a rival for the supremacy of the Mediterranean Sea. Both have powerful fleets, either of which, in conjunction with ours, and aided by torpedoes and infernal machines, would prove more than a match for your boasted navy!

"Hem, sir," said I, "it is very easy and pleasant to talk about these things, but I am of opinion that Russia and France and Italy combined would find their programme impossible. In the first place, I doubt whether the able statesmen at the head of affairs in France and Italy would let themselves be gulled by a 'little Russian diplomacy!' In the second— and supposing that they did,—we can fight as well as you, and have torpedoes and infernal machines as good, if not better, than yours, and I am convinced that it would be your fleets, and not ours, that after a conflict between us would be found reposing harmlessly at the bottom of the sea."

"I am very glad to hear you express those opinions," said he, handing me a cigarette, "and I hope they are shared by your countrymen!"

"To the best of my knowledge and belief they are," replied I, gratefully accepting the proffered smoke.

"Then all I can say is, that the overweening confidence of you Englishmen will be a third and most powerful ally to us. War has its chances, and the mightiest, when most assured of success, have before now come to grief. Mark my words. The very next war you undertake with us or any other great power will place the people of London and Liverpool and Glasgow and your other great cities in absolute distress for want of bread. Any other government than yours, under similar circumstances, would provide public granaries and storehouses, as a necessary precaution, but you English—no, you won't do anything of the kind. Your thick-headed prototype, John Bull, will go on dozing away and enjoying his dream of fancied invincibility and security until he is caught napping, and then it will be too late for him to bestir himself. But here we are at the camp at Deligrad."

We were now challenged by sentries, and our replies and papers being found satisfactory, we were permitted to go to headquarters. Here we had an interview with Colonel Comaroff, General Tchernaieff's second in command. This officer, who was assassinated some months after at Constantinople, informed us that we should have to stay in camp for the night, and could proceed as early as we pleased next morning. It was still early in the evening, so we whiled away the time by strolling quietly about the camp and inspecting its defences. These, in consequence of the untoward result of the recent actions, were being greatly strengthened.

The approach from the Alexinatz side was commanded by heavy artillery brought from Belgrade and other fortresses; all trees interfering with the line of fire had been cut down, dragged into camp, and stripped of their leaves, and then piled up with their branches sharpened and pointing outwards, so as to form an almost impenetrable abattis in parts where such protection was deemed necessary. Winter quarters were prepared by digging large chambers underground and providing them with thick thatched roofs.

As we were returning from our survey, we met a troop of cavalry conducting two prisoners who were seated in a cart into the camp. Both prisoners were bound hand and foot, and seemed to have made a desperate resistance: for round the head of one of them was tied a bloodstained rag, and the clothes of the other were torn and muddy. When we were almost abreast of them my eyes met those of the man whose head was bound up. The effect was electrical, his jaw fell, and a look of the wildest terror spread over his face, as he yelled out, "*Der teufel! der teufel!*" and dropped to the bottom of the car as if he had been shot.

It was Pauloff's accomplice, the Servian. The other prisoner, who had hitherto sat with his chin sunk on his breast, also looked up, and I at once recognised Pauloff. The miserable man started, turned pale, and trembled visibly when he saw me.

"How now, doctor?" said Starvemo inquisitively; "you seem to know those men, and they evidently recognise you."

"I have good cause to know them," replied I. "Would you mind asking their escort what they are charged with?"

Starvemo put the question to the guard, and was told that they were charged with the robbery and murder of two invalided Russian officers. They were to be tried by drumhead court martial, and would probably be shot. The escort then saluted and trotted on with their charge. "Now, doctor," said my companion, "tell me what you know about those men?"

Having no wish to give evidence against them, I exacted a promise of secrecy from Starvemo, and then told him of my adventure in the hut and of my narrow escape. His indignation and astonishment knew no bounds.

"That accounts then, doctor, for their fright at seeing you! Of course, they thought you were burnt. No wonder they took you for the devil! I think you ought to inform Colonel Comaroff of these facts."

I argued that as the men had been caught red-handed in the perpetration of another crime for which they were certain to be shot, the evidence that I could give was not required. The captain shook his head in a dissatisfied manner, and said he knew what he would do under the circumstances, but of course I was the master of my own actions. The next morning, we set out again, reached Paratchin without any mishap, and by nightfall were at Yagodina. Here, for the first time for several weeks, we enjoyed the luxury of sleeping in comfortable beds. We were up at sunrise, and had breakfasted and were well on our way by eight next morning.

About two hours after we started, Starvemo had a violent shivering fit, and complained of feeling very unwell. This alarmed me greatly, as I thought it might be due to some *pyemic* process in connection with the wound in his arm. For want of anything better, I had only applied a water-dressing to the wound in the morning, when it appeared to be progressing satisfactorily, but now, I found, on examination, that it presented a dry and inflamed appearance.

Stopping the driver for a few minutes, I dressed the wound again, and made my patient take a big dose of quinine, the only drug I had at hand. Feverish symptoms, however, developed themselves, and by the time we had reached Semendria (5 p.m.) Starvemo was seriously ill. I drove straight up to the Russian hospital, where Doctors Knifem and Cutemoff, the surgeons in charge, took him into their skilful keeping. They were good enough to ask me to spend the night with them, which I gladly did. We watched by Starvemo's bedside in turns that night, and had the satisfaction to notice a slight improvement in his condition next morning.

Before leaving Semendria I called at the Servian hospital, in the hope of seeing Doctors Ibaum and Stephanovitch, but they had left the place a month since. I then paid a visit to the hospital itself, where Baron Von Tummy's energy had effected a wonderful change. The clumsy and ignorant soldiers were replaced by an efficient staff of nurses, the wards were clean and neat, and the air in them sweet and pure. Altogether, it was completely metamorphosed from the filthy, ill-managed place I had known two or three months before.

Hearing that the steamer for Belgrade was to start at ten that morning, I returned at once to the Russian hospital, bade *adieu* to Captain Starvemo and Doctors Knifem and Cutemoff, and went on board the boat, which left the landing stage a few minutes after.

I now examined my pockets to see how much money was left. To my alarm I discovered that my capital amounted to four *dinars* (four *francs*) only. However, I consoled myself by the hope that my friends in London would have sent me a letter of credit to the Poste Restante at Belgrade. Still, it is not an agreeable thing to find oneself reduced to three-and-fourpence in a foreign country. Whilst I was counting my money, an important-looking young man placed himself opposite to me in an imposing attitude, and said with an unmistakable cockney twang:—

"I presume you are an Englishman."

"I am, sir," said I.

"I presume you are returning to England," said he.

Again, I replied in the affirmative.

"I presume you have no objection to conversing with a fellow-countryman."

"No indeed," replied I, "I am delighted to meet you."

"I presume," said he, "you are a medical man."

"I am a medical student," said I.

"I presume you'll have no objection to taking one of my cards;" and he tendered me a piece of pasteboard.

I accepted the card, and looking at it, read the following inscription:—

Dr. Beazley Smugge,
Green Street, Hackney.

"You are a doctor, I see," said I.

Dr. Smugge nodded in a grave and dignified manner.

"You are very young to have passed your examinations," I remarked.

"No, well, well—no!" said he, stretching out his neck and combing out his beard with his finger.

"You are an M.D., sir, I suppose?" said I.

"Well, no," said he, "I am not exactly an M.D. yet."

"What degrees have you then, doctor?" said I.

"Well, I can't exactly say that I have my degrees yet, but I shall have, very soon. I'm walking a hospital, you know."

"But what does the 'doctor' before your name mean, Mr. Smugge?" I asked.

"Oh, well," replied he, "that's one of my father's cards. He gave me a lot of them, so I'm quite entitled to use them, ain't I?"

"No, I don't think you are," replied I, laughing.

"Oh, but when a man's well up, and knows his work thoroughly, as I do," said he, "it doesn't signify. I am going up for my first college as soon as I get back. I presume you won't mind asking me a few questions in physiology?"

I was a good deal taken aback at this singular request from a stranger, and replied that I was somewhat rusty in my own physiology, but would do the best I could.

Mr. Smugge graciously replied that he would overlook my physiological rustiness; so, I asked him, "What was the normal temperature

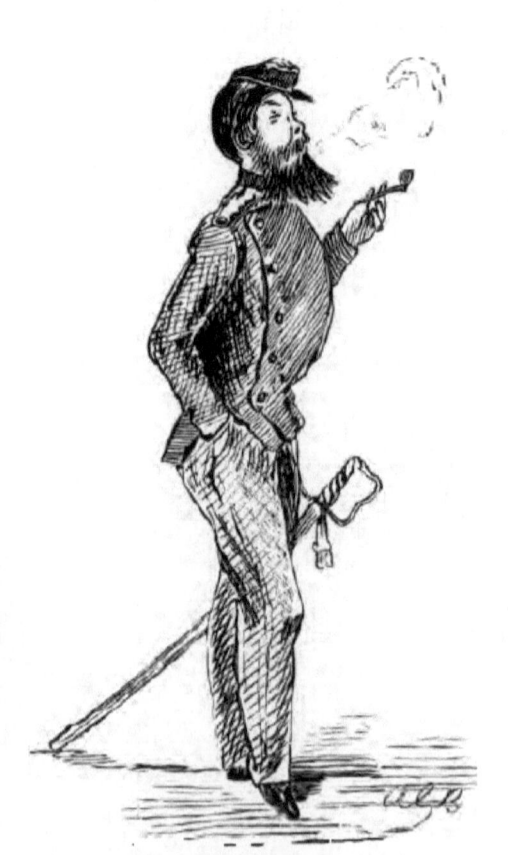

THE IMPORTANT-LOOKING YOUNG MAN WITH A BEARD.

of the blood in man?"

"That's scarcely a fair question, sir," said he, shaking his head deprecatingly, "however, I think I can answer it; 212° Fahrenheit."

This ridiculous reply sent me into a fit of laughter, at which Mr. Smugge became very indignant.

"Mayn't a fellow make a little mistake sometimes without being laughed at?" said he, testily.

"Certainly," replied I, "and I must apologize for my rudeness. But is not 212° rather high?"

"Er—well—perhaps it is a little, but not very much," replied he. "Wait a bit, I know. It's something with a five added to it; let me see—let me see;" and he scratched his nose in his perplexity. "Ah, never mind! I can't think of the exact figure now, but I know that a fellow can't live with his temperature above 900° Fahrenheit."

Again, I burst out laughing, and again my discourtesy excited the ire of Mr. Smugge.

"Er—a fellow needn't laugh, you know. Ask me another question—something straightforward and above-board, you know, not a pottering thing about temperature. If any of the examiners at the college have the cheek—er—to ask me a question about the temperature, I shall say—er—'Oh, go to Bath, and find out!' That's the sort of fellow I am, you know!"

Subduing my inclination to laugh with the greatest difficulty, I complied with Mr. Smugge's request, and asked him another question—*viz*, "At what rate does the blood travel through the arteries?"

"Er—any fool knows that," replied he; "a deuce of a rate—a mile a minute; but that's enough physiology for one day. I presume you've no objection to changing the subject now, sir."

"None whatever, sir," said I.

"Very well, then; we'll talk about something else. Have you done any first-class operations since you came here?"

"No," answered I.

"I did some," said he, "but the fellows have no Stamina, you know, and did not survive the most trifling operation. I was baulked, too, of one beautiful job by Dr. Sharp. You don't know that fellow Sharp. All the better for you; he's not a gentleman. What do you think? I was going to cut off a man's hand for a wound on his little finger, when Sharp had the cheek to remonstrate with me. 'Surely,' said he, 'you are not going to amputate for that?'—'Yes, I am,' said I.—'But it's not necessary,' said he.—'Maybe not,' said I, 'but it's a pretty operation.'—

'A pretty operation,' said he; 'why, you confounded blockhead, who the dickens are you? What qualifications have you got? I shall allow you to do no such thing.' And the fellow made such a deuced row that I had to drop the operation. Wasn't it disgusting, eh?"

"One of the most disgusting things I ever heard of," I replied.

"The profession's going to the dogs, that's what I say. There are a lot of fellows in it nowadays who have no fellow-feeling for a fellow. I was very nearly doing for Dr. Sharp, though. I am not a man to be trifled with, sir; my anger is terrible when roused. I kept my eye on Dr. Sharp after that, and if he had gone a little further and called me a fool, I believe I should have challenged him to fight a duel. If ever you should come across him, you may tell him that Beazley Smugge warns him not to cross his path again!"

As Mr. Smugge spoke these words he folded his arms, knit his brows, and scowled most horribly.

"You surely would not hurt him, Mr. Beazley?" said I.

"Hurt him! *Yah!* (an intensely ferocious whispered snarl); let him look to himself! Let him take care of his back! I would either kick him or bump the back of his head five or six times on the pavement. Hurt him, indeed!" Having thus given vent to his righteous indignation, Mr. Smugge cooled down a bit, and offered me a cracknel biscuit, which I declined with thanks, whereupon he ate it himself, and told me between the mouthfuls that immediately after his arrival at Belgrade he would cross over to Semlin and hurry back to England, to prepare himself for the first College exam, in November.

"I envy you," said I, "the prospect of returning home so speedily. I must stay here until my people send me a remittance—*i.e.*, for about a fortnight." This remarkable young man bade me *adieu* at the Belgrade landing-stage, and went his way.

There was no letter of credit for me at the post-office, and not having sufficient money to pay for a telegram, I wrote a letter to my friends to acquaint them with my impecunious condition. Next, I looked out for some place where I could stay until the remittance arrived—a work of some difficulty, for my unkempt and tatterdemalion appearance went sorely against me, but I at last succeeded in getting a bedroom at the Alexandra Hotel, near the market-place. However, I was not destined to stay there long. The same evening, I had a violent attack of ague, and not being able to get proper attention at the hotel, I applied for admission into the English Ambulance Hospital, where I was immediately received and most kindly treated.

The day after my admission acute dysentery set in, and for three weeks I was confined to my bed.

One day, as I was getting better, some visitors who were being shown through the wards stopped close to my bedside, and began conversing in low tones. I was nearly asleep at the time, but one of the voices aroused me. It was Marie's! She had resumed her proper attire, and was leaning on the arm of a tall, handsome man in the uniform of the Bulgarian legion.

Presently Marie saw me, and coming forward, addressed me in such graceful and sympathetic terms that I quite lost my heart to her again. After speaking to me for a few minutes, she introduced her tall companion to me as her husband, Colonel Nicholas Davorin, of the Bulgarian Brigade. This was a terrible shock! For a minute or two I utterly collapsed; my head swam round, and I could hear nothing in my ears but the words—"my husband!"

When I came to, they had gone.

So great was my disappointment at discovering that Marie was married, that I remember wishing at the time that I might never get better. For one whole day I know that I refused all food, and for a week I resolutely declined taking more than half my allowance. My disgusting constitution, however, survived it all, and three weeks after my last unhappy interview with Marie I was on my way home to England—not, as I had once fondly hoped, a highly distinguished and happily plighted individual, but a nearly extinguished and completely blighted being.

Once arrived in England, however, the kindly faces and hearty greetings of friends and relatives went far to soothe my wounded susceptibilities, and I once more resumed my place at home and my studies at the hospital, a sadder, but it is to be hoped also, a considerably wiser man.

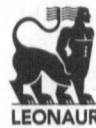

ALSO FROM LEONAUR
AVAILABLE IN SOFTCOVER OR HARDCOVER WITH DUST JACKET

THE WOMAN IN BATTLE by Loreta Janeta Velazquez—Soldier, Spy and Secret Service Agent for the Confederacy During the American Civil War.

BOOTS AND SADDLES by Elizabeth B. Custer—The experiences of General Custer's Wife on the Western Plains.

FANNIE BEERS' CIVIL WAR by Fannie A. Beers—A Confederate Lady's Experiences of Nursing During the Campaigns & Battles of the American Civil War.

LADY SALE'S AFGHANISTAN by Florentia Sale—An Indomitable Victorian Lady's Account of the Retreat from Kabul During the First Afghan War.

THE TWO WARS OF MRS DUBERLY by Frances Isabella Duberly—An Intrepid Victorian Lady's Experience of the Crimea and Indian Mutiny.

THE REBELLIOUS DUCHESS by Paul F. S. Dermoncourt—The Adventures of the Duchess of Berri and Her Attempt to Overthrow French Monarchy.

LADIES OF WATERLOO by Charlotte A. Eaton, Magdalene de Lancey & Juana Smith—The Experiences of Three Women During the Campaign of 1815: Waterloo Days by Charlotte A. Eaton, A Week at Waterloo by Magdalene de Lancey & Juana's Story by Juana Smith.

NURSE AND SPY IN THE UNION ARMY by Sarah Emma Evelyn Edmonds—During the American Civil War

WIFE NO. 19 by Ann Eliza Young—The Life & Ordeals of a Mormon Woman-During the 19th Century

DIARY OF A NURSE IN SOUTH AFRICA by Alice Bron—With the Dutch-Belgian Red Cross During the Boer War

MARIE ANTOINETTE AND THE DOWNFALL OF ROYALTY by Imbert de Saint-Amand—The Queen of France and the French Revolution

THE MEMSAHIB & THE MUTINY by R. M. Coopland—An English lady's ordeals in Gwalior and Agra during the Indian Mutiny 1857

MY CAPTIVITY AMONG THE SIOUX INDIANS by Fanny Kelly—The ordeal of a pioneer woman crossing the Western Plains in 1864

WITH MAXIMILIAN IN MEXICO by Sara Yorke Stevenson—A Lady's experience of the French Adventure

AVAILABLE ONLINE AT **www.leonaur.com**
AND FROM ALL GOOD BOOK STORES

www.ingramcontent.com/pod-product-compliance
Lightning Source LLC
Chambersburg PA
CBHW030218170426
43201CB00006B/129